Prenatal Exposures

Roy P. Martin • Stefan C. Dombrowski

Prenatal Exposures

Psychological and Educational Consequences for Children

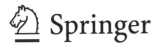 Springer

Prof. Roy P. Martin
University of Georgia
Athens, GA 30602
USA
(706)542-4261
rpmartin@uga.edu

Prof. Stefan C. Dombrowski
Rider University
Lawrenceville, NJ 08648-3099
USA
(609)895-5448
sdombrowski@rider.edu

ISBN: 978-0-387-74397-4   e-ISBN: 978-0-387-74398-1
DOI: 10.1007/978-0-387-74398-1

Library of Congress Control Number: 2007940887

Printed on acid-free paper

9 8 7 6 5 4 3 2 1

springer.com

Preface

Approximately 2 percent to 3 percent of the population of the United States has been diagnosed with severe neurological disabilities (e.g., mental retardation, cerebral palsy, autism, chronic severe mental illness). A far greater percentage (10 percent to 20 percent) has less severe disabilities (e.g. learning disabilities, disorders of attention, episodic mental illness). These neurologically based afflictions result in enormous human suffering and social cost, placing a significant burden on even the most affluent countries in the world. For more than 100 years scientists in a wide range of disciplines (e.g., sociology, psychology, medicine, developmental biology) have attempted to determine the causes of these disabilities. Many factors have been isolated including genetics, nutrition, pollutants, inadequate caretaking and social factors linked to poverty.

It is the belief of the authors of this book that one set of factors, those that alter the neurological development of the child during the fetal period, has not been given the attention that it deserves. The prenatal period of development is particularly sensitive to disruption because it encompasses a precisely timed period when organ systems are formed and rapid growth of neurological structures occurs. During no other period in the life course is the well-being of the individual so dependent on precisely timed biochemical events. As a result, an adverse prenatal exposure can impart immutable damage because of the sensitivity of the developing central nervous system during the prenatal period.

A growing number of specialists are making important discoveries regarding the types of factors that perturb fetal neurological development. These researchers have, in some cases, documented long-term psychological, behavioral and educational sequelae. However, this research is scattered throughout research literatures of a variety of professions (medicine, epidemiology, developmental psychopathology, reproductive biology), is technically challenging for non-specialists and is not readily available to many that do not have access to research libraries or specialized computerized retrieval mechanisms. Thus, it is the purpose of this book to summarize the most important findings regarding prenatal exposures that have been associated with learning and behavior problems of children and adolescents.

This volume is organized into five sections. The first introduces the main themes of the book and, in a separate chapter, presents an introduction to fetal development. This chapter was designed to set the stage for the understanding of how many different types of perturbations result in long-term central nervous system damage that has a continued effect as the child matures. The second section is devoted to low birth weight, preterm birth and asphyxia. These are among the most widely researched markers or indicators that prenatal perturbations have occurred. The remaining three sections are devoted to detailed discussions of the research linking maternal illness, maternal drug use and maternal exposure to pollutants to long-term negative effects on child and adolescent development. We are particularly pleased to be able to summarize many recent findings in the area of air, water and household chemical pollutants as this volume is one of the first to include detailed reviews of this burgeoning area of scientific activity.

It is our hope that having this body of knowledge–compiled for the first time in one volume– will aid researchers, practitioners and policy makers in elevating prenatal events to a more central position in the understanding of learning and behavioral pathologies of children and adolescents. A nuanced understanding of the role of prenatal events is particularly important in today's world, as the number of children with developmental anomalies is increasing, largely due to improved medical care. This book stands to fill a cross-disciplinary conceptual gap and serve as an important resource to the psychological, medical and educational community, setting the context for appropriate prevention and intervention activities that have the potential to foster the developmental well-being of children.

November 2007   Roy Martin and Stefan Dombrowski
                                                Athens, GA   Cherry Hill, NJ

Acknowledgments

This book is dedicated to Janet, Greg and David, the immediate family who has to make the sacrifices of time and attention that a book such as this requires. Thanks for your generosity. In addition, thanks to Claudia (sister) and Claud (father) for your interest and emotional support. Also, Stefan, you have made this project possible; I would not have had the energy or enough ideas to do it without you. Finally, thanks to Susan Sullivan for proofing many of the chapters and helping to compensate for my lack of attention to grammar and punctuation. To all of you, I am very grateful.

R.M.

This book is dedicated to my children, Maxwell and Henry. I look forward to supporting your journey toward a vocation that brings you as much joy and satisfaction as I have found in mine. I would also like to acknowledge the love and support of my parents (Carl and Mary Lee), and my wife (Debbie). Finally, I owe a debt of gratitude to Roy P. Martin, my former major professor who inspired my academic career and remains a mentor to this day.

S.D.

Contents

Section A
Introduction

Human beings have always been concerned and particularly moved by the arrival of babies who looked abnormal. Cave paintings and petrogylphs from the prehistoric era suggest that, since the dawn of recorded history, humans have contemplated why babies are born with deformities. In antiquity, these deformities were thought to be divinely inspired and to portend future events. The Greek and Roman civilizations produced works based upon birth defects that continued to be referenced until the 17th Century. These sources cataloged birth defects providing an indication for each one of its divine meanings. Some societies viewed the arrival of a child with a birth defect in a harsh manner. In Sparta babies born with noticeable physical deformities were thrown off a cliff because they would not be able to contribute to the war effort in that bellicose society.

Within the last 150 years the study of birth defects has assumed a more scientific basis, moving away from its linkage to theology, philosophy and divination. Based on epidemiological studies isolating the variables that could predict where and in what populations birth defects were most likely, the field moved a long way from its historical roots. The beginning of modern scientific epidemiological has been traced to the efforts of John Snow and Henry Whitehead in their efforts to find the source of a cholera epidemic in London in 1854. These researchers discovered that one particular pump had been tainted with sewage. While this seminal investigation was not aimed at birth defects, it documented stillbirths of women who had taken water from the affected pump (Johnson 2006). Though not as rigorous as the effort of Snow and Whitehead, as early as 1787, William Prefect observed a greater prevalence of "insanity" among those exposed prenatally to a particularly virulent influenza epidemic. At the turn of the 20th Century, Emil Kraeplin (1919) commented that infections during pregnancy might have a relationship with schizophrenia, or as he referred to it, dementia praecox.

In addition to early epidemiological studies, experimental studies began to shed light on the biological explanations for adverse pregnancy outcomes. These studies used animal models of human pathology. For example, in 1877, Dareste exposed pregnant fowl to nonlethal heat and found that hyperthermia produced congenital anomalies in offspring (Warkany 1986).

During the past 150 years the greatest strides have been in isolating maternal conditions and environmental factors that produce a visable malformation in the infant at the time of birth. A name was given to events or conditions that produced structural malformations of the newborn or of the fetus; they were called teratogens. Teratology is that branch of science concerned with production, development, anatomy and classification of malformed fetuses (Dirckx 1997).

Within the last 30 years a subset of this field has emerged that focuses on what has come to be known as behavioral teratology. Behavioral teratology is that branch of science that studies the abnormal behavioral sequelae of environmental events that occur during the prenatal period. Behavioral teratology is not limited to behavioral manifestations of structural abnormalities of the fetus or newborn, although such behaviors are of interest. The primary focus is on long-term behavioral outcomes that result from prenatal perturbations that are often so subtle they are not observable in the clinic examination of the newborn, or even in detailed imaging of the structure of the central nervous system of the infant. Yet, as child development progresses, abnormalities may begin to appear that can be linked to events that occurred during fetal development. This book is intended to be one of the first compendia of the growing literature in human behavioral teratology.

Purpose and Organization of this Book

Investigations of prenatal insults that may result in subtle central nervous system malformation are increasing. Further, links to developmental problems of children are becoming increasingly clear (Dombrowski and Martin, 2007). However, this research is scattered throughout the literature of various professions (medicine, epidemiology, developmental psychopathology, reproductive biology), is technically challenging to read for non-specialists and is not readily available to many that do not have access to research libraries or online journals in a wide range of disciplines.

Not having ready access to this information has unfortunate consequences for a variety of disciplines. For researchers, lack of access limits theory building and research design. For practitioners, lack of access to this knowledge results in communicating faulty etiological models to patients and clients and, in some cases, inappropriate treatments. These problems are particularly apparent for trainers of professionals, as they influence both the research and practice communities. Thus, it is the purpose of this book to summarize the most important findings regarding prenatal insults to normal development that result in learning and behavior problems of children and adolescents.

The bulk of this book, then, is devoted to bringing together in one place some of the most commonly studied prenatal factors that have been shown to be linked to behavior and learning problems of children. For many environmental events or conditions of the mother during pregnancy, no long-term follow-up studies that implicate learning and behavior problems are available. Events or conditions that have been shown to result in structural, physiological or developmental problems of the neonate or infant will be reviewed if there is evidence of a link between these neonatal or infant abnormalities and learning problems. For example, a maternal hypertension may be linked to low birth weight, but there may be no long-term studies of the effect of this medical condition in childhood. Since low birth weight is known to have adverse effects on development, the literature on the maternal condition that resulted in low birth weight infants will be reviewed.

The book begins with a discussion of the importance of behavioral teratology. It examines why prenatal events have been slow to assume their rightful place in the manifold explanations of abnormal behavior. This introductory chapter also presents the viewpoints of the authors, including our guiding principles and our biases.

After this introductory chapter, the authors outline the essential features of normal fetal brain development. Conditions that are associated with abnormal development of the central nervous system are the primary focus of this book. Thus, through this introduction to normal fetal brain development the reader will come to understand not only some of the essential processes of brain development, but also the vulnerability of the developing brain when these processes are disturbed. The remainder of the book is divided into five sections, four of which review specific sets of factors known to perturb prenatal development. The first is devoted to the perinatal events of low birth weight, preterm birth (Chapter 3) and anoxia/hypoxia (Chapter 4). Many of the perturbing factors that are the primary focus of behavioral teralogy investigations result in a cascade of events that are manifest in abnormal conditions that can be observed at the time of birth. These conditions include low birth weight, preterm delivery and perinatal anoxia/asphyxia. These perinatal conditions have been widely researched, and this research will be reviewed prior to a discussion of the more distal perturbing factors. These perinatal events are the subject of Section B.

Sections C, D and E are devoted to those factors that are often associated with the onset of this cascade of negative developmental events. Section C is devoted to maternal illnesses or conditions that are most associated with adverse neonatal development, including infections (Chapter 5), chronic illnesses of the mother (Chapter 6), maternal malnutrition (Chapter 7) and stress (Chapter 8). Section D describes the highlights of the literature on maternal recreational drug use and pregnancy outcomes. Topics reviewed are maternal smoking during pregnancy (Chapter 9), use of alcohol (Chapter 10) and maternal use of illicit drugs (Chapter 11). Section E describes the recently developing literature on environmental toxic substances (pollutants) that seem to be associated with perturbed fetal development. The topics covered include air and water pollution (Chapter 12) and heavy metal and household pollutants (Chapter 13).

The final section of the book includes some of the authors' thoughts about the history and future of research on prenatal factors that adversely affect human fetal development. The book also includes a brief dictionary of medical terminology so that individuals with little or no exposure to the specific terminology related to fetal development and birth can readily utilize this book.

Chapter 1
Themes and Purpose

The level of developmental pathology among children is alarming to parents, policy makers and mental health experts. Medical authorities have estimated that 10 to 20 of every 1,000 (1 percent to 2 percent) infants born in the United States will have clinically significant mental retardation, two per 1,000 (0.2 percent) will have cerebral palsy and 1.9 per 1,000 (0.19 percent) will have severe hearing or visual impairment (Gortmaker, Walker, Weitzman and Sobol 1990; American Psychiatric Association 1994). A far greater number of children are afflicted with less severe dysfunctions, including attention deficits (about 10 percent) and learning disabilities (4 percent to 7.5 percent, depending on definition) (Gortmaker, et al. 1990; American Psychiatric Association 1994).

Severe and persistent mental illness in adulthood (predominantly schizophrenia) affects two to four persons per 1,000 per year, depending on diagnostic criteria, and the country in which the diagnosis is applied (Ruggeri, Leese, Thornicroft, Bisoffi and Tansella 2000). Estimates of the lifetime risk of mental illness and behavior disorders include especially large numbers of individuals. For example, the lifetime risk of a major depressive disorder in adult community samples is about 5 percent to 9 percent for men, and 10 percent to 25 percent for women (American Psychiatric Association 1994).

Educational records provide additional data on the prevalence of disability in the population. During the 2003-2004 school year 6,634,000 children were designated as disabled and received services in federally supported programs *(http://nces.ed. gov/programs/digest)*. This was 13.7 percent of the enrollment in public schools. As this figure does not include those in private educational systems, the number of disabled students is higher, although these data are unknown. Further, the special education enrollment is rapidly increasing. From the 1990-1991 to the 2003-2004 school year there was a 38.5 percent increase in special education enrollment.

Broadly speaking, then, a reasonable estimate is that 2.5 percent of the population has severe neurological disabilities (e.g., mental retardation, cerebral palsy, autism, chronic severe mental illness), and 13 percent to 20 percent (depending on the diagnostic definition that is used) have less severe disabilities (e.g., learning disabilities, disorders of attention, episodic mental illness). These estimates are consistent with those of Rutter (1989) who estimated 14 percent to 22 percent of all children

R.P. Martin and S.C. Dombrowski, *Prenatal Exposures: Psychological and Educational Consequences for Children.*
© Springer 2008

have a significant disability. The cost of diagnosis and treatment of children with significant learning, behavior and emotional problems places an enormous burden on even the most affluent countries in the world. For example, the cost to the federal budget for special education services in 2002 in the United States was over seven billion dollars *(http://nces.ed.gov/programs/digest)*.

We believe that a sizeable percentage of developmental disabilities and mental disorders have their roots in the prenatal period. Further, we believe that many health, mental health, and educational professionals (e.g., physicians, teachers, parents) do not fully appreciate the role that prenatal disturbances of development, particularly of neurological development, play in many aspects of child pathology. This book was written because there is a growing body of research indicating that prenatal conditions that are less then optimal greatly increase the risk of behavioral and learning problems during childhood and beyond.

Why have health professionals, social scientists and the public been slow to appreciate the effects of prenatal perturbations of development on learning and mental health outcomes? The answer seems to be that each group has had a primary set of causative factors on which they focus their theoretical and research activities. Mental health professionals, particularly psychologists, have traditionally focused on caretaker-child relationships as the primary determinants of childhood and adolescent pathologies. Medical professionals, particularly during the past three decades, have placed primary etiological focus on genetic factors. Although all types of professionals acknowledge genetic and environmental factors as playing a role in abnormal behavior of children and adolescents, we believe that the prenatal environment has received less attention than is warranted, given the data that is available. Before we describe this data, which is the primary purpose of this book, a brief review of current thinking about the etiology of child psychopathologies will be described in more detail.

Etiology of Childhood and Adolescent Psychopathology

Research into the determinants of childhood and adolescent psychopathology has focused on five primary types of factors: genetics, characteristics of the caretaker-child relationships, physical contaminants that result in somatic and central nervous system damage, social/cultural issues and the prenatal environment (Mash and Barkley 2003). Due to recent advances in molecular biology, the public and many in the research community are placing primary emphasis on genetics as the quickest and most fundamental path toward an understanding of psychopathology. Gene variants have been found that affect risks for cancer, diabetes and some infectious and immunologic disorders (Khoury 1997). Further, almost every month in the popular press a new gene has been found to be associated with schizophrenia, autism or attention-deficit/hyperactivity disorder.

The association of genetic variation to learning disabilities, and particularly to dyslexia, will serve to illustrate progress in linking genetic factors to developmental pathologies. Dyslexia is a language-based reading disorder characterized by difficulties in the development of accurate and fluent single word decoding skills, usually associated with poor phonological processing skills. Phonological processing refers to the use of the sound structure of oral language for processing written information (Lyon, Fletcher and Barnes 2003). Reading problems clearly run in families. If a child's parent is dyslexic, they have an eight times higher probability of being dyslexic than members of the general population (Pennington 1999). In studies involving monozygotic and dizygotic twins, DeFries and Fulker (1985) found that 50 to 60 percent of the variance in reading achievement was attributable to heritable factors. Finally, in linkage studies in which the presence of specific genes in families with high levels of reading disability are studied, findings have been reported linking gene variants on chromosomes 1, 2, 6 and 15 (Lyon, et al. 2003), although several studies have failed to replicate these findings.

Highly publicized research outcomes such as these have provided hope that behavioral, emotional and many forms of cognitive disabilities will yield to similar efforts. However, progress has been slower than originally anticipated. Failures can be attributed to a lack of consensus on phenotypic definitions of disorders, complex modes of inheritance, strong environmental effects including environmental effects during the prenatal period, gene-environment interactions and polygenic inheritance (Merikangas 2000). The slow progress on the genetic front should not be misconstrued as indicating that genetic predispositions do not play a role in psychopathology. In fact most current thought about the etiology of these conditions includes a place for direct genetic effects, as well as for predispositions that interact with specific environmental insults to produce pathology. In fact there is no behavior (normal or pathological) in which genetic factors do not play a role. However, the question is this: how do specific environmental perturbations affect development given a specified genetic makeup? The ability to answer this type of question remains in the future.

The second most obvious place to look for factors that contribute to childhood and adolescent disability is the influence of caretakers (parents, extended family, teachers). Associations have been repeatedly documented between parental caretaker behaviors and behavior and learning problems (Coie and Dodge 1998), parental characteristics such as parental depression and a variety of negative childhood outcomes (Downey and Coyne 1990; Field 1992), and the socialization techniques used by caretakers, such as harsh disciplinary practices and the probability that the child will engage in antisocial behaviors (Patterson 1982).

The literature on developmental sequelae of early childhood institutionalization provides a particularly vivid model of caretaker behavior. This literature is compelling because it offers extreme examples of the effects of child neglect in the form of communication (verbal, tactile), and poor caretaker responsiveness to child needs. Johnson (2000) documented a variety of negative developmental outcomes for children from Romanian orphanages during the 1990s. This research is particularly revealing because the participants had been adopted into homes in the United States and were receiving appropriate to excellent parenting at the time of the study. Johnson found that these children had unusually high rates of motor skill delays, language delays, problems of impulse control, difficulties in making transitions from one activity to another and impaired cognitive skills. With regard to general cognitive skills, of those children who had spent two years or more in institutional care, the mean overall IQ was 69, with a range from 52 to 98 (population mean is 100). Thus, there is no doubt that the postnatal care-taker environment can play a role in childhood pathology. Again, the most important questions involve determination of which environmental event for which types of children are most pathogenic.

Toxic characteristics of the physical environment that might damage important physiological systems of the developing child, particularly the rapidly developing central nervous system, constitute another broad class of etiological factors for psychopathology. Included in this category are environmental toxins ingested through the lungs (e.g., carbon monoxide), via drinking water (e.g., insecticide runoff from agricultural fields), in food (e.g., polychlorinated biphenyls-PCBS-found in fish) and other toxins ingested orally that are not food (e.g., lead paint). The negative effects of heavy metals are a clear example in this category of etiological factors. Lead, for example, has been present in the air, and continues to be present in dust due primarily to the combustion of lead-based additives in gasoline (Shannon 1996). Lead is also present in food, usually at very low levels, due to processes used to preserve some foods (e.g., canning). Lead pipes in older buildings also deposit lead into the water supply and airborne lead is eventually deposited in soil. Infants are particularly vulnerable to lead intoxication, partly because of their tendency to place materials in their mouth, but also due to the physiological factors related to this developmental period. For example, infants and preschool-aged children absorb five times more of the lead they ingest than do adults (Anderson, Pueschel and Linakis 1996). After absorption lead is deposited in blood, soft tissue and bone. One soft tissue site for deposits is the central nervous system. Physiological measures of brain activity have revealed that the electrical activity of the brain is altered when lead levels are high (Anderson, Pueschel and Linakis 1996). A review by Bellinger (1996) demonstrates associations between blood lead levels and measured intelligence, academic achievement, learning disabilities, hearing problems and hyperactivity. Studies on this one type of heavy metal poisoning illustrate the vulnerability of the young child to environmental toxins, and the relationship to pathopathology is clear.

The fourth set of etiological factors that have been found to be associated with psychopathology in childhood and adolescence is characteristics of the general (non-familial) social environment. A wide range of variables could be included in this, set including inadequate housing, crowding, deviant peer and adult models, poorly educated peers and adult models, lack of access to adequate health care and minority status. The classic research variable in this category is socioeconomic status (SES). Lower SES is associated with attention-deficit/hyperactivity disorder (Szatmari, 1992), conduct and oppositional defiant disorders (Capaldi and Patterson 1994), depression (Costello, et al. 1996), childhood-onset schizophrenia (Bromet and Fennig 1999) and mental retardation (Hodapp and Dykens 2003), to mention only the most well-documented examples.

The Underestimated Importance of the Prenatal Environment

Given the progress that has been made in understanding all these contributions to child psychopathology, it is not surprising that the medical, psychological and sociological communities continue to look to these areas for further advances. However, it is possible that many researchers are guilty of the same problem that afflicts the man who loses his keys while walking home from the pub at night. He looks only under the lamp post because that is where the light is.

To be sure, some light has been shed on the effect of the prenatal environment on developmental psychopathology. Most medical and mental health professionals know something about the negative effects of smoking during pregnancy and have been introduced to the concept of fetal alcohol syndrome. However, we believe that prenatal development does not have a sufficient time afforded to it during the training of the majority of developmental experts. Thus, we in psychology, sociology, education and medicine tend to underestimate the range of factors that can perturb development in the prenatal period, and underestimate the extent of these effects. Our belief in the importance of the prenatal period in developmental psychology are based on the increasing quantity and quality of research findings linking perturbations during prenatal development with medical, psychological and psychiatric outcomes for children. It is also based on five assumptions about development.

First, we subscribe to the notion that the development of the child is most easily disturbed by adverse events that occur during the period of most rapid development. In particular, insults to the CNS have their greatest impact upon cell populations, structures and processes that are in a period of rapid development at the time of the insult. This principle is a restatement of the Dobbing hypothesis outlined several decades ago (Dobbing and Smart 1974). During the second trimester and to a lesser extent during the third trimester of fetal development, the structure of the brain undergoes very rapid development. Cells proliferate, migrate and organize themselves at an astonishing rate. Axons grow, dendrites proliferate and myelination begins during the prenatal period, although these processes continue well into childhood and perhaps adolescence.

Aylward (1997) posits that brain development is more vulnerable to insult during the prenatal period than during infancy and early childhood, because insults during the fetal period result in damage to the developing architecture of the brain. During infancy and later in childhood, the structures are in place, but functions have not become crystallized. Thus, if one region of the CNS is damaged during childhood, another region might assume this function. Functional reorganization is more difficult if the construction of the basic structural elements of the brain have been disturbed.

Second, we believe there are higher levels of central nervous system compromise at the time of birth than has been recognized. Estimates by neuroscientists indicate that about 25 percent of conceptions are affected by developmental central nervous system disturbance (Aylward 1997). A portion of these disturbances results in fetal and infant death. Of those infants that survive, but are damaged, the risk of pathological outcomes is substantially increased, particularly if caretaker behaviors and sociological factors are less than optimal.

There is good reason to believe that the rate of CNS disturbance of infants that appear healthy at birth is higher than expected. The most highly developed research on birth defects is focused on those factors that produce physical anomalies (structural defects) that can be observed at birth. Most of these defects are the result of some problem that occurs during the first three months of pregnancy (see website of the Centers for Disease Control, *http://www.cdc.gov/ncbddd/bd*). The literature on early-occurring anomalies of pregnancy such as neural tube defects, for example, is substantial and rich in detail (Moore and Persaud 1993; Norman and Armstrong 1998). However, insults to the developing brain that occur during the later stages of fetal development (trimester two and three) are much less likely to be accompanied by readily observable physical anomalies. These less obvious CNS perturbations result in so called 'sleeper effects,' effects on behavior that may not appear until the child begins to engage in higher-level cognitive functions (speech, reading, social cognition). Often, these problems do not become obvious until the first few years of schooling.

Third, there is evidence that a large portion of prenatal disturbance to fetal development is environmental and is not due directly to genetic anomalies. The well-known negative effects on fetal CNS development of infections (e.g., toxoplasmosis, cytomegalovirus, rubella), of maternally ingested drugs (e.g., alcohol, dioxins) and hypoxia (oxygen deprivation) that are to be described more fully in this volume illustrate such environmental perturbations.

Fourth, there is a high level of comorbidity among psychopathologies. Comorbidity refers to the phenomenon whereby a single child is found to evidence symptoms at a level warranting diagnosis in more than one diagnostic category (Sroufe 1997). A disturbance during prenatal development may be responsible for central nervous system anomalies that manifest themselves as multiple psychopathologies, rather than as a single disorder. Angold, Costello and Erbani (1999) conducted a meta-analysis of 25 published studies on comorbidity and calculated median odds ratios for some of the most common co-occurring psychiatric disorders of childhood. They found a median odds ration of 10.7 for Attention-deficit/ Hyperactivity Disorder (ADHD) and Conduct Disorder (CD), meaning that if a child was diagnosed with ADHD, the child would be almost 11 times more likely to be diagnosed with a CD than if the child did not have a diagnosis of ADHD. High levels of violence, emotional and behavioral disorders, substance abuse, delinquency and learning difficulties have been observed in the same individuals in many samples (e.g., Greenbaum, Prange, Friedman and Silver 1991). Another common pattern is the comorbidity of anxiety and depression. Angold, et al. (1999) found that the median odds ratio for anxiety and depression in their meta-analysis was 8.2 and 6.6 for CD and depression. Seligman and Ollendick (1998) have also reported high comorbidity between anxiety and depression, and Willcutt and Pennington (2000) have documented high comorbidity for anxiety, depression and reading problems.

The pervasiveness of comorbidity suggests similar processes of malfunctions are involved in the array of seemingly heterogeneous symptoms (Angold, Costello and

Erbani 1999). The mechanism by which a heterogeneous set of symptoms occurs from a common neuro-architectural anomaly is not difficult to understand. A maternal viral infection, for example, might cross the placental barrier infecting the fetus. The resulting damage to the developing CNS would depend on the level of infection (mild, severe), the particular regions of the CNS that were most exposed to the infection and those regions that were most rapidly developing at that time. Since a number of brain structures are rapidly developing during any one week during the second trimester of pregnancy, damage to a variety of structures and biochemical processes could occur simultaneously. Further, any one structure subserves many different neurological functions.

The outcomes of infection by the cytomegalovirus (CMV) are illustrative. The virus has a particular affinity for rapidly growing germinal cells in the area of the lateral ventricles. This results in lesions in the region of the ventricles, cell death and calcifications. It may also result in cyto-architectural anomalies such as polymicrogyria (Aylward 1997). CMV infections result in a diverse set of somatic and brain anomalies that, in turn, result in fetal death, intrauterine growth retardation, microcephaly, seizures, mental retardation, prematurity, retinal pathologies, hearing pathologies and learning disabilities (Gershon, Gold and Nankervis 1997). Also, it is estimated that 90 percent of infected babies have no symptoms of the disease at birth, even though problems in hearing and learning are common later in development (Aylward 1997). It is noteworthy that almost all individuals are exposed to this virus during their lifetime (Gershon, et al. 1997). After exposure the infection may continue to reside in the infected individual for the remainder of their life, often in a dormant state. However, if the immune system becomes compromised (pregnancy may compromise the immune system), then the infection may become active again.

The final reason that prenatal factors play such a critical role in the development of psychological and behavioral problems of children is that the status of the CNS at the time of birth sets parameters for the influence of the other factors that affects the child throughout development. Consider the simplified model of development that we have described. First, genetic and prenatal factors, both singularly and in interaction, influence the development of the child. Further, the effect of environmental perturbations on fetal development is influenced by the genetic predispositions of the fetus. For example, male fetuses (a genetically determined characteristic) are more susceptible to many kinds of prenatal perturbations than females. Of course, a series of postnatal influences, of which most have strong reciprocal influences, also affect development (e.g., caretaker behavior). The principle point for the current discussion is that the prenatal influences that may alter the CNS of the fetus continue to have effects not only on the individual, but also on the social interactions of the child with caretakers, interactions with the physical environment and interactions with the social environment. Thus, if the child's cognitive abilities have been compromised by prenatal influences, these lessened abilities will influence caretaker behavior (e.g., parents and teachers may have to repeat socialization experiences many more times before the child learns a behavior), will have an influence on the broader social interactions of the child (e.g., may impact the economic resources of caretakers due to costs of remedial activities) and will have an influence on the environmental toxins to which the child is exposed (e.g., reduced intellectual capacity increases the likelihood of eating non-edible substances that may be contaminated). Thus, abnormalities of the child's CNS occurring in the prenatal period typically have a broad range of negative consequences that further perturb postnatal development.

This simplified model of development should not be interpreted to indicate that the authors view the CNS of the child as set on a given developmental path at the time of birth. In fact vast CNS development takes place during the first two years of life and structural changes continue through adolescence. Further, the function of the CNS is strongly influenced by caretaker behaviors and other factors (e.g., see Lyon, et al. 2003 for an example of CNS changes after reading instruction). Still, the evidence is compelling that environmental influences occurring during the prenatal period set probabilistic parameters for future development.

It is troubling that the prevalence of disrupted fetal CNS development has increased during the past 20 years and may increase in the near future. This is primarily due to two factors. First, more premature and very low birth weight infants are being saved through enhanced neonatal interventions than ever before. Allen, Donohue and Dusman (1993) now estimate that the lower limit of viability for premature infants is approximately 500 grams (14.2 ounces) (3,000 to 3,500 grams is typical) and 23 weeks gestation (37 to 40 weeks is typical). Children at these birth weights and levels of prematurity have very high risks of psychopathologies (Hack and Fanaroff 1999). Plural births (twins, triplets, etc.), also greatly enhance the rate of pregnancy complications, including low birth weight and prematurity. Due to improved technology for treating infertility there has been a steady increase since 1990 in the rate of plural births. This may further add to the rate of infants with mild to severe psychopathology. Thus, new and developing technologies have significantly decreased fetal and infant death, and have increased human fertility. These technologies are implemented at some cost. That cost is that there is a likely increase in the number of children with learning and behavior problems.

Summary

Approximately 2.5 percent of all children and adolescents born today will have severe behavioral, emotional and cognitive pathologies such as schizophrenia, mental retardation and autism. An additional 25 percent will exhibit less severe pathologies such as clinically significant anxiety, depression, conduct problems, learning disabilities and speech and language pathologies. The costs of these cognitive, behavioral and emotional problems are enormous, contributing significantly to medical, educational and penal burdens on society. The number of factors that contribute to these pathologies is large, but can be classified into genetic, prenatal environmental, postnatal caretaker, social environmental and physical environmental categories. Environmental factors occurring during the prenatal period have profound effects on development and these effects are not well understood by clinicians, researchers and policy makers. Prenatal influences are particularly important since (a) environmental perturbations have their greatest effect on systems that are in the state of most rapid development, making the CNS particularly vulnerable during the prenatal period; (b) estimates of CNS compromise may have underestimated the level of abnormality present because most research has been directed toward disease processes that resulted in easily observable physical anomalies at the time of birth; (c) there is strong evidence for specific adverse effects on the CNS of infections, maternally ingested toxins, maternal disease and perinatal events (e.g., hypoxia) on fetal CNS development; (d) the level of comorbidity among the emotional, social and cognitive psychopathologies of childhood strongly suggest similar processes or malfunctions are involved in these pathologies, and prenatal effects on the CNS represent likely candidates; and (e) prenatal CNS anomalies influence the affects of postnatal contributors to psychopathology, such as caretaker behavior, social responses to the child and exposure to environmental toxins.

Chapter 2
Prenatal Central Nervous System Development

This chapter provides an overview of the major stages of prenatal central nervous system (CNS) development. CNS development plays the central role in the primary argument of this book. That argument is that the prenatal CNS is particularly vulnerable to environmental perturbations because it is rapidly developing during that time period. Further, we argue that many of the learning and behavioral problems that occur in childhood and adolescence have their origins in these prenatal perturbations of CNS development.

This chapter sets the stage for exploring the relationship between prenatal exposures and later behavioral and/or psychological pathology by elucidating the normal course of prenatal brain development.

Prenatal CNS Development

To help conceptualize fetal CNS development, Nowakowski and Hayes (1999) metaphorically link the development of the CNS to the construction of a house. In the same way that a blueprint guides house construction, an individual's genome serves as a blueprint for the brain. Some of the DNA in the genome creates proteins that build structures, while others are 'timing genes' that manage the sequencing of the building process. Neurons and glial cells function as the foundational materials of bricks, wood and cement. Axons, dendrites and synaptic connections among neurons serve as the wiring for electricity and the telephone.

The construction of this elaborate communication structure we call the brain is complex, but there are some general principles that guide the process. First, while genes provide the blueprint, CNS development is a complex process that results from the interplay of genetically governed biological processes and a number of experiential/environmental factors (Capone 1996; Hynd and Willis 1989). Second, despite this complex genetic and environmental interaction, the formation of brain regions occurs according to a precisely sequenced schedule with more phylogenetically primitive regions (e.g., limbic system, forebrain) developing before more complex structures (e.g., cerebral cortex). Third, within these regions, brain development is most vulnerable to insult during periods of most rapid growth and development (Dobbing and Sands 1979). Thus, the timing of an insult may be more important than the dose or nature of the insult in influencing the pattern of malformation. The fourth guiding principle is that of all organs in the body, the brain is most vulnerable to teratogenic disruption because of the extended amount of time it requires for development (Capone 1996). Fifth, although this chapter discusses prenatal brain development, birth does not mark a particular milestone in the development of the brain. The brain continues to develop throughout the lifespan (Bayer, Yackel and Puri 1982), although the most significant development occurs early in development during the fetal period and the first years of life (Aylward 1997; Nowakowski and Hayes 1999). With these general principles in mind, the following discussion highlights the most important developmental processes occurring in the CNS.

First Trimester Development

Following fertilization of the ovum and subsequent rapid cell division, the embryonic disc emerges. The embryonic disc comprises three layers of cells: the ectoderm, mesoderm and endoderm. The inner layer (endoderm) will transform into the internal organs (e.g., digestive and respiratory systems) of the body while the middle layer (mesoderm) will form the musculature and skeletal systems. The outer layer (ectoderm) evolves into a variety of structures including the Central Nervous System (CNS). The central process through which the ectoderm forms the initial structure of the CNS is neurulation. Neurulation commences toward the end

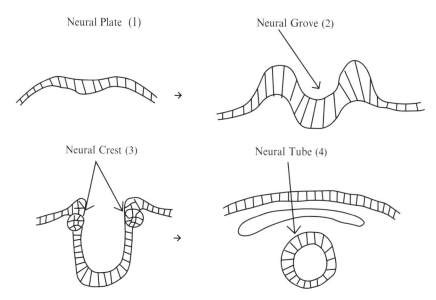

Fig. 2.1 Folding of Neural Tube

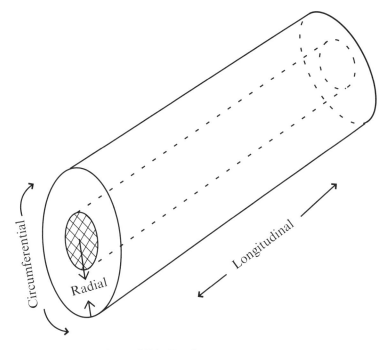

Fig. 2.2 Three Dimensional Neural Tube Development

of the third week of gestation when the outer layer of the embryo (the ectoderm) begins to fold upon itself to form the neural tube (see Figure 2.1).

The neural tube has a cylindrical (e.g., pipe-like) shape and develops along the three dimensions (longitudinal, circumferential and radial) that are typically used to describe a cylinder. Differentiation along these three dimensions determines the major structural aspects of the nervous system. Aylward (1997) and Nowakowski and Hayes (1999) provide a synopsis of this development. The head portion of the neural tube becomes the brain while the middle portion becomes the brain stem. The head or cephalic portion further differentiates into the forebrain, midbrain and hindbrain. In turn, these structures differentiate such that the rudiments of the adult brain are recognizable by the fifth week of gestation. For instance, by about the fifth week, the neural tube differentiates into the three primary structural units of the brain: the proencephalon (forebrain), the mesencephalon (midbrain) and the rhombencephalon (hindbrain). By the seventh week two additional structures are formed, creating the five primary units that will become the mature brain (Crossman and Neary 2000). The two additional structures are created when the prosencephalon and the rhombencephalon divide in two. The prosencephalon divides into the telencephalon and the diencephalon, while the rhombencephalon divides into the metencephalon and the myelencephalon. This developmental progression is illustrated in Fig. 2.3. Table 2.1 indicates the mature structures that develop for each of these five basic units of the CNS.

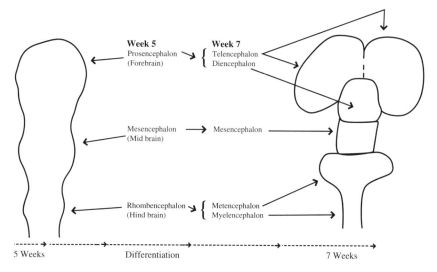

Fig. 2.3 Three & Five vesicle stages of brain development reference

Table 2.1 Sequence of CNS Development

Three-Vesicle Stage (Primary Brain Vesicles)	Five-Vesicle Stage (Secondary Brain Vesicles)	Mature Structure
Forebrain (Prosencephalon)	Telencephalon	Cerebral cortex, basal ganglia, hippocampus, amygdala, olfactory bulbs
	Diencephalon	Thalamus, hypothalamus, optical tracts, retinae
Midbrain (Mesencephalon)	Mesencephalon	Midbrain
Hindbrain (Rhombencephalon)	Metencephalon	Pons, cerebellum
	Myelencephalon	Medulla oblongata
Caudal part of neural tube	Same	Spinal cord

From: Crossman and Neary (2000). *Neuroanatomy: An illustrated color text*. New York: Churchill Livingstone.

Disruption to neural tube development during the first few weeks often produces severely teratogenic outcomes. These typically involve structural anomalies of the CNS, such as a complete failure to develop major structural elements (e.g., anencephaly), to more minor structural flaws (e.g., myelomeningocele, encephalocele). Structural failures produced at this early stage of development frequently have catastrophic functional outcomes ranging from fetal death to serious mental and motor dysfunctions (Layde, Edmonds and Erickson 1980; Lynberg, Khoury, Lu and Cocian 1994; Milunsky, et al. 1992; Shiota 1982).

Although the rudimentary brain structures appear very early in life via differentiation of the neural tube along the longitudinal and circumferential dimensions, significant development along the radial dimension continues to occur throughout the prenatal period. Development along the radial dimension involves the processes of cell proliferation, migration and differentiation. Fig. 2.4 illustrates the timing of these processes.

Cell Proliferation

Cell proliferation is the molecular process by which the two types of cells (e.g., neurons and glia) that comprise the nervous system are created. Cell proliferation begins within the germinal matrix following closure (or "zipping") of the neural tube. The germinal matrix is comprised of ventricular and subventricular proliferative zones of cells that are, in turn, responsible for creating all the remaining structural and functional cells of the nervous system (Rakic 1992). Cell proliferation begins around the 40th embryonic day and is almost complete by the sixth month of gestation (Sidman and Rakic 1973), although cell proliferation continues in a few areas (cerebellar and hippocampal areas) even after birth (Bayer, Altman, Russo and Zhang 1993). Nonetheless, most of the neurons of the adult CNS are produced during the middle third of gestation (Nowakowski 1987). In the cerebral cortex, for instance, cell proliferation ends by about day 120 of gestation (week 17 of a 40 week gestation; see Fig. 2.5) (Rakic and Singer 1988).

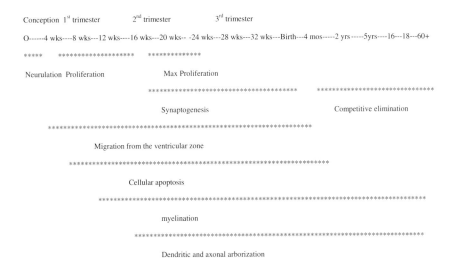

Fig. 2.4 Timing of CNS Cellular Development. From: Giedd, J. N. (1997). Normal Development. *Child and Adolescent Psychiatric Clinics of North America*, 6(2), 265-282

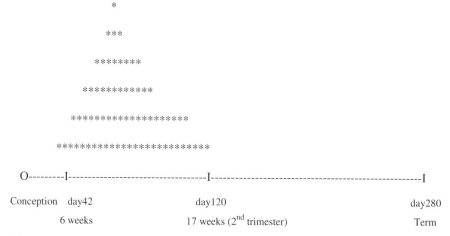

Fig. 2.5 Cell Proliferation in the Cerebral Cortex

All parts of the developing CNS have a ventricular zone. In some parts of the developing CNS there is an additional proliferative zone called the subventricular zone. This zone differs in several ways from the ventricular zone. Most of this difference is associated with the behavior of proliferating cells and the type of cells ultimately produced. Within the ventricular zone, for instance, there is substantial movement of the nuclei to and from the ventricular surface to the border of the ventricular zone with the subventricular zone and back again (Caviness, et al. 2003). This movement is depicted in Fig. 2.6.

On the other hand, proliferating subventricular zone cells do not move (See Nowakowski and Hayes 1999 for a more in-depth discussion of the cell cycle within the ventricular zone). Based in part on such behavior, it is thought that the subventricular zone primarily produces glial rather than neuronal cells (Nowakowski and Rakic 1981; Takahashi, Nowakowski and Cavines 1995). It has also been speculated that the subventricular zone is an evolutionarily newer cortical structure, compared to the ventricular zone (Sidman and Rakic 1973). Research typically posits that all of the neurons of the major subdivisions of the hippocampus (areas CA1, CA2 and CA3), an evolutionarily old cortical structure, are derived from the ventricular zone (Nowakowski and Rakic 1981). In contrast, the subventricular zone is believed to contribute large numbers of cells to the neocortex, the evolutionarily youngest structure in the brain (Sidman and Rakic 1982).

Cell Migration

Cells migrate from the two ventricular zones to their final positions. The timing of these events and ultimate destination of these neurons appears to be genetically

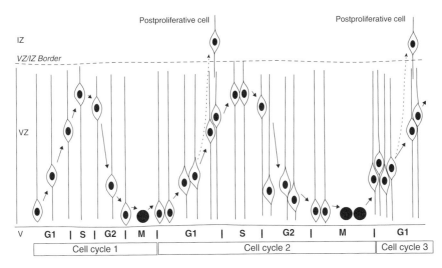

Fig. 2.6 Discussion of the Cell Cycle in the Ventricular Zone This diagram illustrates the up-and-down movement of the nuclei of the cells comprising the proliferative ventricular epithelium of the ventricular zone (VZ). With each pass through the cell cycle the nucleus of a single cell moves from its starting position at the ventricular surface at the beginning of G1 to the border of the VZ where it enters S. During G2, the nucleus again moves down the ventricular surface, where it enters M and divides to form two cells. With each pass through the cell cycle some postmitotic neurons are produced. The postmitotic neurons migrate away from the VZ to produce the structures of the adult brain (in this case the cerebral neocortex). (Copied with permission of Cambridge University Press from Nowakowski and Hayes 1999)

predetermined. The primary migrational activity occurs during weeks eight to 16 of gestation, with lesser activity continuing until week 25 (Kuzniecky 1994). There appear to be two forms of neuronal migration: passive and active (Hattan 1999; Hatten and Mason 1990; Nowakowski and Hayes 1999). Passive migration (cell displacement) occurs when cells are simply pushed away from where they originated by more recently generated cells (see Figure 2.7). In turn, these older cells are passively moved outward away from the proliferative zone. The result is that the oldest cells are located farthest from the proliferative zone. Passive migration is thought to lead to midline structures like the thalamus, dentate gyrus and regions of the brain stem (Altman and Bayer 1980; Bayer, Yackel and Puri 1982; Nowakowski and Rakic 1981).

Active migration requires that cells play a much more active role in reaching their final position. In contrast to passive migration, active migration occurs when younger cells move past older cells to the external regions of the brain, including the cerebral cortex (Rakic 1972; Sidman and Rakic 1973). Thus, the newly generated cells are located farthest from the proliferative zone, resulting in an inside-to-outside spatiotemporal gradient (see Fig. 2.8). Active migration is a big

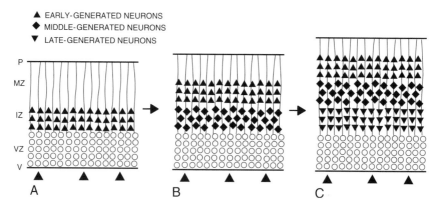

Fig. 2.7 Discussion of Passive Migration Some cells migrate only a short distance from the outer edge of the proliferative zone. When new cells are produced, the older ones are displaced outward away from the proliferative zone by the newly produced cells. (A through C) This sequence of events is illustrated as follows: (A) The first neurons to leave the ventricular zone are shown as triangles. (B) The next neurons to form (shown as diamonds) move away from the ventricular zone, displacing the earlier generated ones outward. (C) Finally, the last neurons to form (shown as inverted triangles) move away from the ventricular zone and displace both populations of earlier generated neurons. This sequence of events results in a specific distribution of neurons generally known as an outside-to-inside spatiotemporal gradient. V = Ventricular surface; VZ = ventricular zone; IZ = intermediate zone; CP = cortical plate; MZ = marginal zone; P = pial surface (Copied with permission of Cambridge University press from Nowakowski and Hayes 1999)

contributor to the development of the structures of the cortex, with different layers containing neurons with different migrational timetables (Nowakowski and Hayes 1999; Nowakowski, Cavines, Takahashi and Hayes 2002; Takahashi, Nowakowski and Cavines 1995). Migration is ultimately responsible for transforming the four fundamental layers of the telencephalic wall into the six-layered adult cerebral cortex. During the fifth gestational month, cerebral convolutions (e.g., sulci and gyri) appear. By the seventh month of gestation, all gyri appear and secondary and tertiary sulci become evident.

With an understanding of the mechanics of passive and active migration in mind, one understands that the final position of a neuron is linked to its time of origin. Researchers do not agree upon the actual mechanism by which cells "know" the location to which they should migrate. One of the more widely accepted theories suggests that radiating glial fibers direct migration to genetically predetermined regions of the brain in a complicated process that consists of at least three phases (Rakic 1978). At the beginning of a cell migratory phase a young neuron starts migrating by linking to a radial glial fiber. During the second or locomotor phase of migration the neuron moves along the surface of the radial glial cell. In the last phase of migration the neuron arrives at its final destination, detaches from the radial glial cell and is now ready for the process of differentiation. Recent research has focused attention on how

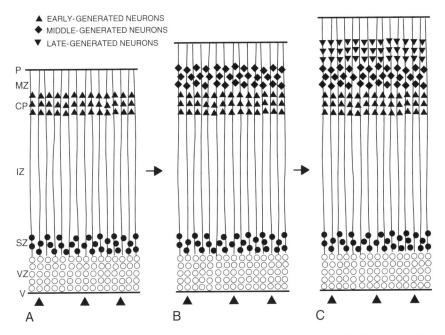

Fig. 2.8 Discussion of Active Migration Some cells may migrate a considerable distance from the proliferative zone. For example, in the cerebral cortex the later-generated cells bypass the earlier-generated cells and assume a position even farther from the proliferative zone. This is illustrated as follows: (A) The first neurons to leave the proliferative zones are shown as triangles. These cells form a cortical plate between the intermediate and the marginal zones. (B) The next neurons to form (shown as diamonds) leave the proliferative zones and migrate across the intermediate zone and past the previously generated cells to the top of the cortical plate. (C) The final neurons to reach the cortical plate are shown as vertical triangles. These cells have also migrated across the intermediate zone and past the previously generated cells to the top of the cortical plate. This sequence of events results in a specific distribution of neurons generally known as the inside-to-outside spatiotemporal gradient. V = Ventricular surface; VZ = ventricular zone; SZ = subventricular zone; IZ = intermediate zone; CP = cortical plate; MZ = marginal zone; P = pial surface. (Copied with permission from Cambridge University press from Nowakowski and Hayes, 1999)

reelin, a cell surface molecule, aides in directing neurons to their final position (Fatemi, et al. 1999; Nowakowski 1987). Additional research at the cellular and molecular levels is required to more precisely elucidate the mechanism of migration.

Cell Differentiation

Once neuronal and glial cells have migrated to their final positions these cells begin the process of differentiation. This starts by about the 25th month of gestation and does not finish until adolescence (Sidman and Rakic 1982). During the differentiation stage axonal and dendritic properties become fine-tuned as cells transform into committed members of specialized systems. As a result relevant connections among neurons become established and begin to function. Axons involve presynaptic functioning while dendrites involve postsynaptic activity. Dendrites grow out and form an arborization (e.g., tree-like) pattern depending upon cell class. Dendritic growth begins after the completion of the migration phase (25 to 30 weeks), and continues at a relatively slow rate through adolescence. Synapses are over-produced up until about three years of age; thereafter, synapses are eliminated such that by adolescence, synaptic density is only about 60 percent of the maximum density that was achieved at age two (Aylward 1997).

Axonal development progresses via pioneer axons. Pioneer axons establish a chemical marker by which other axons recognize and produce selective contact with specific neurons and systems. These chemical markers are thought to be present only at selective periods during fetal development and guide the development and differentiation of the axon to its ultimate site. Although axon growth seems to occur primarily prenatally, axon development has been observed to occur postnatally in certain brain structures such as the corpus collosum, at least into early childhood (Nowakowski and Hayes 1999). There is some debate within the neuroscience community regarding the growth and evolution of axons. Some researchers suggest that axonal growth is genetically programmed while others indicate that environmental and experiential factors influence the connections that are formed and eliminated (Schore 2001). For instance, lack of environmental stimulation significantly disrupts dendritic growth (Kolb and Fantie 1989; Kolb and Gibb 1999).

Neuronal differentiation is also important for a number of formative processes, including the later formation of neurotransmitters and specific receptor cells at postsynaptic sites. Each differentiating neuron must distinguish which neurotransmitters it will ultimately use. Similarly, postsynaptic sites must express the receptors they will need to receive input from presynaptic sites.

Myelination

During neuronal differentiation the axonal myelination process begins (around six months gestation), but will not be completed until adolescence. Myelination refers to the process of covering the axon with a fatty substance (myeline) that serves the function of insulating axons. Myelination promotes rapid and efficient transmission of nerve impulses, like the insulation on an electrical wire enhances the transmission of electricity in your home. Prior to myelination the communication between neurons is approximately 50 to 100 times slower than what it is after myelination.

Alyward (1997) discusses several general rules by which axons myelinate. First, proximal pathways myelinate before distal pathways. Second, sensory pathways myelinate prior to motor pathways. Third, projection pathways experience myelination prior to association pathways. As an example, corticovisual pathways necessary for the visual-smile response experience myelination by the third postnatal month, while motor cortex axons are myelinated by the first year of life. Fine motor development, as well as the maturation of the frontal lobes, is intimately linked to the myelination process.

Around the sixth month of gestation glial cells also begin the process of differentiating into oligodendrocytes and astrocytes. Oligodendrocytes are important for the genesis of myelin, while astrocytes have diverse functioning within the CNS, including repair of damaged tissue and removal of waste (Montgomery 1994). In the brain glial cells vastly outnumber neurons (10 to 50 times more).

Cell Death (Apoptosis)

During proliferation the number of cells created exceeds that which is needed within the mature CNS (Rakic, Bourgeois, Eckenhoff, Zecevic and Goldman-Rakic 1986). Some cells must be removed. This process has two distinct mechanisms: axonal retraction and neuronal pruning (Nowakowski and Hayes 1999). Axonal retraction involves recession of the collaterals of a neuron's axon or by a shrinking of the terminal arborization of the axon. Other connections are removed through selective cell death in which neurons die as a result of failing to establish appropriate connections (Hynd and Willis 1988). The retraction of axons and the death of cells are critically important to fetal brain and CNS development. Abnormalities in each process, selective cell death in particular, have been shown to lead to severe developmental abnormalities in experimental animals (Kuida, et al. 1996). Some research indicates that certain areas of the brain may experience up to 50 percent cell death (Oppenheim 1991). It is suggested, therefore, that neurons without appropriate connections become redundant and are eliminated according to a "use it or lose it" phenomenon. Cell death (apoptosis) is critically important for appropriate brain development (Zaidi, et al. 2001).

Summary

Within this chapter, we presented an overview of prenatal CNS development, emphasizing the processes occurring during the second and third trimester of pregnancy. The most important of these are cell proliferation, cell migration, cell differentiation, myelination and cell death. This discussion sets the stage for understanding the mechanisms by which the fetal brain may become perturbed, resulting in psychological and behavioral outcomes. Within each of the next chapters we discuss the mechanisms by which various factors such as smoking, illness, stress or infection can disrupt the developing fetal CNS.

Section B
Perinatal Meditors and Markers of Disturbances of Fetal Development: Introduction

Section B is devoted to three related topics: low birth weight, preterm birth and perinatal anoxia/hypoxia. These three related perinatal risk factors represent a significant public health concern. In addition to costly Neonatal Intensive Care Unit (NICU) stays, each condition has been linked to persistent health problems throughout the lifespan. For instance, babies born with low birth weight are at risk for a host of later medical complications including cerebral palsy, coronary heart disease, Type 2 diabetes and osteoporosis (Barker 1998). One study reported that the cost of low birth weight exceeds that of AIDS and approaches that of alcoholism (Lewit, Baker, Corman and Shiono 1995).

Effects of low birth weight and preterm birth are discussed together in Chapter 3, as these phenomena are typically highly correlated. That is, infants born prematurely are almost always of lower birth weight than those born at term. This chapter will also discuss consequences and issues of infants who have a birth weight that is lower than expected based on gestational age. In the case of small-for-gestational-age babies, the association between birth weight and birth age is more complex. Regardless of the type and causes of low birth weight, more has been written on the long-term learning and behavioral consequences of this variable than any other pre- or perinatal risk factors.

Chapter 4 summarizes some of the most relevant literature on oxygen deprivation in the perinatal period. It has been known for centuries that the transition from the fetus obtaining oxygen from the blood supply of the mother, to the infant obtaining oxygen from the air, is particularly difficult. Historically, much infant mortality took place at the time of birth because the physiological processes that are necessary for the infant to make this transition were poorly understood and few interventions were available. In the past five decades tremendous strides have been made in reducing infant mortality and morbidity due to perinatal anoxia. However, in the current medical environment, partly because of great strides in neonatal intensive care, anoxia and hypoxia continue to be major concerns of obstetricians because these improvements in medical technology have increased the number of extremely premature and very low birth weight babies that survive.

Both chapters are presented in this section for two reasons. First, the phenomena discussed in each chapter are related. Preterm birth is associated with increased risks of perinatal anoxic or hypoxic events. There is a second reason for combining these two chapters in one section. Very often low birth weight, preterm delivery and hypoxia are just one step in a cascade of events that began much earlier in pregnancy. Thus, these risk factors can be viewed in part as markers or mediators of a set of earlier risks to the health and development of the fetus.

Low birth weight, preterm birth and anoxia/hypoxia, of course, produce their own risks, independent of the factors that lead to these events. Leaving the environment of the uterus before all physiological systems are prepared, for example, creates a variety of hazards that can lead to further compromises of health and psychological well-being. Even some of the treatments used to sustain the viability of preterm infants are known to increase risks of pathology later in development. One example is the link between the use of oxygen and mechanical ventilation and malformations of the lungs, referred to as bronchopulmonary dysplasia (see Chapter 4).

One of the great difficulties of the vast literature on developmental outcomes of low birth weight is that it is unclear to what extent the effects observed are due to the perinatal condition of preterm birth or to the prior occurring events that lead to preterm birth. Given the current state of the literature, it is imperative that the reader keep in mind that the cause of the developmental pathology is most likely the result of a number of factors. The perinatal event being assessed is simply one of the most observable outcomes that occur at the time of birth. The reader should also understand that low birth weight and preterm birth have been studied as much as they have because the data necessary for the research is readily available. That is, records of birth weights are kept in hospital registries and other databases because these data are easily obtained and have been recorded for decades in most industrialized countries. In fact, birth weight is more easily assessed than length of gestation, so the majority of outcome studies are on low birth weight rather than preterm birth.

The emphasis in these two chapters is on definitions, physiological mechanisms and developmental outcomes of these perinatal conditions. Much less time will be devoted to the demographic, psychological, sociological, medical or environmental factors that are associated with low birth weight, preterm delivery or hypoxia. The remainder of the book reviews many of these more distal factors that are precursors to these perinatal events.

Chapter 3
Low Birth Weight and Prematurity: Effects on Child Developmental Outcomes

Low birth weight (LBW) and preterm birth are related phenomena about which more has been written with regard to child outcomes than any other set of variables in the pre- and perinatal literature. With a literature of thousands of articles related to the etiology and associated economic, sociological, psychological and medical correlates, this literature is difficult to summarize. This chapter is specifically devoted to outcomes for children and will not directly address the etiology of low birth weight or prematurity. Etiology is in large part what the remainder of this book is about since each of the conditions described under the heading of maternal medical complications, maternal substance abuse and maternal exposure to pollutants during pregnancy results in low birth weight and preterm delivery. But even limiting this chapter to outcome studies associated with children's learning and behavior problems, the available literature is far too large to be summarized here. Thus, the chapter will review only the most important trends in this literature. Further, primary consideration will be given to LBW. This is done for two reasons. First, LBW is easier to measure than premature birth; thus it is the subject of far more important studies than prematurity. Second, the correlation between premature birth and LBW is very high (greater than .80), so much of this review applies to premature birth.

The purpose of this chapter is to present an overview of the LBW outcomes in relation to intelligence, specific cognitive abilities, behavior and academic performance. In addition, this chapter will discuss the pathophysiological mechanisms by which LBW relates to such outcomes. Prior to embarking on such review, it is important to define LBW and distinguish it from preterm birth and intrauterine growth restriction (IUGR).

Definitions

The World Health Organization (WHO) has defined low birth weight (LBW) as a weight at birth of less than 2,500 grams (WHO 1980). However, birth weight is routinely categorized as normal (2,500 grams or more), low (less than 2,500 grams, about 5.5 pounds) or very low (less than 1,500 grams, about 3.3 pounds). LBW is further categorized in some contexts into three subgroups: moderately low (1,500 to 2,499 grams), very low (1,000 to 1,500 grams) and extremely low (less than 1,000 grams).

R.P. Martin and S.C. Dombrowski, *Prenatal Exposures: Psychological and Educational Consequences for Children.*
© Springer 2008

Included among the definition of LBW is a group of infants who have experienced intrauterine growth retardation (IUGR). The IUGR subgroup is comprised of infants below the 10th percentile in gender-specific birth weight for gestational age. They are sometimes referred to as 'small for gestational age' (SGA). All low birth weight babies are born either preterm or with IUGR. Most very low birth weight babies are born preterm. Preterm babies general are defined as those born at less than 37 weeks gestation.

IUGR represents a separate and discrete phenomena and can be considered as a sub-group of the LBW infants. There is a distinct literature devoted exclusively to IUGR. Whenever possible, therefore, researchers prefer to distinguish babies born with IUGR and adjust for their inclusion in the analysis. However, this often is difficult because information on gestational age is either unavailable or inaccurate.

One other area of definitional confusion exists. The terms LBW and premature birth have been and continue to be used interchangeably; this is due to their close statistical and clinical relationship. It was not until 1961 that the World Heath Organization (WHO) made the distinction between low birth weight and preterm birth. This distinction was clearly necessary because LBW births sometimes included babies born at term, but who are small for gestational age, as well as those born preterm. Still, the legacy of using these terms interchangeably persists, in part because of the high correlation between LBW and preterm birth (about .80). The confusion also persists because the outcomes associated with LBW are sometimes thought to be related to a disruption of neurological development caused by the premature birth. The disruptions could be the result of some intrusive medical intervention (ventilation) or psychosocial stress (lack of contact from caregivers; intrusive and painful medical procedures) associated with preterm birth, or could be a result of direct complications of premature birth (e.g., underdeveloped pulmonary function). Babies born with very low birth weight (<1,500 grams) are almost always born preterm, and these babies are the subject of much of the relevant literature.

These terms and their corresponding rates of birth are provided in Tables 3.1 and 3.2. These tables summarize natality data in the United States compiled by the Center for Disease Control and Prevention (CDC). Table 3.1 reveals that 7 to 8 percent of all babies have birth weights less than 2,500 grams. Further birth weight is related to ethnicity in the United States; African American women give birth to LBW babies at twice the rate of other ethnic groups. Table 3.2 documents that approximately 12 percent of all births are preterm, and again shows that African American mothers having a disproportionate percentage of these babies.

Outcomes

Historical Account of Adverse Outcomes

Prior to World War II, LBW research tended to be qualitative, sometimes even anecdotal. It rarely utilized standardized measures of intelligence, academic achievement and behavior (Benton 1940). Yet the conclusions reached from these early studies

Table 3.1 Birthweight for Three Major Ethnic/Racial Groups

Birth Weight	White Non-Hispanic	Black Non-Hispanic	Mexican	Total
2001				
>=2,500 grams	93.23	86.93	93.92	92.32
<2,500 grams	6.79	13.07	6.08	7.67
2,500-1,500 grams	5.60	9.99	5.03	6.23
<1,500 grams	1.17	3.08	1.05	1.44
<1,000 grams	0.54	1.70	0.50	0.71
2002				
>=2,500 grams	93.09	86.61	93.84	92.12
<2,500 grams	6.90	13.39	6.16	7.88
2,500-1,500 grams	5.73	10.24	5.09	6.35
<1,500 grams	1.17	3.15	1.07	1.46
<1,000 grams	0.54	2.10	0.52	0.72

Table 3.2 Gestation Length for Three Major Ethnic/Racial Groups

Birth Weight	White Non-Hispanic	Black Non-Hispanic	Mexican	Total
2001				
>=37 weeks	89.19	82.37	88.78	88.06
<37 weeks	10.81	17.63	11.22	11.94
36 weeks	4.23	5.53	4.12	4.41
32-35 weeks	5.02	8.05	5.51	5.58
28-31 weeks	1.04	2.27	1.06	1.22
<28 weeks	0.52	1.75	0.53	0.73
2002				
>=37 weeks	89.02	82.34	88.59	87.92
<37 weeks	10.98	17.66	11.41	12.08
36 weeks	4.23	5.55	4.25	4.49
32-35 weeks	5.10	8.06	5.54	5.63
28-31 weeks	1.02	2.25	1.06	1.22
<28 weeks	0.43	1.80	0.56	0.74

were generally consistent with conclusions resulting from research since that time. The early studies depicted a linear negative relationship between birth weight and child outcomes: that is, the lower the birth weight, the greater the risk of learning or behavior problems. LBW children were found in these early studies to experience increased difficulties in the areas of concentration and attention. Also, LBW children were found to display higher levels of irritability, shyness, fearfulness and emotional reactivity than their peers with normal birth weight. For all these outcomes the lower the birth weight, the more adverse the outcome.

Prior to the 1940s children born prematurely were often left with little or no neonatal intervention which tended to exacerbate developmental outcomes. Between 1940 and 1960 some interventions were instituted, with varying effects on the later development of the baby. Some interventions, such as hyper-oxygenation of incubators, strongly contributed to the adverse affect of preterm birth and LBW. High levels of oxygen were found to increase the chances of brain damage, retinopathy and deafness. As a result, the medical community often ascribed the negative developmental outcomes observed to prematurity or LBW. This attribution was reinforced by the available literature of the day, in which two-thirds of children with LBW were found to have a disability, particularly if they were born with VLBW. As an example, one study of very low birth weight children born between 1947 and 1950 found that 44 percent of these children had intelligence quotients under 70, and only one-third escaped any disability (Lubchenco, et al. 1963). The outcomes were better for moderately low birth weight infants (1,500 to 2,499 grams), but still worse than for their normal birth weight counterparts. During this time period, children born below 1,000 grams (or less than 28 weeks gestation) usually died. If they survived, these children experienced higher levels of physical, psychological and cognitive disability (Hack, Klein and Taylor 1995). Many of the studies focused on more profoundly disabling outcomes such as cerebral palsy, mental retardation and disabilities such as visual or hearing impairment. Very little research investigated more subtle psychological, educational and behavioral outcomes that would not have necessarily been evident at birth.

After the advent of neonatal intensive care in the 1960s the field has witnessed increased survival of even the smallest infants. At present the lower limit of viability of an infant is around 450 grams or 23 weeks gestation, though there have been reports of "micro-premies" weighing less who have survived (Allen, Donohue and Dusman 1993; Picard, Del Dotto and Breslau 2000). Furthermore, the field has experienced a concomitant decrease in the level of cerebral palsy, blindness and deafness, due in part to advances in neonatal and obstetrical technology such as improved delivery room care, ventilation, surfactant therapy, intravenous fluid therapy, umbilical artery catheter placement to monitor oxygenation, improved neonatal monitoring of cardiac and respiratory functioning and phototherapy to treat jaundice. These medical interventions all helped to reduce mortality levels, resulting in a larger percentage of survival of extremely low birth weight babies. However, surviving micro-premies generally experience a higher percentage of severe developmental outcomes such as cerebral palsy. As a result the overall level of severe developmental delay has remained nearly constant despite improved neonatal and perinatal technology.

Very low birth weight babies constitute about 15 percent of low birth weight births, but are the subject of the majority of developmental outcome studies. The next section will provide a synopsis of this large and expanding research by presenting an overview of the cognitive, academic and behavioral sequelae of LBW. Studies based upon regional and national cohorts are summarized in Tables 3.3 to 3.5.

Outcomes of Low Birth Weight

Medical and psychological researchers have contributed the largest number of studies documenting the association between low birth weight and various child outcomes. However, this literature is broad and includes researchers from education, nursing

Table 3.3 Relationship Between Birth Weight and Intelligence Test Scores

Authors	Cohort Description	Age	Birth Weight Range (grams) (Percent with IQ <70 and IQ 70 to 84; Mean IQ test score)					
			<750	750 to 1,000	<1,000	1,000 to 1,499	1,500 to 2,499	>2,500/NBW
Saigal et al. 2005	Regional (Ontario)	12-16	<70 22.5% 70-84 25.0 Mean IQ=86					<70 0% 70-84 8.1% Mean IQ=102
Anderson et al. 2003	Regional (Australia)	8		Mean IQ=91	Mean IQ=95.5			Mean IQ=104.9
Doyle et al. 2001	Regional (Australia)	14			<70 20.2% 70-84 25.3% Mean Verbal IQ=90.1			<70 2.4% 70-84 14.3% Mean Verbal IQ=103.2
Taylor et al. 2000	Regional (Cleveland)	12-16	<70 37% Mean IQ=83.5	15.0% Mean IQ=96.8				<70 6% Mean IQ=106.2
Stjernqvist et al. 1999	Regional (South Sweden)	10			<70[a] 15% 70-84 28% Mean IQ=89.8			<70 0% 70-84 4% Mean IQ=106.5
Wolke et al. 1999	Regional (South Germany)	6				<70[b] 23.5% 70-84 26.1 Mean IQ=84.8		<70 0.8% 70-84 12.5% Mean IQ=99.7
Horwood et al. 1998	National (New Zealand)	7-8			<85 36.2%	24.7%		<85 10.7%
Hall et al. 1995	National (Scotland)	8			<70 – <70-84 27% Mean IQ=90.4	4% 19% 93.7		<70 0.4% <70-84 10.0% Mean IQ=101.1
McCormick et al. 1992	Regional	8-10			<70 13% 70-84 29% Mean IQ=87.9	5% 19% 96.5	5% 17% 96.3	<70 0% 70-84 13% Mean IQ=103.1
Saigal et al. 1991	Regional (Ontario)	8			<70 8% 70-84 25% Mean IQ=91.1			<70 1% 70-84 4% Mean IQ=103.8

[a] Birthweights range from 500 to 1,480; mean = 1,042
[b] Birthweights are < 1,500 grams.

Table 3.4 Relationship Between Birth Weight and Academic/School Performance

Authors	Cohort Description	Age	Measure	Birth Weight Range (grams)					
				<750	750 to 1,000	<1,000	1,000 to 1,499	1,500 to 2,499	>2,500/NBW
Saigal et al. 2005	Regional (Ontario)	12-16	WRAT Reading						
			<70	38.2 %	18.4%				<70 2.4 %
			70-84	20.6 %	18.4%				70-84 8.9 %
				Mean = 96	Mean =94				Mean = 102
			Arith <70	50.0 %	32.0 %				<70 4.8 %
			70-84	26.5 %	35.9 %				70-84 24.2 %
				Mean =84	Mean =84				Mean = 94
			Repeat Grade	25 %	N/A				6 %
			Special Education	49 %	N/A				10 %
			School Difficulty	72 %	53 %				13 %
Breslau et al. 2004	Regional (Detroit)	11	WJ Reading					Mean =106.2[c]	111.1
			WJ Math					Mean =105.7	112.1
		17	WJ Reading					Mean =104.6	108.0
			WJ Math					Mean =100.8	104.7
Granau et al., 2004	Regional (British Columbia)	17	WRAT Math <1 Std Dev	43 %					10 %
Anderson et al. 2003	Regional (Australia)		WRAT Reading			Mean=96.6			103.3
			Spelling			Mean=94.4			100.0
			Arithmetic			Mean=89.2			98.0
Finnstrom et al. 2003	Regional (South Sweden)	9	School Problems	School Problems			32.8 %[b]		11.1 %[b]
		12		School Problems			39.1 %[b]		12.3 %[b]
Elgen et al. 2002	Regional (Norway)	11		CBCL School Problems			17 %[b]		7 %[b]
Taylor et al. 2000	Regional (Cleveland)	12-16	WIAT Reading WJ	Mean =87.7	96.4				Mean = 102.4
			Letter/Word ID WJ	88.8	101.0				105.6
			WJ Math	Mean= 78.9	98.1				103.2

Table 3.4 (continued)

Birth Weight Range (grams)

Authors	Cohort Description	Age	Measure	<750	750 to 1,000	<1,000	1,000 to 1,499	1,500 to 2,499	>2,500/NBW
Wolke et al. 1999[a]	Regional (South Germany)	6	KABC Achievement						
			Serious Impairment			<72 [b]	23.5 %	<72	1.9 %
			Mild Impairment			<86	25.0	<86	10.6 %
						Mean = 84.6		Mean = 100.9	
Horwood et al. 1997	National (New Zealand)	7-8	Below Avg						
			Reading			23.9 %	29.3 %		15.6 %
			Writing			37.1 %	37.4 %		20.3 %
			Spelling			41.3 %	40.7 %		21.3 %
			Math			37.5 %	37.0 %		15.9 %
			P.E.			32.9 %	24.3 %		9.2 %
			Special Education			26.7 %	22.9 %	9.4 %	
Hall et al. 1995	National (Scotland)	8	Learning Support			55 %	39 %		18 %
			Retained			11 %	45 %		0.4 %
McCormick et al. 1992	Regional	8-10	Learning Problems				25 %[b]	19 %	13 %

[a] Birthweights range from 500 to 1,480; mean=1,042

[b] Birthweights are <1,500 grams

[c] Birthweights <2,500; used suburban outcomes data from study

Table 3.5 Relationship Between Birth Weight and Behavior

Authors	Cohort Discription	Age	Measure	Birth weight range (grams)							
				<750	750 to 1000	<1000 P	<1000 T	1000 to 1499	1500 to 2499	>2500/NBW P	>2500/NBW T
Anderson et al. 2003	Regional (Australia)	8	BASC								
			Externalizing			50.0	48.8			48.9	47.6
			Internalizing			50.1	52.4			47.2	50.3
			Behavior Symptoms Index			51.2	51.2			48.7	48.5
			Adaptive Skills			48.0	47.3			50.7	51.2
Grunau et al. 2004	Regional (British Columbia)	17	Achenbach CBCL (%=Clin sig problems)								
			Total	23%						7%	
			Internalizing	30%						7%	
			Externalizing	19%						0%	
Taylor et al. 2000	Regional (Cleveland)	12-16	Achenbach CBCL								
			Total Prblms-Parent	51.9	48.2 [a]					49.7	
			Total Prblms-Teacher	54.1	51.9					50.1	
			Attention-Parent	58.5	55.2					52.4	
			Attention-Teacher	56.8	55.1					53.7	
			Behavior Compet	43.0	45.6					47.7	
			Social Skills-Teach	94.9	97.9					96.7	
			Child Depression Inv	47.9	46.7					44.9	
Stjernqvist et al. 1999	Regional (South Sweden)	10	Achenbach CBCL								
			Total Problem			26.1 [a]				15.5	
			Internalizing			7.8				3.8	
			Externalizing			8.5				6.0	
			Social Competence			2.9				0.7	
			Attention			4.0 (24% ADHD)				1.6 (8% ADHD)	

Table 3.5 (continued)

Authors	Cohort Discription	Age	Measure	Birth weight range (grams)						
				<750	750 to 1000	<1000	1000 to 1499	1500 to 2499	>2500/NBW	
Horwood et al. 1997	National (New Zealand)	7-8	Behaviour Problems (Combined Conner's/ Rutter Scale)							
			Inattention/hyperactivity			21.3%	22.1%		7.4%	
			Conduct Problems			12.0%	18.0%		8.1%	
			Anxiety/Withdrawal			25.3%	17.9%		7.1%	
McCormick et al. 1992	Regional	8-10	Behavior Problems			29%	28%%	29%	21%	

[a] Birthweights range from 500 to 1480; mean = 1042
[b] Birthweights are <1500 grams
[c] Birthweights <2500; used suburban outcomes data from study

and epidemiology. Researchers from different disciplines often used different methods, making comparisons across studies somewhat difficult. For example, the majority of the medically oriented studies are case-control investigations that allow for analysis of smaller sample sizes and control of confounding variables through sample selection. The data from these studies is often analyzed using logistic regression techniques, with the main outcome being an odds ratio. The odds ratio indicates the relative risk of the 'case' outcome when compared to the 'control.' The psychological community typically favors univariate or multivariate statistical procedures that allows for the control of confounding effects via statistical covariation. This approach also provides for a comparison of means (e.g., full scale IQ) or other statistical parameters.

Cognitive Outcomes. Shenkin, Starr and Deary (2004) indicated that there are more than 3,000 citations with the keywords birth weight and intelligence. Regardless of type of research design, this literature clearly indicates a gradient relationship between LBW and intelligence, even when SES is accounted for. Although many LBW babies have few deleterious effects, the risk of scores in the below average or mentally retarded range of intelligence increases with decreasing birth weight (See Table 3-3). Such deficiencies become increasingly evident in the smallest of LBW children (< 1,000 grams), the so-called extremely low birth weight (EBLW) babies.

Several studies indicate that from 32 to 49 percent of extremely low birth weight children (< 1,000) will experience below average (< 85) IQ test scores. This compares with approximately 16 percent of the population of normal birth weight children (McCormick, Gortmaker and Sobol 1992; Saigal, Szatmari, Rosenbaum, Campbell and King 1991; Stjernqvist and Svenningsen 1999; Teplin, Burchinal, Johnson-Martin, Humphrey and Kraybill 1991). Differences in IQ between low birth weight and normal birth weight children persist even when children with obvious neurological abnormalities (e.g., cerebral palsy) are excluded from analyses. Saigal, et al. (2005) report a mean IQ of 86 among adolescents who weighed < 750 grams at birth. These authors noted that babies born with birth weights of 750 to 1,000 grams had average IQs of 91, compared to NBW peers of 102. Taylor, Klein and Hack (2000) reported average IQs of 83.5, 96.8 and 106.2 in children with birth weights of less than 750 grams, 750 to 1,000 grams and normal birth weights, respectively.

VLBW research suggests that the adverse cognitive effects persist beyond childhood into adolescence and adulthood (Hack, et al. 1992; Hack, et al. 1991; Hack, et al. 2002; Taylor, Klein and Hack 2000; Taylor, Klein, Minich and Hack 2000). In essence, the research suggests stability of IQ test score performance starting around childhood and persisting into adulthood. Furthermore, the limited available research in relation to gender suggests that females fare better than males, although not all studies have reported such gender effects.

The literature on the cognitive outcomes of moderately low birth weight (MLBW; 1,500 to 2,499 grams) is sparse. It often is included in VLBW studies in an ancillary fashion, with the outcomes from the VLBW babies receiving primary consideration. Still, data with respect to MLBW babies indicates a similar gradient relationship such that the higher birth weight babies tend to manifest higher IQ test scores (Shenkin, Starr and Deary 2004).

Bhutta, Cleves, Casey, Cradock and Anand (2002) present the results of an interesting meta-analysis investigating 15 case-control studies of children born preterm who were assessed after their fifth birthday. These researchers conducted a MEDLINE search and their review initially included 227 studies. Of these, 15 studies with cognitive data were selected for inclusion. Sample sizes of the cases ranged from 15 to 255, and sample sizes of controls ranged from 15 to 500, with control populations matched with the cases on at least one demographic characteristic (e.g., gender, ethnicity, socioeconomic status). The authors used fairly stringent inclusion criteria and limited their review to only case-control studies, omitting studies that employed multivariate methods. Using a random-effects meta-analysis model, Bhutta, et al. (2002) reported results consistent with that of the LBW literature. They reported a weighted mean difference between the mean cognitive scores of the cases and the controls of 10.9 in favor of the controls. In other words, children born preterm were likely to have an IQ score approximately 10.9 points lower than normal birth weight children matched for sociodemographic characteristics. Moreover, the mean cognitive test scores were significantly correlated with birth weight ($R^2 = 0.51$; $p < 0.001$). The authors of this meta-analysis concluded that preterm birth is clearly associated with lower cognitive scores. Limitations of this particular meta-analysis involved its inability to determine the specific impact of demographic variables on the measured cognitive outcomes because of the type of methodology employed (case-control). Also, the review did not distinguish low birth weight from very low birth weight.

Overall, whether the variable under investigation is birth weight or preterm birth, the relationship with cognitive ability clearly indicates a gradient relationship with decreasing intelligence test scores following decreasing gestational age or birth weight. These findings have been replicated internationally in data sets ranging from small case control studies to large nationally based studies from New Zealand or Scotland. Unfortunately, data regarding gender and ethnicity moderation of this relationship LBW is poor. The limited available research suggests that LBW males experience greater adverse impact with respect to IQ test scores, but not all research has produced this result. The research in relation to ethnicity is surprisingly sparse, but does suggest a gradient relationship between birth weight and IQ test performance. (Dombrowski, Noonan and Martin, 2007)

Specific Cognitive Abilities. The vast majority of researchers who have looked at the outcomes for preschool and school-aged children of LBW have used a global measure of cognitive ability. With the possible exception of measures of language development, measures of specific cognitive abilities have been rare. Research into the specific abilities or skills that LBW children have failed to develop is important, because it allows for a better understanding of why general cognitive ability has been adversely affected.

Memory and processing speed are two specific abilities that play a role in molar cognitive ability. In a recent series of studies Rose and colleagues have found that LBW infants and school-aged children obtained poorer memory scores and scores on measures of processing speed than their age-matched full term peers (see Rose and Feldman 2000 for a review). Of particular interest is the work of this group with VLBW infancy. They found that memory and processing speed deficits assessed at six months were stable through the first year of life, and accounted for much of the difference between VLBW infants and age-matched controls on a general cognitive measure. Preterm infants with respiratory distress syndrome (RDS) in particular performed more poorly on measures of memory. This finding was also obtained in a school-age follow-up. RDS occurred for about 76 percent of the LBW infants in the study. In most cases they required mechanical respiratory ventilation for at least one day. Such infants, despite attempts to maintain oxygenation, are likely to suffer hypoxic-ischemic episodes, or disturbances of cerebral blood perfusion. In all such cases the brain is deprived of oxygen. It is known that the neurons of the hippocampus, an area of the brain particularly involved in short-term memory, is especially vulnerable to oxygen deprivation (Rose and Feldman, 2000). Thus, Rose and Feldman tentatively believe that perinatal oxygen deprivation may account for memory differences observed for children with RDS.

Academic Achievement and School-Related Functioning. There is a sizeable body of research documenting that LBW is associated with increased learning difficulties, below average standardized achievement performance, grade repetition and special education placement (Carran, Scott, Shaw and Beydoun 1989; Hack, Taylor, Klein and Eiben 1994; Hunt, Tooley and Harvin 1982; McCormick, Brooks-Gunn, Workman-Daniels, Turner and Peckham 1992; Schreuder, et al. 1992) (See Table 3.4 for a tabular summary of these and other related studies). For instance, several regional and national birth cohort studies have revealed that increased rates of special education or learning support services are provided for students who had low birth weight (Hall, McLeod, Counsell, Thomson and Mutch 1995; Horwood, Mogridge and Darlow 1998; Saigal, et al. 2005). These studies indicate that approximately one-half of children with very low birth weight received learning support for special education services. A smaller sample size hospital-based study revealed that nearly one-third of very low birth weight (<1,500 grams) children either experienced special education placement (15 percent) or grade repetition (17 percent) compared with 14 percent of normal birth weight matched controls (11 percent repetition; 4 percent special education), even when accounting for socioeconomic status (McCormick, et al. 1992). This compares with a respective rate of 17 percent and 5 percent for grade repetition and special education placement for moderately low birth weight children. Carran, et al. (1989) indicated a 25 percent rate of special education placement among very low birth weight children, compared to a rate of 13 percent for the moderately low birth weight and normal birth weight children. A recent study by Saigal, et al. (2005) indicated that 49 percent of the babies with ELBW (<750 grams) received special education support as children. Further, one-fourth experienced a grade repetition.

Additional studies have shown that ELBW and VLBW children utilize special education services and other services for slow learners at a particularly high rate. One of the strongest was by Hall, McLeod, Counsell, Thomson and Mutch (1995). They investigated a national birth cohort from Scotland. These researchers found that VLBW and ELBW children experienced a greater percentage of grade retentions (11 percent and 9 percent, respectively) compared with a normal birth weight control (0.4 percent). Further, ELBW (55 percent) and VLBW (39 percent) utilized learning supports in school at a higher rate than normal birth weight control (18 percent).

A national birth cohort study out of New Zealand produced similar results (Horwood, Mogridge and Darlow 1998). Compared to a nationally representative control group, children born with very low birth weight and extremely low birth weight produced more adverse findings across all outcomes studied. This study revealed a 6.3 and 5.6 relative risk of enrollment in special education for the ELBW and VLBW groups, respectively. The relative risk of below average school performance for both the ELBW and VLBW groups was found to be 2.0 for reading, 2.3 for written expression, 2.6 for spelling, tripled for mathematics and nearly quadrupled for physical education.

The Saigal, et al. (2005) study indicated that mathematics performance was a particularly affected academic area with over three-fourths of ELBW babies scoring in the below average range. This is consistent with other literature that reports greater difficulty in mathematics among child with LBW (Breslau, Paneth and Lucia 2004). For example, Breslau, et al. (2004) found that LBW youth at age 17 had a 50 percent greater likelihood for scoring below a standard score of 100 on measures of mathematics and reading when compared to their NBW counterparts. However, these authors found a stronger relationship with mathematics than with reading. Breslau, et al. (2004) and Johnson and Breslau (2000) indicated that LBW boys tend to be more affected than girls.

Another recent study focused on birth weight differences between monozygotic twins (Asbury, Dunn and Plomin 2006). This research design allowed for the control of some environmental and genetic factors not controlled in most studies. Significant associations were obtained between birth weight differences between twins and academic performance. Differences were particularly strong at the extremes of discordance in birth weight of the twins. This study also clearly implicated the early child rearing environment of the twins, and the interaction with birth weight.

In summary, the research indicates increasing special education, learning support and grade repetition with decreasing birth weight. Furthermore, the rates of special education participation appear to accelerate as the children advance in age, and cognitive and learning activities become more demanding (Carran, et al. 1989). In fact, recent research suggests that the difficulties found in childhood linger through age 17 (Breslau, Paneth and Lucia 2004).

Behavioral Outcomes. Children with low birth weight have been found to have higher levels of behavioral and emotional difficulties than their age-matched normal birth weight peers (See Table 3.5). Most of the studies regarding behavioral correlates have been conducted on VLBW cohorts. Four regional and national low birth weight studies are compiled in Table 3.5 and demonstrate that LBW children displayed greater symptoms of ADHD, total behavior problems and behavior problems categorized as internalizing and externalizing. Taylor, et al. (2000) reported that LBW children had higher scores on the Child Depression Inventory than controls. Similarly, ratings on the Achenbach Child Behavior Checklist (CBCL) revealed higher ratings of inattention, behavioral incompetence and total CBCL problems in an ELBW (< 1,000 grams) population. Stjernqvist, et al. (1999) investigated the relationship of VLBW (< 1,500 grams) in relation to ratings on the CBCL and diagnoses of ADHD in a regional cohort from southern Sweden. This study revealed that 24 percent of VLBW children were diagnosed with ADHD, compared with 8 percent of the NBW children. Similarly, this study found increased ratings of behavioral problems (total score, internalizing, externalizing) within the VLBW group. In a national birth cohort study, Horwood, et al. (1998) found greater levels of inattention/hyperactivity, conduct problems and anxiety/withdrawal in a national birth cohort from New Zealand. This study revealed that VLBW babies displayed problems at nearly three times the rate of NBW children. Horwood, et al. (1998) also found a gradient relationship with behavior problems, both internalizing and externalizing, such that ELBW babies experienced greater behavioral problems than VLBW babies in the areas of inattention/hyperactivity and anxiety/ withdrawal. Likewise, McCormick, Gortmaker and Sobol (1992) reported increased behavioral problems across all LBW categories studied (< 1,000 g, 1,000 to 1,499, 1,500 to 2,499). Consistent with the preponderance of the research evidence, Sommerfelt, Ellertsen and Markestad (1993) reported greater conduct and emotional difficulties in VLBW males from a regional cohort from Norway on the Personality Inventory for Children (PIC). This study, along with several others, points toward a propensity for VLBW males, compared to VLBW females, to experience greater behavioral difficulties (Sommerfelt, Ellertsen and Markestad 1996); however, not all studies have found such a relationship.

Bhutta, et al. (2002) conducted a meta-analysis of case control studies of preterm births that looked at behavioral functioning. Their meta-analysis investigated whether children born preterm were likely to have different outcomes on measures of internalizing and externalizing behaviors, and measures of ADHD. Children born preterm were found to experience greater difficulty in either internalizing or externalizing behaviors in 81 percent of the 16 studies. Further details regarding the nature of these difficulties were unavailable from this study. However, this meta-analysis underscores the finding that some children born preterm with LBW are described as having disruptive behavior in some studies, and in other studies they are described as being more withdrawn and less socially competent (Hoy, Sykes and Bill 1992). The six studies reviewed for differences in ADHD revealed a pooled 2.64 relative risk of an increase in ADHD following preterm birth.

A recent study of monozygotic twins by Asbury, et al. (2006) studied the differences in behavior ratings of twins as these were related to differences in birth weight at age seven. They found that anxiety, hyperactivity, conduct problems, peer problems and academic achievement correlated significantly with monozygotic differences in birth weight and early family environment. Associations increased at the extremes of twin discordance in birth weight. Effect sizes ranges from 2 to 12 percent of the variance. Higher risk families showed stronger associations. This research design allows for important controls of a large number of variables and helps put into perspective the effects of birth weight on behavior. One take home message is that the effects of birth weight are moderated by issues of family chaos, maternal depression and general socioeconomic circumstances. Under optimal conditions, these effects need not be large, except in extreme cases of LBW.

Pathophysiological Basis of LBW

There is increased evidence that preterm birth is a singularly significant risk factor for later adverse developmental outcomes. This evidence has accumulated from neurological studies using brain imaging techniques such as cranial ultrasound or MRI technology. Studies comparing the brains of preterm and full-term children have identified morphological patterns in children who manifested developmental sequelae. For instance, neurological studies of babies born premature with LBW have revealed a thinner corpus callosum, a reduction in grey matter and a reduction in brain volume that results in larger ventricles containing more cerebrospinal fluid. In addition, the sensorimotor cortex, amygdala and hippocampus also are often reduced in size. These morphological outcomes are probably the result of brain hemorrhage including bleeding into the germinal matrix and the lateral ventricles (Paneth, Rudelli, Kazam and Monte 1994).

Forfar, et al. (1994) suggest that there are three pathophysiological mechanisms by which brain damage occurs in the preterm/low birth weight infant. This includes periventricular leukomalacia, perinatal telencephalic leukoencephalopathy and periventricular hemorrhage. Periventricular leukomalacia is a condition of prematurity that results in softening and subsequent damage to the white matter of the brain around the ventricles. The white matter in this region is responsible for transmitting information between the nerve cells and the spinal cord, and can affect the nerve cells that control motor movements. Babies afflicted by periventricular leukomalacia, particularly those born before 30 weeks gestation, are at greater risk of developing cerebral palsy as well as cognitive and learning deficits.

Telencephalic leukoencephalopathy is another type of brain damage associated with prematurity. Like periventricular leukomalacia, telencephalic leukoencephalopathy results in destruction to the white matter of the brain responsible for transmission of information in the telencephalon. This condition also leads to a spectrum of neurological abnormalities and developmental sequelae.

One of the most important and extensively studied etiological factors is periventricular hemorrhage (PVH). This condition is sometimes referred to as germinal matrix hemorrhage or intraventricular hemorrhage. The germinal matrix is located within the periventricular regions of the head of the caudate nucleus of the thalamus where active neuronal synthesis occurs (Grant 1986). Containing a very fragile network of capillaries whose function is to support neurogenesis, the germinal matrix is an ephemeral structure that disappears between the 32nd to 34th weeks of gestation. As a result infants born at term generally escape germinal matrix hemorrhaging. Similarly, infants born beyond 32 weeks gestation have a reduced risk of PVH since, by this point in gestation, the germinal matrix has begun the process of involution. Since the germinal matrix is located just beneath the ependymal layer of the ventricles, bleeding very often spreads into the ventricles. As such, this type of brain hemorrhaging also has been referred to as intraventricular or subependymal hemorrhage. For nearly 130 years scientists have recognized the link between brain hemorrhaging and subsequent motoric handicapping conditions such as hemipelegia (McNutt 1885). Recent research also has begun to associate germinal matrix hemorrhaging not only with conditions such as hemipelegia or cerebral palsy, but also with more subtle educational and behavioral outcomes (Paneth, et al. 1994).

Conclusion and Future Research Directions

The preponderance of the research suggests a linear relationship between LBW and developmental outcomes. Research documents a wide range of deficits in cognitive ability, academic attainment, psychosocial and behavioral functioning. More of the profound developmental outcomes are found among infants with very low birth weight or extremely low birth weight. An increasing longitudinal research base suggests that many of these outcomes persist through childhood into adulthood. Furthermore, the observed outcomes are not mitigated when controlling for socioeconomic status, although LBW babies born into poverty face a double jeopardy of socioeconomic disadvantage, in addition to the biological consequences of LBW birth.

As the school curriculum advances and places increasing demands on the cognitive, behavioral and emotional capacities of children, children with low birth weight might manifest difficulties with learning, behavior and social competence that they had not previously displayed. Thus, babies who were initially thought to escape the deleterious effects of low birth weight may now require professional support. Finally, although the LBW literature is voluminous with respect to VLBW outcomes, there is a paucity of research that has investigated moderately LBW outcomes. Future research in this area is important, particularly since MLBW births comprise nearly 85 percent of all LBW births.

In addition, there is need for research that investigates gender-based LBW outcomes, particular outcomes stratified by ethnicity. For instance, the prevalence of African-American preterm/LBW births at 14 percent suggests that this phenomenon is nothing less than a public health crisis. Yet, we know very little about specific African-American LBW outcomes and the effects of gender on these outcomes. In addition, future research should attempt to control for variables that have been associated with adverse developmental outcomes, such as cigarette smoking and substance abuse. If left unaccounted for, these factors might distort the true effect of LBW on developmental outcomes. Finally, it will be important in future studies to exclude children born at term, but small for gestational age (<2,500 grams). These children tend to suffer adverse developmental outcomes, but have an etiology that is distinct from the LBW. We have made significant strides in understanding the role of LBW in producing producing childhood pathology. However, we still have need for additional research that more fully explicates the more subtle relationships between low birth weight and educational, cognitive and behavioral outcomes.

Chapter 4
Pre- and Perinatal Anoxia and Hypoxia

Damage to the human brain that occurs around the time of birth is attributable to a variety of proximal causes. These include hemorrhage, infection, metabolic difficulties and hypoxia/anoxia. Of these, hypoxia and related conditions constitute the majority of perinatal injuries. Hypoxia can result from conditions related to the mother or the fetus. For example, hypoxia can result from a decreased concentration of oxygen in the air breathed by the mother as might occur at high altitude. It can also result from a decreased blood flow due to rupture or obstruction (referred to as ischemia) of blood vessels of the mother or fetus. Further, it can be the result of reduced cardiac (abnormal valve functioning of the heart) or pulmonary functioning (e.g., pulmonary disease of the mother; hyaline membrane disease of the infant).

In the perinatal period the predominant cause is 'birth asphyxia' which is technically referred to as critically impaired intrapartum gas exchange. This may result from many factors such as umbilical cord prolapse, abruption placentae or immaturity of the lungs. In the prenatal period the most commonly encountered problem of oxygen exchange is prolonged hypoxia due to placental inadequacies; this form of hypoxia often results in babies who are abnormally small for gestational age.

Several terms are used to denote a condition in which the mother or the fetus experience inadequate oxygen. Hypoxia is the term used to indicate a deficiency of oxygen. A related term that is often used in relation to perinatal brain injury is anoxia, meaning without oxygen. Asphyxia refers to the physiological results of hypoxia or anoxia.

Hypoxia and the Preterm Infant

Preterm infants are particularly vulnerable to hypoxia. This results from three interrelated problems. First, infants delivered at less than 32 weeks gestation are not prepared for the transition from obtaining oxygen from the blood of the mother via the placenta, to obtaining oxygen directly from the air. This transition requires increased quantities of red blood cells to carry oxygen, the development of alveolar structures of the lungs which increases the surface area of the lungs and several other processes. Thus, the severely preterm infant is at risk of hypoxia simply due to the inadequacy of lung development.

R.P. Martin and S.C. Dombrowski, *Prenatal Exposures: Psychological and Educational Consequences for Children.*
© Springer 2008

The inadequate lung development of the preterm infant has been widely understood by attending physicians for decades. Yet a sizeable percentage of preterm infants experience some level of respiratory distress. In a recent study by Rose and Feldman (2000), 76 percent of their preterm sample was diagnosed with respiratory distress syndrom (RDS). This diagnosis required both the presence of clinical evidence of respiratory distress in the first hours of life and characteristic roentgenograms (tracings of the action of the heart as determined by the use of X-ray). RDS typically requires mechanical ventilation, with the severity of the RDS being roughly categorized by the length of time mechanical ventilation is used.

Unfortunately, the use of oxygen and/or mechanical ventilation can result in the second hypoxia risk of the preterm infant. The use of oxygen and mechanical ventilation can interfere with or inhibit the alveolar and vascular development of the lung. This interference can result in a condition known as bronchopulmonary dysplasia (Jobe and Bancolari 2001). Currently, due to advances in neonatal care, many cases of bronchopulmonary dysplasia are avoided. However, it remains a particular problem for severely preterm infants (less than 30 weeks) with very low birth weight (less than 1,200 grams).Current estimates indicate that about 30 percent of the infants with birth weights less than 1,000 grams and gestations of less than 36 weeks will have this condition (Jobe and Bancolari 2001).

Bronchopulmonary dysplasia is associated with inflammation of the lung tissue, with reduced surface area of the lungs and with dysmorphic pulmonary vasculature. All these can result in obstructive airway disease and increased airway reactivity. These are symptoms generally referred to as asthma. Some of the symptoms may be reduced by the third or fourth year of life, but some of the symptoms of brochopulmonary dysplasia continue into adulthood. These long-term effects can obviously reduce the stamina and exercise capability of a child or adolescent, and might result in learning or behavioral problems during childhood due to being excluded from some social circumstances (e.g., sports).

Another risk to the preterm infant due to hypoxia is that low birth weight and preterm delivery may have resulted from a prolonged hypoxia. This can result from uterine insufficiency or other factors that are the cause of the preterm birth. One of the factors often associated with preterm delivery is bacterial infection of the chorioamnion (the innermost lining of the placental sac) and the amniotic fluid. In fact there is a negative correlation between colonization on these structures by bacteria and the length of the gestation of the fetus. In one study 73 percent of the women with spontaneous preterm births occurring prior to 30 weeks gestation tested positive for chorioamnion infections (Andrews, et al. 1995).

In summary, the preterm infant is at much greater risk of hypoxia/anoxia than term infants. This results from the inadequate development of the lungs, the negative developmental changes that can be produced by use of oxygen and mechanical ventilation and by other factors that may have produced the preterm delivery (e.g., infection). Thus, the large and growing literature on the developmental outcomes of premature delivery and low birth weight are, in part, directly attributable to consequences of hypoxia. Unfortunately, it is not known how much of the effect of preterm birth and low birth weight can be attributed to this effect.

Mechanisms by Which Hypoxia Produce Neurological Damage

The damage to the developing CNS produced by anoxia or hypoxia are different, depending on when they occur. In particular, different types of cells are damaged in infants delivered preterm and in infants delivered at term. Several authorities agree that hypoxic injury in the preterm infant most often occurs to white matter, or the oligodendroglial cells in the periventricular region of the brain. In the term infant, most of the injury occurs to the neuronal cells of the cerebral cortex, while periventricular injury may also occur (Volpe 2001).

In preterm infants there is evidence that the hippocampus, an area of the brain involved in short-term memory, is particularly susceptible to damage from hypoxia/anoxia. In animal studies quantifiable neuropathology has been documented to specific regions of the hippocampus (Davis, Tribuna, Pulsinelli and Volpe 1986). Rose and Feldman (2000) also discuss the possibility that hypoxic-ischemic injury may impair or delay the development of myelin, which in turn slows the conduction of nerve impulses. This may occur because hypoxia is associated with intraventricular hemorrhage in the preterm infants. Such hemorrhage is destructive of the germinal matrix with results in either a loss of the oligodendroglial progenitor cells that produce myelin, or may disrupt the migration of these cells.

The events which directly cause cell death in hypoxic and anoxic conditions are oxygen and glucose deprivation. This leads to anaerobic glycolysis (the dissolution or hydrolysis of sugar), depletion of high-energy phosphate reserves and loss of cell membrane functions, which further results in the accumulation of lactic acid, calcium, free radicals and neurotoxic, excitatory neurotransmitters such as glutamate outside the cell wall (Higgins, et al. 2006). This process leads to acute or primary cell death. Interestingly, much cell death occurs after the restart of blood flow to the region (referred to as reprofusion). As blood flow begins to reoccur in the region, glutamate receptors are activated and calcium accumulates in the cell setting off a cascade of events that lead to the secondary phase of cell death (for details see Volpe 2001). These processes may evolve over days or weeks after the hypoxic injury.

In large scale studies a hypoxic-ischemic event is indicated for full-term babies when the Apgar score is <5, at five or 10 minutes after birth. Another index that is sometimes used is the need for continual resuscitation at five or 10 minutes after birth. A third indication of a hypoxic event is a pH of <7.0 (a measure of the acidity of the blood) in umbilical blood or venous blood within 60 minutes of birth. Finally, an EEG can be used to detect moderate to severe hypoxic-ischemic encephalopathy.

One of the most promising developments for the amelioration of cell damage after hypoxia is the discovery that placing the infant in a hypothermic (e.g., low temperature) condition can slow the biochemical cascade that occurs when blood begins to flow back into the regions previously deprived. The infant temperature is reduced to 32 C (90 degrees Fahrenheit) within two hours after injury for 48 to 72 hours. In one study the percentage of infants who had died or had moderate/severe disability at 18 months was calculated for a group of children who had been treated at birth with hypothermia. Results were compared to a group of similarly hypoxic infants who had not been treated. Forty-four percent of the hypothermia treated group had died or were moderately to severely impaired, while 62 percent of the control group were similarly afflicted. When only the mortality rate was studied, it was 24 percent in the hypothermia group and 37 percent in the control group (Shankaran, et al. 2004).

Perinatal Hypoxia/Anoxia and Developmental Outcomes

Health Outcomes

As we have seen with several types of prenatal perturbations of development described in this volume, there is growing evidence that prenatal events can create a predisposition for diseases that are not manifested until adulthood. One interesting example is the effect of hypoxia on lung growth, which in turn has been linked to chronic obstructive pulmonary disease and pulmonary hypertension in adulthood. During the last stages of pregnancy the circulatory system of the lungs undergoes important structural and functional changes to allow for the transition from gas exchange by the placenta to gas exchange by the lungs. These changes lead to an approximate 10-fold increase in blood flow through the lungs and a corresponding decrease in pulmonary vascular resistance (the resistance experienced by the blood as it goes through the arteries and veins of the lungs) (Sartori, et al. 1999). It has become clear in recent years that perinatal events can alter lung development during this critical period and place the individual at increased risk throughout life.

Most of this work has been done with animals. For example, Caslin, Heath and Smith (1991) found that hypoxia in infancy increased the rate of vasoconstrictive pulmonary vascular disease in adult laboratory rats. This implies that the expected lungs had not developed their vascular structure appropriately to allow the blood to flow through the lungs in an unrestricted fashion. In humans Sartori, et al. (1999) tested healthy young adults who had experienced transient hypoxia during the perinatal period and a matched set of controls in a high-altitude exposure. At low altitude pulmonary-artery pressure was similar in the two groups. However, 24 to 36 hours after arrival at high altitude (approximately 4,500 meters), those persons who had perinatal hypoxia had a significantly higher increase in pulmonary-artery pressure than the controls.

While the mechanism is still unclear, a recent study has shown that a brief perinatal hypoxic experience can alter the functioning of the heart and lungs in laboratory animals. Tang, le Cras, Morris and Abman (2000) put newborn rats in a reduced oxygen chamber for three days after birth. They found that, compared to controls, hypoxic rat pups tested two weeks later had altered cardiac functioning as well as altered cardiac and pulmonary structure. With regard to lung structure, the hypoxic rats had a reduced alveolar count and reduced density of pulmonary arteries. This is another example that supports the Barker (1998) hypothesis that prenatal disruptions of development are the bases for some types of adulthood diseases and subclinical disorders.

The connections of hypoxia during the perinatal period to measure lung capacity and response to stressors (e.g., exercise) during childhood and adolescent have not been done. But it appears likely that some children who experienced hypoxia in the prenatal period may have pulmonary difficulties that limit the ease with which they can participate in exercise. As sports play such a large role in social interactions in elementary and middle school, reductions in the ability to participate could have far-reaching effects beyond those directly related to the physiological disability. The physiological disability could reduce opportunities to practice social skills and could impair the development of a positive self-image. Both factors have the potential to affect classroom performance and social adjustment.

Neurological Outcomes

There is no doubt that severe asphyxia can cause damage to the CNS. This has been well established in classic laboratory studies in fetal monkeys (e.g., Myers 1972) and fetal lambs (e.g., Gunn, Parer, Mallard, Williams and Gluckman 1992). Human postmortem research with stillborn fetuses and research on early neonatal deaths have demonstrated neuropathology that was attributed to asphyxia (Burke and Tannenberg 1995).

In cases in which the infant survives, a number of investigators have looked at the short-term effects of birth asphyxia on a variety of neonatal indicators of neurological abnormality. For example, Azzopardi, et al. (1999) studied continuous electroencephalography (EEG) soon after birth (within 12 hours) of 22 infants suspected of having suffered birth asphyxia and 11 healthy controls. All infants were assessed for developmental outcomes at one year of age. All control infants had normal EEG and sleep/awake cycles at 12 hours, and had normal outcomes at one year. Seventeen of those suspected of asphyxia had normal neurodevelopmental outcomes at one year. These infants also had normal EEGs. Of the five infants who died or who had developmental anomalies at one year, all had abnormal EEGs. This research supports the contention that anoxia at birth can cause abnormal electrical activity of the brain and this abnormality is diagnostic of long-term negative developmental outcomes.

The most common clinical manifestation of asphyxia in the neonate is seizures. One of the controversies in neonatal neurology is whether seizures contribute further damage to the already compromised brain tissue of the infant who has experienced hypoxia or anoxia during the prenatal period. Data from animal studies are somewhat unclear on this issue (Holmes and Ben-Ari 2001). However, the consensus is that seizures independently contribute additional damage to that sustained due to hypoxia.

Miller, et al. (2002) studied 90 infants who had indications of having suffered asphyxia (e.g., Apgar score ≤ 5). These infants varied in the amount of seizure activity they experienced from none to severe recurrent seizures. At an average age of six days the infants were given MRIs to study the amount of brain injury that had occurred. These researchers found that seizure scores predicted several indicators of neonatal brain injury. They concluded that severity of seizures in human newborns with perinatal asphyxia is independently associated with brain injury. Thus, anoxia/hypoxia can set off a chain reaction and some of these reactions (e.g., seizures) can produce further damage.

It is an established finding that anoxia is often associated with peripheral nerve damage that results in hearing loss. A study by Jiang (1995) was particularly important in this literature because it demonstrated different effects on hearing that were related to the timing of the anoxia experience. Jiang examined one group of children who had suffered perinatal asphyxia and another group that had experienced postnatal asphyxia. In the perinatal asphyxia group hearing loss occurred in 17 percent of the cases that also exhibited residual neurodevelopmental deficits, and in 6 percent of those who did not. However, among children who survived severe postnatal asphyxia and exhibited neurodevelopmental deficits, there was no indication of hearing loss. This study supports the importance of a critical period of sensitivity to damage when the peripheral nervous systems that support the auditory system is developing, sometime in the last trimester of pregnancy, and perhaps extending a few months into the postnatal period.

Learning and Behavior Outcomes

With regard to neurological functioning, a number of studies have shown that hypoxia is associated with neurological morbidity. Long-term effects of hypoxia/anoxia on learning and behavior problems have rarely been studied. Of those studies that have been published, the results are mixed.

Long-term effects on development seem to be most clearly related to the severity (duration and amount of oxygen deprivation) of the hypoxia. Handley-Derry, Low, Burke, Waurick, Killen and Derrick (1997) studied 43 children who had mild intrapartum fetal asphyxia. The level of asphyxia was assessed biochemically at delivery. Newborn assessments indicated no or minor encephalopathy. The purpose of the study was to determine if there were long-term effects of this mild intrapartum asphyxia. Measures of motor and cognitive development were obtained at four to eight years of age. Particular emphasis was placed on measures of memory (paired associate memory, digit span, spatial memory) as some animal studies had revealed that experimentally induced asphyxia in animals had produced lesions in the hippocampus, a region of the brain known to be involved in a variety of memory processes. In addition measures were obtained of general cognitive ability (McCarthy General Cognitive Index), motor functioning (McCarthy motor score) and child behavior (Achenbach Behavior Problem Checklist as rated by parents and teachers). The results of the study were consistent across all measures. The performance of the mild asphyxia group was indistinguishable on any measure from that of matched controls.

In contrast to the findings of this study, Rose and Feldman (2000) have followed a sample of preterm infants who experienced hypoxic events ranging from mild to severe. The sample was assessed in infancy, in early childhood and again in late childhood. In one investigation of this sample, relationships between pre- and perinatal complications and specific aspects of psychological functioning were studied. These researchers found that most medical risk factors were unrelated to later neuropsychological outcomes. However, there were statistically and clinically significant associations between the diagnosis of Respiratory Distress Syndrome (RDS) and memory functioning assessed both in infancy and at 11 years of age. As was noted earlier, 76 percent of this preterm sample experienced RDS. Of those with RDS most required mechanical ventilation. Based on this observation, the researchers developed a scale of severity of RDS such that those infants who had no ventilation were categorized as mild, those who were ventilated for one to three days as moderate, and those who were ventilated for more than three days as severe. This scale was significantly correlated with seven-month visual recognition memory, six-year digit span performance and two measures of memory obtained at 11 years. Further, other indicators of respiratory problems were found to be associated with memory functioning. These included days receiving oxygen and days of continuous positive airflow pressure.

The Rose and Feldman (2000) research is particularly noteworthy because of the quality of the measurements obtained, the repeated assessments of the sample at different stages of development and the attention to specific measures of neuropsychological functioning, as opposed to relying on one general measure such as IQ. Their research also strongly supports the animal research which indicates that the hippocampus is particularly vulnerable to hypoxia/anoxia, and that hypoxia/anoxia at moderate to severe levels often results in compromised memory functioning.

Some recent studies have implicated hypoxia/anoxia as a risk factor for childhood psychopathology. Amor, et al. (2005) studied several perinatal risk factors thought to predict Attention-Deficit Hyperactivity Disorder (ADHD). Previous studies had implicated both genetic and nonshared environmental factors (factors experienced by one member of a family) as causes of ADHD. In order to better understand the nonshared environmental component, these researchers studied families of at least two children in which one had a diagnosis of ADHD (n = 70) and the other did not (n = 50). The unaffected child closest in age to the child with ADHD was chosen as the control. The children with ADHD had significantly higher rates of neonatal complications, compared to their unaffected siblings. Neonatal complications associated with anoxia (being in an incubator, oxygen therapy) played an important role in the differences between groups. The findings are consistent with research on animals indicating that neonatal hypoxia can result in increased locomotor activity later in life (e.g., Brake, Sullivan and Gratton 2000).

Hypoxia can be chronic as in the case of inadequate blood flow through the umbilical artery from the mother to the infant. Hypoxia can also be acute, as in birth asphyxia. Hypoxia that is chronic often results in IUGR, which poses risks for all of the learning and developmental problems of low birth weight babies (see Chapter 3). However, not all IUGR is due to chronic hypoxia. A study by Berg (1989) helped elucidate the consequences of IUGR caused by hypoxia and IUGR attributed to other causes. Berg studied a large sample of seven-year-old-children (n = 4,545) with IUGR. He demonstrated that intrauterine growth retardation was not associated with neurological problems of children, unless it occurred among children who had also experienced a perinatal hypoxia-related event. This study demonstrated that neurological problems can result from hypoxia-related IUGR. It also demonstrated that the causes of IUGR may be more important in affecting learning and behavior than IUGR considered in isolation.

The results of a similar investigation were reported by Weinerroither, Steiner, Tomaselli, Lodendanz and Thun-Hohenstein (2001). They studied 38 growth-restricted fetuses and a control group matched on week of delivery. All children studied came from the same hospital. The control group had no signs of IUGR or abnormal blood flow during development. Outcomes were assessed at age six with the Kaufman Assessment Battery for Children and a variety of neuromotor assessments. The IUGR study group had lower Kaufman IQ scores at age six than the controls. However, those infants with reversed diastolic blood flow (an indicator of prolonged hypoxia) in the umbilical artery had the worse outcome both in the neonatal period and at age six. The reversed diastolic blood flow was indicative of long-term abnormal fetoplacental blood flow due to placental insufficiency.

Summary and Conclusions

In summary, severe hypoxia is clearly associated with severe morbidity or mortality. Somewhat less severe hypoxia is associated with long-term somatic health problems, particularly health problems associated with pulmonary functioning. Moderate to severe hypoxia is also associated with significant neurological pathology that can be diagnosed in early infancy. The neurological damage is not limited to the central nervous system; for example, peripheral nerve damage resulting in hearing loss is a common outcome of moderate to severe hypoxia. In some cases hypoxia sets off a cascade of events that further exacerbates neurological dysfunction. A classic example is the link between hypoxia and seizures occurring in the neonatal period. There is evidence that the seizures can produce further neurological damage independent of the initial neurological damage caused by the hypoxia. Also, moderate-to-severe hypoxia has been associated with childhood psychopathologies that affect learning and behavior. The link between hypoxia and ADHD serves as one example. However, mild hypoxia has seldom been found to predict abnormal development in any sphere, whether somatic health, learning or behavior.

Section C
Maternal Illness: Introduction

The management of pregnancy and childbirth is the specialty of the obstetrician. A good portion of this practice and the underlying science deals with the management of maternal illness or preexisting conditions during the pre- and perinatal period in order to protect the health of the mother and optimize the opportunites for the fetus to develop appropriately. The great textbooks in obstetrics (e.g., Williams Obstetrics; Cox, Werner, Hoffman and Cunningham, 2005) are primarily concerned with this topic. Further, hundreds of articles dealing with specific techniques for the management of maternal illness during pregnancy are published each year.

For these reasons Section C of this volume is a brief and selective review. Our review is limited to discussion of the most common health problems of pregnant women that have been shown to have adverse effects on fetal and/or child development. Our review will not deal with how these conditions are managed, with rare exceptions. Because of space limitations, many topics of interest were eliminated from consideration. Among the most important are effects of pharmacological substances administered during pregnancy to manage maternal and fetal health.

The topics we have reviewed include maternal infections (Chapter 5), with particular emphasis on influenza, Rubella, mumps and measles, chicken pox, cytomeglavirus infection, herpes simplex 2 and toxoplasmosis. Chapter 6 is focused on chronic maternal illness, focusing on maternal diabetes, obesity, heart and pulmonary disease. The next chapter in this section (Chapter 7) reviews the literature on maternal nutrition during pregnancy. Protein-energy malnutrition, iron deficiency and vitamin deficiencies of various kinds are described with regard to their long-term influence on child behavior and learning. The final chapter in this section, Chapter 8, summarizes the research on stress during pregnancy. This is an area of increasing interest to researchers and an area that opens many new avenues of research connecting the psychological world to the biological in transgenerational context.

Chapter 5
Prenatal Infections

For over 200 years it has been conjectured that prenatal infection results in adverse physical and developmental outcomes for children. In 1787 William Perfect wondered whether a particularly virulent influenza epidemic occurring during that year was responsible for an increase in insanity among those gestationally exposed. In 1845 Esquirol commented that insanity is more prevalent during epidemic years and this increase seems to be independent of moral causes. At the turn of the 20th Century Emil Kraeplin (1919) commented that "infections in the years of development might have a causal significance" for dementia praecox (p. 240). After the 1919 influenza pandemic, which killed more people than World War I, Karl Menninger speculated that the infection may be causally related to schizophrenia. Menninger (1928) later retracted his statement.

In 1941 Sir Norman Gregg, an Australian pediatric ophthalmologist, discovered that mothers who contracted rubella during pregnancy had offspring with severe eye cataracts and other physical deformities. Gregg (1941) reported that of the 78 children born in the first few months of 1941 who came to see a doctor in the Sydney area for cataracts, 68 had been prenatally exposed to Rubella, two to three times the usual congenital rate. This research increased professional interest in the relationship between viral infections, and profound physical and neurological outcomes that were clearly evident at birth.

It was not until 1988 when researchers turned their gaze toward prenatal infection in relation to more subtle psychological and behavioral outcomes. This interest was inaugurated following Mednick, Machon, Huttunen and Bonnett's (1988) reported association between the 1957 influenza pandemic and increased risk of schizophrenia in a sample from Finland. Since this study, more than three dozen articles have appeared that have investigated this issue. The majority have found a significant association between infection and schizophrenia. Since the early 1970s other prenatal infections including Rubella, measles, mumps, cytomegalovirus, chicken pox, toxoplasmosis and herpes simplex 2 have been sporadically investigated for their possible association with psychopathology. The research base on these infections in relation to psychological and behavioral outcomes is sparse compared to that of influenza.

R.P. Martin and S.C. Dombrowski, *Prenatal Exposures: Psychological and Educational Consequences for Children.*
© Springer 2008

Within this chapter we broadly review the extant literature regarding some of the more commonly experienced prenatal infections in relation to adverse developmental outcomes. We have further limited the discussion primarily to psychological and behavioral effects.

Influenza

Influenza is the most extensively studied prenatal infection in relation to possible psychological and behavioral outcomes. A secondary body of research as it relates to other psychiatric outcomes is available but less abundant. This includes influenza's possible association with affective disorders and autism. A body of research has investigated influenza's link to congenital anomalies following first trimester exposure. This literature will be discussed first, followed by outcome research in regard to psychiatric outcomes.

Influenza's Association with Congenital Anomalies

Since the 1957 A2 (Asian) influenza pandemic, the association between gestational influenza exposure and observable abnormalities at birth has been debated (Hanshaw and Dudgeon 1978). Several studies, primarily in the first 10 years after the 1957 epidemic, reported a significant association (Coffey and Jessop 1959; Hakosalo and Saxen 1971; Hardy, Azarowicz, Mannini, Medearis and Cooke 1961; Lynberg, Khoury, Lu and Cocian 1994). However, an almost equal number of studies reported no association (Ingalls 1960; Korones, Todaro, Roane and Sever 1970; Wilson, Heins, Imagawa and Adams 1959). Commonly associated congenital anomalies include anencephaly, cardiovascular defects, congenital limb defects, neural tube defects, spina bifida and orofacial clefts (Acs, Banhidy, Puho and Czeizel 2005; Coffey and Jessop 1959; Hardy, et al. 1961; Lynberg, et al. 1994). All of these studies, except the study by Acs, et al. (2005), relied on clinical observation or retrospective report. The Acs, et al. study is unique in that it presented data on serologically confirmed influenza infection, timing of exposure and magnitude of a febrile (e.g., fever) episode. Control of fever is important. Several researchers have hypothesized that maternal fever within influenza exposure may have been the agent that contributes to teratogenesis (Dombrowski, Martin and Huttunen 2003; Edwards 2006). Consistent with this hypothesis, Acs, et al. (2005) found a higher prevalence of isolated cleft lip/palate, neural tube defects and cardiovascular congenital anomalies in offspring who were gestationally exposed to influenza during the second and third months of pregnancy. However, these authors concluded that the effect is likely caused by fever rather than by the influenza virus since the association was not found in mothers who received anti-febrile intervention.

Influenza's Association with Affective Disorder

Machon, Mednick and Huttunen (1997) investigated a possible relationship between the 1957 (Asian) influenza epidemic and later onset of affective disorders in adulthood. They found a significant association for individuals exposed to influenza, but only during the second trimester of gestation. The effects were greater for males than for females. Further analyses indicated that the significant association with affective disorders was due to an elevation in the number of unipolar subtypes of depression.

The results of this study are consistent with those reported by Cannon, et al. (1996). Using a sample from Dublin, Cannon, et al. (1996) compared the number of subjects exposed in utero to the influenza virus with those who remained unexposed. Studying cases of schizophrenia, bipolar disorder/mania, neurotic disorder and depressive disorder, the only association was with depressive disorder.

Takei, Sham, O'Callaghan, Glover and Murray (1993; 1994) examined general influenza outbreaks in England and Wales between 1938 and 1965. These authors reported that in utero influenza exposure during the second trimester may be responsible for diverting females who would have been diagnosed with an affective disorder toward schizophrenia. This interpretation may explain the excess of males with affective disorders as a result of influenza exposure found by Machon, et al. (1997). Although the above noted studies found an association, Morgan, et al. (1997) did not find evidence for an association with affective disorders in a large cohort from Australia.

Influenza's Association with Schizophrenia

Over the past 20 years a significant body of research has emerged supporting the association between maternal exposure to influenza during gestation and schizophrenia in progeny. There has been intermittent conjecture for the past 200 years on this possible association. One of the first modern researchers to suggest this association was Karl Menninger who made his observation following the 1918-1919 influenza pandemic (Crow and Done 1992). Menninger (1928) initially believed that approximately one-third of those exposed to influenza in utero had characteristics of schizophrenia. As a result he suggested that schizophrenia might be caused by the virus. Following Menninger, other researchers dabbled with the notion of an association between influenza and schizophrenia (Crow 1983; Goodall 1932; Torrey and Peterson 1973); however, it was not until 1988, when Mednick, Machon, Huttunen and Bonnet (1988) published data from the greater Helsinki region on the 1957 A2 (Asian) pandemic, that intense interest in this topic arose.

Currently, well over four dozen articles have been published documenting the association between the risk of schizophrenia and season of birth (Boyd, Pulver and

Stewart 1986; Bradbury and Miller 1985). These studies suggested that individuals with schizophrenia are more likely to have late winter and early spring birthdays than other seasonal birthdays. These studies prompted researchers to turn their efforts toward uncovering the possible reasons for the season of birth association. A number of hypotheses were considered, including statistical artifact, cold exposure and influenza infection. The possible influenza effect has stimulated most of the research activity. Much of this research is summarized in Table 5.1.

A majority of studies finding this association point to infection in the second trimester of gestation as having the greatest effect. Others indicate a range from the third to the seventh month of gestation. A preponderance of the studies found an association with the 1957 A2 Asian influenza pandemic, although associations were also found for the 1968 to 1972 Hong Kong influenza pandemic, and for various flu outbreaks between 1910 and 1965 (Brown, et al. 2004). The results also suggest that there may be a gender effect, particularly for the greater incidence of females with schizophrenia following in utero exposure to influenza (Takei, et al. 1993, 1994; Venables 1996).

Although the majority of studies have been conducted in the northern hemisphere, researchers have also found a positive association in southern hemisphere studies (McGrath, Pemberton, Welham and Murray 1994). Venables (1996) examining data from the 1968-1972 Hong Kong influenza epidemic found elevated schizophrenism scores in female offspring following a fifth month gestational exposure in the population of Mauritania.

Finally, Brown, et al. (2004) discusses the association with schizophrenia in serologically confirmed cases of influenza. To date, this remains the only research article that has used serological confirmation of gestational exposure to influenza. This study reported a three-fold increased risk of schizophrenia following exposure during the first half of pregnancy, and a seven-fold increased risk following first trimester exposure.

Despite the success of studies demonstrating an association between influenza and schizophrenia, numerous researchers in several countries have failed to find this relationship. Three of these studies used a population-based sample (e.g., all children born during epidemic years in an entire country). Several studies conducted on the 1957 A2 Asian influenza epidemic did not find evidence for an association (e.g., Cannon, et al. 1994; Cannon, et al. 1996; Crow and Done 1992; Erlenmeyer-Kimling, et al. 1994; Selten and Slaets 1994; Susser, Lin, Brown, Lumey and Erlenmeyer-Kimling 1994). In addition, studies conducted on general influenza outbreaks from both the northern and southern hemispheres did not find an association (e.g., Morgan, et al. 1997; Takei, Van Os and Murray 1995; Torrey, Rawlings and Waldman 1988). Finally, several studies investigating the 1918-1919 influenza pandemic did not find evidence for an association (e.g., Kendell and Kemp 1989; Adams, Kendell, Hare and Munk—Jorgenson 1993).

Overall, a majority of the influenza-schizophrenia research has been conducted in relation to the 1957 A2 Asian flu outbreak, the 1918-1919 influenza pandemic, and the 1968-72 Hong Kong influenza epidemic. Unfortunately, while many reports of significant associations have been published, an almost equal

Table 5.1 Maternal Influenza and Schizophrenia

No	Date	Journal	Title	Author (s)	Type of Flu	Geographic Regions	Size (N)	Statistical Analysis Employed	Description of Association	Significance	Hypothesis of Mechanism	Further Comments
Northern Hemisphere Studies												
1957 A2 (Asian)												
1	1988	Arch Gen Psychtry 45 189-192	Adult schizo-phrenia following prenatal exp to an influenza epidemic	Mednick, Machon, O'Huttunen and Bonnet	1957 A2 (Asian)	Uusimaa Conty Finland	1781	Compared proportion of schiz births in index year vs control years using chi-sq analysis	2nd trimester for MandF combined	$p<01$	Exp in 2nd or 3d tri casuses CNS damage	Schizophrenia=Dx at any point in Px history
2	1989	Arch Gen Psychtry 46: 878-882	Maternal influenza in the etiology of schizophrenia	Kendell and Kemp	1957 A2 (Asian)	1) Edinburgh Psych Case Register	National Sample	Compared the # of Schiz born in a 12mnth period with the # born in the corresponding period in each of the 2 preceding yrs using a chi-square analysis.	a) MandF 6th month and b) 6 to 8 month combined	$p<05$	Fetal brain damage as a result of viral infection	Association for Edinburgh data, but none for Scottish National sample. Study employed narrow Dx criteria: Schizophrenia Dx made only if ICD-9 Dx at discharge. See section 2b for 1918-19 analysis
						a) Edinburgh	a) Indx=15 Cntrl=27		MandF 6th	$p<05$		
						b) Scotland	b) Indx=21 Cntrl=49		NONE			
						c) United Kingdom	c) Indx=26 Cntrl=63		NONE			
						d) Born Elsewhere	d) Indx=30 Cntrl=71		NONE			

(continued)

Table 5.1 (continued)

No	Date	Journal	Title	Author(s)	Type of Flu	Geographic Regions	Size (N)	Statistical Analysis Employed	Description of Association	Significance	Hypothesis of Mechanism	Further Comments
						2) Scottish National Data	2) National Sample Indx=227 Cntrl=525					
3	1991	The Lancet 337 1248-50	Schizophrenia after prenatal expos to 1957 A2 influenza epidemic	O'Callaghan, Sham, Takei, Glover and Murray	1957 A2 (Asian)	England and Wales	National Sample Indx = 339 Cntrl =1331	Compared # of index and control patients for each month. Index=Aug 15,1957 to Aug 14, 1958; Ctrl=Avg of corresponding 2 yrs before and after.	Females in 5th month	p=.011	Distrubed migration in entorhinal region in 5th month	# of births of individuals who later developed schiz was 88percent higher than the avg # in the corresponding 2 yr before and after.
4	1992	Br J Psychtry 161, 390-393	Prenatal exposure to influenza does not cause schizophrenia	Crow and Done	1957 A2 (Asian)	England, Wales and Scotland	National sample of 16,266	Conducted ANOVA (2x2) to compare infected vs. non-infected mothers. 2nd trimester = Sept to Nov. 1957	NONE	broad p=.63 narrow p=1.00 affec ill p=.11	n/a	Case-control: Determined who contracted infection in large population Unique as a result.
5	1992	Schiz Research 6:98-99	Schiz in Afro-Caribbeans in the U.K. following prenatal expos to the 1957 A2 influenza epidem	Fahy, Jones, Sham, Takei and Murray	1957 A2 (Asian)	Afro-Caribbeans in the U.K.	white=537 1st gen =208 2d gen=145	Using gen linear model, compared the observed number of schiz births in each mnth from 1931-1970 to values predicted by the model	2nd trimester (March 58)	n/a		Lack of flu exposure in Afro-Caribbeans incrsd incidence of schiz births

#	Year	Journal	Title	Authors	Strain	Location	Sample	Statistic	Month	M and F	Mechanism	Notes
6	1993	Br J Psychiatry 163: 522-534	Epidemiological evidence that maternal influenza contributes to the aetiology of schizophrenia	Adams, Kendell, Hare and Munk-Jorgenson	Asian 1957 A2	Scotland Denmark England	National Sample N1 = 16,960 N2 = 18,723 N3 = 22,021	T-value [index (7/57-8/58) vs cntrl (56-59)] T-value [index (7/57-8/58) vs cntrl (56-59)] T-value [index (7/57-8/58) vs cntrl (56-59)]	mnth 4 mnth 4 and 6 mnth 4	$p<.05$ F $p<.05$ MandF $p<.05$	Flu interferes with cellular migration process in fetal brain	See 6b and 6c for 1932-60 and 1911-65 analyses.
7	1994	Am J Psychtry 151(6): 922-924	No relation between risk of schizophrenia and prenatal exposure to influenza in Holland	Susser, Lin, Brown, Lumey and Erlenmeyer-Kimling	1957 A2 (Asian)	Holland	National sample of approx 20K exposed monthly vs. approx 80K not exposed	Used standardized methods for estimating 95 percent CI of those exposed [born 1958] vs not-exposed [born 1956, 57, 59, 60 combined]	NONE	n/a	n/a	Entire birth cohort studied. Denominator = number of births in given month; numerator = number of schizophrenic births
8	1994	Schiz Bulletin 20 (2): 263-7	Prenatal influenza and adult schizophrenia	Mednick, Huttunen and Machon	1957 A2 (Asian)	Helsinki, Finland	71	Compared 2nd trimester with 1st and 3rd using Fisher's exact t-test	Males and females	$p<.01$	Neural development impacted	86.7 percent of schizo patients had infection in 2nd trimes vs. 20 percent who were exposed during 1st and 3rd. Lends support for 2nd trimester pathogenesis.

(continued)

Table 5.1 (continued)

No	Date	Journal	Title	Author (s)	Type of Flu	Geographic Regions	Size (N)	Statistical Analysis Employed	Description of Association	Significance	Hypothesis of Mechanism	Further Comments
9	1994	Am J Psychiatry 151 : 1496-98	Schizophrenia and prenatal exposure to the 1957 A2 influenza epidemic in Croatia	Erlenmeyer-Kimling, Folnegovic, Hrabak-Zerjavic, Borcic, Folnegovic-Smalc and Susser	1957 A2 (Asian)	Croatia	National Sample Index=348 cntrl=3761	Chi-sq to compare schiz in index year to those in control year:Entire pop index yr n=348 of 77,662 births vs. control 1,468 of 326,230 births. Two comparison periods [1955-57 and 58-60]	NONE	n/a	n/a	Entire birth cohort from Croatia
10	1994	Br J Psychiatry 164 : 674-676	Evidence against maternal influenza as a risk factor for schizophrenia	Selten and Slaets	1957 A2 (Asian)	Netherlands	National Sample Index=873 \control=3761	Compared # of schizph in index yr with avg of schiz in 4 control years	NONE	n/a		Obtained birth info of all Dutch born patients admitted b/w 1978 and 1991 for ICD-9 Dx of schizophrenia. Huge study. Dutch use notorious narrow schizophrenia defn.
11	1995	Am J Psychiatry 152 (3) : 450-452	Schiz following in utero exp to the 1957 influ epidemic in Japan	Kunugi, Nariko, Takei, Saito, Hayashi and Kazamatsuri	1957 A2 (Asian) and (A/B Mixed)	Tokyo, Japan	index=260 cntrl=1024	Chi-sq to compare # of schiz in index yr (6/57-5/98) vs to # schiz 2 yrs before and after index year	Females in 5th month	$p<.05$	n/a	No definite info on when exposed or if exposed. Did not use preterm patients or those in remission.

#	Year	Citation	Title	Authors	Virus	Location	Final size	Method	Exposure timing	Result		Comments
12	1996	Br J Psychiatry 168 : 368-71	Prenatal exposure to the 1957 influenza epidemic and adult schizophrenia:a follow-up study	Cannon, Cotter, Coffey Sham, Takei, Larkin, Murray and O'Callaghan	1957 A2 (Asian)	Dublin, Ireland	Final size of 525 expd = 238, not expd = 287	Odds ratio to compare exposed to non-exposed	NONE	1.10 (95per-cent CI 0.41-2.95)	n/a	Retrospective birth cohort study. Increase in depression among exposed=1.59 (95percent CI 1.15-2.19)
13	1998	Schiz Research 30 : 101-103	Prenatal exposure to influenza and schiz in Surinamese and Dutch Antillean immigrants to The Netherlands	Selten, Slaets and Kahn	1957 A2 (Asian)	Netherlands	N = 57 Dutch Antilleans; N = 16 Surima-mese	Used standardized methods for estimating 95percent CI of those exposed vs not-exposed	NONE	n/a	n/a	No evidence following 2nd trimester exposure
14	1999	Schiz Research 38 : 85-91	Prenatal exposure to the 1957 influenza pandemic in the Netherlands	Selten, Brown, Moons, Slaets, Susser and Kahn	1957 A2 (Asian)	Netherlands	Expd = 275/78, 557; Not expd = 1084/317, 789	Simple Odds ratio	NONE	expd Rel Risk=1.0; Not expd RR=1.1	n/a	Very large study
15	1999	Bio Psychiatry 46 : 119-24	Schiz and the 1957 Flu epidemic in Japan	Izumoto, Inoue and Yasuda	1957 A2 (Asian)	Japan	Index = 188/22, 754; Control = 753/93, 297	Calculated Relative Risk	2nd Trimester for Female	RR=2.86 (95percent CI 1.37-5.26)	n/a	Addressed methological problems of previous ecological stuies–included both inpatient and outpatient schizophrenia

(continued)

Table 5.1 (continued)

General Influenza Outbreaks

No	Date	Journal	Title	Author(s)	Type of Flu	Geographic Regions	Size (N)	Statistical Analysis Employed	Description of Association	Significance	Hypothesis of Mechanism	Further Comments
6b	1993	Br J Psychiatry 163: 522-24	Epidemiological evidence that maternal influenza contributes to the aetiology of schizophrenia	Adams, Kendell, Hare and Munk-Jorgenson	General b/w 1911-60	Scotland Denmark England	N1 = 16,960 N2 = 18,723 N3 = 22,021	Method 1: simple regression method 2: regression formula method 3: compare months w/highest incidence of flu with remainder	Eng (6 to 7th) Eng (6 to 7th) Eng (6 to 7th)	$p<.05$ $p<.05$ $p<.05$	Flu interferes with cellular migration process in fetal brain	5 to 7th month implicated for measles and varoster.
16	1988	Schiz Research 1: 73-77	Schizophrenic births and viral diseases in two states	Torrey, Rawlings and Waldman	General b/w 1920-55	United States (Connecticut and Massachusetts)	7526 CT = 2519 MA=5007	Time series using spectral analysis. Sig level >=coherence of .0964(0.002)	non for schiz measles (both) polio (CT) varzoster (CT)	0.956 0.967-72 0.965 0.971	Immune dysfun	
17	1990	Arch Gen Psychtry 47:869-8740	Exposure to influenza epidemics during gestation and adult schizophrenia: a 40-year study	Barr, Mednick and Munk-Jorgensen	General 1911 to 1950	Denmark	National sample of 7,239 schiz patients	Using (1) deviation scores and (2) trichotomized months to compare # of schiz with influenza rates	Males and females	$p<.01$ (6th) $p<.01$ (6th) $p<.05$ (7th)	Fever causes microvascular damage leading to hemorrhage	Data from Danish Ministry of Health; Adjusted for seasonality
18	1992	British J Psychiatry 160: 461-466	Schizophrenia following prenatal exp to influenza epidemics between 1939 and 1960	Sham, O'Callaghan, Takei, Murray, Hare and Murray	General b/w 1939 and 1960	England and Wales	14830	Used a generalized linear model with a Poisson-dependent variable and a logarithmic link to a linear predictor.	3rd to 7th month	n/a	Perturbs fetal brain development	1.4percent increase in the # of schiz births for every 1,000 deaths attrib to flu.

#	Year	Citation	Authors	Population	Country	N	Method	Sex effect	p-value	Mechanism	Findings
19	1993	Acta Psychi Scanda 88. 328-336	Takei, O'Callaghan, Sham, Glover and Murray	Does prenatal influenza divert susceptible females from later affective psychosis to schizophrenia?	General b/w 1938 and 1965	England and Wales	6982	Poisson regression analysis using a quintic polynomial model.	Females	$p<.007$ 5ht month	Disruption of neuron migration	Inverse relationship b/w schiz and affec disorder; 6.9percent increase in schiz incidence in those exposed in 5th month.
20	1993	Schiz Research 9, 137	Morris, Cotter, Takei, Walsh, Larkin, Waddington and O'Callaghan	An association between schiz births and influenza deaths in Ireland in the yrs 1921-1971	General b/w 1921 1971	Ireland	2846	Applied generalized linear model.	Exists, but not specified.	$p<.01$		
21	1994	Am J Psychiatry 151, 117-119	Takei, Sham, O'Callaghan, Murray, Glover and Murray	Prenatal exposure to influenza and the development of schiz is the effect confined to females?	General b/w 1938 and 1965 except 1958	England and Wales	3827	Poisson regression analysis using a quintic polynomial model.	Females	$p=.02$ 5th month	n/a	Replication of 1993 study (see number 19); 14 percent incid in # Births of schizoph.
22	1995	J Psych Res v 29, No 6	Takei, Van Os, and Murray	Maternal exposure to influenza and risk of schizophrenia: a 22-yr study from the Netherlands	1947 to 1969 Netherlands except 1958		10115	Compared # of schiz with # of flu deaths in respective yr using graphical analysis and Poisson regression analysis.	none	$p=.11$	n/a	n/a

(continued)

Table 5.1 (continued)

No	Date	Journal	Title	Author(s)	Type of Flu	Geographic Regions	Size (N)	Statistical Analysis Employed	Description of Association	Significance	Hypothesis of Mechanism	Further Comments
23	1995	Am J Psychiatry 152, 1714-1720	Maternal influenza, obstetric complications and schizophrenia	Wright, Takei, Rifkin and Murray	General	London	121	Compared # of women infected during 2nd trimester with those infected during combined 1st and 3rd trimesters using odds ratios and t-test	Males and females 76.9percent M 23.1 percent F	$p=.004$ 2nd trimester	n/a	No control of moms of non-schiz children in 2nd trimester; schiz are 5X more likely to have birth complications
24	1996	Biological Psych 40, 817-824	Relationship b/w in utero exp to influenza epidemic and risk of schiz in Denmark	Takei, Mortensen, Klaening, Murray, Sham and O'Callaghan	General b/w 1915 and 1970	Denmark	9462	Used Poisson reg anal to compare # of schiz births with # of influz deaths.	6th month			1.4percent increase in the # of schiz births for every 1,000 deaths attrib to flu.
25	1997	Schiz Reserch 26: 121-125	Mat Exp to Flu and Paranoid Schizophrenia	Grech, Takei and Murray	1923 to 1965	England and Wales	17247	Chi-Square and Logistic Regression	none	n/a	n/a	
26	2000	J of Psychiatric Reserch, 34(2), 133-138	No relationship b/w schizophrenia births and flu in Japan	Mino, Oshima, Tsuda and Okagami	1957/1958, 1962 and 1965	Japan	1957n=1137 1962n=844 1965n=734	Chi-square and Odds Ratio	none	n/a	n/a	
27	1999	Arch Gen Psychtry v 56: 993-998	Exp to prenatal flu and child-hood infections and the risk of Schizophrenia	Westergaard, et al.	General b/w 1950 and 1988	Denmark	2669	Logistic regression producing Odds ratio	none	n/a	Maternal infection	# of siblings associated with schizophrenia via increased infection exposure

#	Year	Citation	Author	Title	Sample	Location	N	Method	Results	Significance		Notes
28	2003	Acta Psychi Scanda 107(5), 331-335	Limosin, Rouillon, Payan, Cohen and Strub	Prenatal exp to flu as a risk factor for adult schizophrenia	General b/w 1949 and 1981	France	974	Mantel-Hanzel method producing Odds ratio	OR=2.64 (95percent CI 1.49-2.35) for 5th month exposure	n/a	n/a	Only study to produce serological confirmation. Although results say 7 fold increase, not stat sig.
29	2004	Arch Gen Psychiatry 61(8), 774-780	Brown, et al.	Serologic evidence of prenatal flu in the etiology of schizophrenia	General b/w 1959 and 1966	Alameda County, California	Cases=64 Controls=125	Mantel-Hanzel method producing Odds ratio	First half of preg OR=3.0 (95percent CI 0.9-10.1)	$p=.052$	Maternal infection	

1968-1972 Hong Kong

#	Year	Citation	Author	Title	Sample	Location	N	Method	Results	Significance		Notes
30	2002	Schiz Research 54: 7-16	Machon, et al.	Adult schizotypal personality and prenatal influenza	Hong Kong 1969	Finland	Wk 21 n=60; wk 22 n=39; wk 23 n=72; wk 24 n=62	Pearson Chi-Square analysis	Month 6 ; Week 23	$P<.003$; $P<.005$		Used Schizotypy MMPI code profile (2-7-8)

Southern Hemisphere Studies
1957 A2 Asian

#	Year	Citation	Author	Title	Sample	Location	N	Method	Results	Significance		Notes
31	1998	Med J of Australia 168(20): 421-422	Allen and Nero	Schiz and influenza in Palau	1957 A2 Asian	Palau	60	T-test	Higher schizophrenic births during 1957			Very small sample; One page study

General Influenza Outbreaks

#	Year	Citation	Author	Title	Sample	Location	N	Method	Results	Significance		Notes
32	1994	Schiz Research 14, 1-4	McGrath, Pemberton, Welham and Murray	Schizophrenia and the influenza epidemics of 1954, 1957 and 1959: A southern hemisphere study	General in 1954, 57 and 59	Queensland, Australia	7858	Compared ratio of schiz births to ratio of non-sch births using z-scores.	mnth 4- 1954M mnth 5- 1957 F none- 1959	$p<0.001$ $p<0.05$		Southern hemisphere study

(continued)

Table 5.1 (continued)

No	Date	Journal	Title	Author (s)	Type of Flu	Geographic Regions	Size (N)	Statistical Analysis Employed	Description of Association	Significance	Hypothesis of Mechanism	Further Comments
33	1997	Schiz Research 26, 25-39	Influenza epidemics and incid of schiz affective disorders and mental retardation in West Austr no evid of a major affect	Morgan, Castle, Page, Fazio, Gurrin, Burton, Montgomery and Jablensky	General b/w 1950 and 1960	Western Australia	1852	Used relative risk ratios for individual epidemics. Poisson regression analysis, and a proportional hazards model	none			No assoc w/schiz, affec psych, and neur depress. Assoc in 1st and 2nd trimest males for ment retard
1968-1972 Hong Kong												
34	1996	J Abnormal Psych v 105, No 1, 53-60	Schizotypy and maternal exp to influenza and to cold temp the Mauritius study	Venables	1968-1972 Hong Kong	Mauritas Island in southern hemisphere	1800	Measured schizotypy with 2 factors: schizophrenism and anhedonia: MANOVA using Sz and Ah as dep var yielded (p=.058) Univariate t-tests sig for Sz (p=.004) for females rather than males. No sig assoc for Ah	Females for schizo-phrenism	Females (p=.004) 5th month	Neron migration in 2nd tri-mester	May suggest that schiz exists on continuum Venables (1997) corrob results examining electrodermal response to cold and flu: flu=hyper=pos cold=hypo=neg schiz scores

Northern Hemisphere Studies
1918-1919 Influenza Pandemic

	Year	Journal	Title	Authors	Event	Location	N	Method		Mechanism	Findings
2b	1989	Arch Gen Psychiatry 48, 878-882	Maternal influence in the etiology of schizophrenia	Kendell and Kemp	Pandemic of 1918-1919	Scotland	16,317	Compared # of schiz births in 1918-19 with yrs b/w 1913 and 1922.	none	Fetal brain damage as a result of viral infection	Increased incidence of Parkinson's in those exposed to 1918-1919 pandemic. Re-analysis by Mednick et al (1990) revealed assoc for 1919
6c	1993	Br J Psychiatry 163, 522-24	Epidemiological evidence that maternal influenza contributes to the aetiology of schizophrenia	Adams, Kendell, Hare and Munk-Jorgenson	Pandemic of 1918-1919	Denmark	index=14260 cntrl=18723	T-tests [index (6/18-12/19) vs cntrl (16-21)]	none	Flu interferes with cellular migration process in fetal brain	If pathogenic mechanism depends on maternal flu, pregnant women should be given immunization; if depends on immune response, this is contraindicated.

number of published reports have failed to find an association. For example, researchers studying the most virulent epidemic this past century—the 1918-1919 influenza pandemic—did not provide evidence for an association in Denmark and Scotland. Less emphasis should perhaps be placed upon these studies due to methodology issues that have been raised about this research. However, some of the more rigorously controlled and methodologically sound studies of other epidemics have also not found an association. In the studies that found an association, it appears that the second trimester of gestation has been primarily implicated, although the first trimester through month seven have also been targeted as a period of potential vulnerability. Several research reports suggest that there may be a higher incidence of schizophrenia in females following influenza exposure. Additional research related to gender effects is warranted.

Several research studies have concluded that influenza exposure during gestation may be associated with later onset of affective disorders. This line of research deserves further study. In addition, although conceptual articles based mostly upon experimental animal models have suggested a possible association with autism, the only study to investigate this possible association did not find any association (Dassa, Takei, Sham and Murray 1995).

Other Prenatal Infections

What follows is a discussion of the literature involving some of the more common infectious illnesses, other than influenza, experienced by mothers during pregnancy. All of these infections have been associated with profound physical and neurological outcomes. Few investigations report data regarding more childhood or adolescent psychological and behavioral outcomes.

Congenital Rubella

Prenatal rubella occurring during pregnancy was one of the first viral infections to be studied with regard to affects on children. In 1941 Gregg, an ophthalmologist, described that children exposed to rubella developed congenital cataracts that led to blindness. Approximately a quarter of a century later, Menser, Dods and Harley (1967) reported similar results in a 25-year follow-up of 50 congenital rubella patients in Australia: 96 percent were deaf, 52 percent had cataracts, 50 percent were of small stature and 22 percent had heart defects.

First trimester maternal rubella infection commonly results in offspring with congenital rubella syndrome, the results of which include hearing loss, mental retardation, cardiac malformations and eye defects (Freij, South and Sever 1988). Maternal rubella infection primarily exerts its harmful impact on the fetus during the first 16 weeks of gestation (Miller, Cradock-Watson and Pollack 1982).

Infection after the 16th week of gestation results in transmission to the fetus, but development of sequelae seems to be rare (Grillner, et al. 1983).

For instance, Miller, et al. (1982) investigated over 1,000 women with confirmed rubella infection at different stages of pregnancy. The likelihood of manifesting symptoms after maternal exposure was more than 80 percent if exposure occurred during the first 12 weeks of pregnancy, 54 percent if exposure was from 13 to 14 weeks and 25 percent if exposure occurred at the end of the second trimester. Follow-up two years after birth indicated that defects, primarily heart and hearing, occurred in all infants infected before the eleventh week of gestation. In 35 percent of those infected between the 13th and 16th week, deafness resulted. No malformations were found in children who were exposed in utero after the 16th week of gestation.

Zgorniak-Nowoseilska, Zawilinska and Szostek (1996) investigated 310 pregnant women from southern Poland who were exposed to rubella during the 1985-1986 epidemic in that country. None of these women had been vaccinated against rubella. Consistent with previous studies, the results of this study indicated greatest teratogenic impact during first trimester exposure. Only 22.7 percent of women who were infected during the first trimester gave birth to healthy babies, compared to 66.7 percent of women who were infected during the second trimester of gestation.

The rubella virus crosses the placental barrier and has been isolated in the fetuses of accidentally vaccinated pregnant mothers (Bologonese, Corson, Fuccillo, Sever and Traube 1973). There are two primary hypothesized pathogenic mechanisms associated with the rubella virus. The first involves a direct viral effect whereby the virus inhibits cell replication. The second involves an immune response in which permanent physical and brain damage is inflicted via inflammatory mechanisms, including immune cytolysis (e.g., destruction of somatic cells by immune cells), interruption of blood supply by inflammation of vascular walls and scarring (South and Sever 1985). It is noted that fever is often a by-product of immune reactions in general and may be a tertiary mechanism by which teratogenesis is induced.

In addition to adverse physical and neurological outcomes, several studies have reported an association with later psychiatric conditions. In fact, Gregg (1941) reported that two of his 50 subjects (4 percent) received a diagnosis of schizophrenia and conjectured that gestational exposure might be linked to autism. Chess, Korn and Fernandez (1971) investigated a cohort of children prenatally exposed to the 1964 rubella epidemic in New York City. The study included participants with serologically confirmed exposure. The results provided evidence for an increased risk of autism, separation anxiety disorder and impaired social skills in children exposed during the prenatal period. In a follow-up study Chess (1977) quantified the increased prevalence of autism, reporting that 8 to 13 percent of children born during the rubella pandemic of the early 1960s developed autism.

In 1988 Torrey, Rawlings and Waldman investigated the relationship between schizophrenic births and viral diseases in Connecticut and Massachusetts on a sample of 7,526 patients. The time period under investigation for Massachusetts was 1920 to 1932, while that analyzed for Connecticut was 1920 to 1955. The authors compared time series using spectral analysis and examined the coherence between the series. No evidence for an association with rubella was found. Similarly, O'Callaghan, et al. (1994) did not find evidence for a relationship between gestational rubella exposure and later psychological or behavioral outcomes.

More recently, the work of Alan Brown and colleagues have reported an association between serologically documented gestational rubella exposure and later onset of schizophrenia in exposed offspring. Brown, et al. (2001) found that offspring exposed during the prenatal period had a 20 percent increased risk of developing later schizophrenia spectrum disorders in adulthood. Brown, et al. (2001) also commented that prenatal exposure produces increased behavioral anomalies and neuromotor dysfunction in childhood. Brown, Cohen, Greenwald and Susser (2000) also reported a five-fold increased risk for non-affective psychosis in adulthood following clinical and serological confirmed gestational rubella exposure.

In summary, several epidemiological studies have not found evidence for an association between prenatal rubella exposure and mental illness. However, all three of the studies that had serological documentation of prenatal rubella exposure found a significant association. These findings suggest that there may be an association with later psychiatric outcomes including schizophrenia, autism and affective disorders.

Measles/Mumps

Measles during pregnancy has known harmful effects on the developing fetus. Measles has been linked to prematurity, spontaneous abortion and stillbirth (Chiba, Saito, Suzuki, Honda and Yaegashi 2003). One of the more frequently studied outcomes is in relation to autism. Singh and colleagues (Singh, Lin and Yang 1998; Singh, Lin, Newell and Nelson 2002; Singh and Jensen 2003) performed a series of tests for the presence of measles antibodies in children with autism spectrum disorders. This group found that the children with autism, compared to controls, had elevated anti-measles serum antibodies. Uhlmann, et al. (2002) found a similarly high level of anti-measles antibodies in the guts of children with autism. Gut tissue was positive for the presence of the measles virus in 75 of the 91 affected children, whereas only five of 70 controls were positive for measles virus antibodies. However, Deykin and MacMahon (1979) did not find evidence for an increase in autism cases following measles exposure. These antibody studies suggested that a possible subclinical or altered immune response to measles exposure may be linked to later developmental outcomes.

Research on mumps during pregnancy is sparse. In one study dating back to the 1960s, mumps infection during the first trimester of pregnancy was linked to adverse fetal outcomes, including spontaneous abortion (Siegel, Fuerst and Peress 1966). Several studies have since failed to document this association between prenatal mumps exposure and congenital anomalies (Shepard 1998; Siegel 1973). One study has documented a possible cardiac defect (Ni, et al. 1997). In regard to possible psychological outcomes, only Deykin and MacMahon (1979) have reported an association with gestational mumps exposure (increased risk of autism). Additional gestational mumps exposure studies are needed prior to arriving at any conclusions regarding its impact on developmental outcomes in offspring.

Varicella-Zoster (Chicken Pox)

Maternal infection with varicella-zoster virus (chickenpox) can result in children with congenital defects including brain damage, skin scars, abnormal limb development and numerous ophthalmological defects: cataracts, microphthalmus, Horner syndrome (e.g., insult to eye muscle and eye sympathetic nervous system), anisocoria (e.g., pupils are different sizes), optic atrophy, nystagmus (e.g., involuntary movement of eyes) and chorioretinitis (e.g., inflammation of chorioid and retina) (Hollier and Grissom 2005; Jones, Johnson and Chambers 1994). There appear to be two critical time periods for varicella infection: the first trimester and zero to four days before delivery. First trimester exposure is linked to the above described abnormalities. Perinatal infection within four days of birth manifests in neonatal death in approximately 30 percent of the cases (Fuccillo 1988).

Despite the well-known teratogenic effects of varicella-zoster exposure in utero, the incidence of symptoms in the progeny of infected pregnant women remains unknown (Jones, Johnson and Chambers 1994). Estimates indicate that there is an approximate 4 percent chance of congenital anomalies when infection takes place during the first trimester. In a recent study of women who became infected, only two of 146 live births had features consistent with fetal varicella syndrome described above. In addition, six of the fetuses were spontaneously aborted, seven were therapeutically aborted and two were stillborn (Jones, et al. 1994).

In the only comprehensive study of psychological and behavioral outcomes in children prenatally exposed to varicella, Mattson, et al. (2003) concluded that maternal varicella infection during pregnancy does not pose a risk for adverse neurobehavioral outcomes in children who do not display clinical features of fetal varicella syndrome. This result of no effect is consistent with other studies which did not report an association with psychological and behavioral outcomes following varicella infection (e.g., Deykin and MacMahon 1979). Mattson, et al. (2003) concluded that the risk of structural abnormalities in children prenatally exposed is small (<2 percent). Knobloch and Pasamanick (1975) found the only positive association with a behavioral outcome when they reported an increased risk of autism following postnatal varicella encephalitis, suggesting a possible role in the etiology of autistic spectrum disorders following prenatal exposure. Overall, the

pathogenic mechanism remains unknown, although direct viral effects are postulated to cause pathogenesis.

Cytomegalovirus infection (CMV)

CMV is the most common viral infection experienced by women during pregnancy and the most common infectious cause of brain damage in the fetus
(Burny, Liesnard, Donner and Marchant 2004; Persaud 1985). Congenital CMV
infection occurs in approximately 0.5 to 3 percent of all newborns and often
results in significant neurological sequelae (Ross and Boppana 2005). Children
with congenital CMV infection following first trimester maternal infection are
more likely to have CNS sequelae, especially sensorineural hearing loss, than are
those who were infected later in pregnancy. However, some degree of CNS
impairment can follow even late gestational infection (Pass, Fowler, Boppana,
Britt and Stagno 2006).

With regard to the effects of the timing of the infection, Persaud (1985)
indicated that the greatest risk occurs during the first and third trimester, with
minimal risk associated with second trimester infection. Research indicates that
first trimester CMV infection results in the greatest teratogenic effects for the
fetus (Preece, et al. 1983), although the risk of intrauterine infection during this
time period is less than what it is during later gestational trimesters (Kumar and
Prokay 1983).

Of those who become infected, approximately 10 percent develop cytomeg-
alic inclusion disease shortly after birth (Nelson and Demmler 1997), resulting
in outcomes ranging from death (20 to 30 percent of the time) to physical
defects. The associated pathology includes microcephaly, blindness, hearing
loss, mental retardation, lower birth weight, physical disabilities and developmental delay (Hedrick 1996; Persaud 1985). The majority of infected infants
are asymptomatic at birth. Of the asymptomatic group of infants, it is estimated
that 5 to 15 percent will experience some neurodevelopmental complication
during childhood (Alford, Stagno, Pass and Britt 1990; Fowler, et al. 1997;
Wong, Tan, Tee and Yeo 2000). For instance, several case reports indicate that
CMV infection is associated with autism spectrum disorder (Stubbs 1978;
Markowitz 1983; Ivarsson, Bjerre, Vegfors and Ahlfors 1990; Sweeten, Posey
and McDougle 2004).

One study by Williamson, Desmond, LaFevers, Taber, Catlin and Weaver
(1982) reported that CMV infection is associated with learning disabilities.
Some authorities believe that congenital CMV infection is believed to be the
most common infectious cause of learning disabilities in children (Fowler,
et al. 1997; Fowler and Boppana 2006). However, research that has tested
this hypothesis in clinically asymptomatic infants suggests that offspring are not
at increased risk for any cognitive deficits (Ivarsson, Lernmark and Svanberg
1997; Kashden, Frison, Fowler, Pass and Boll 1998; Kumar, Nankervis, Jacobs

and Emhart 1984; Pearl, Preece, Ades and Peckham 1986; Temple, Pass and Boll 2000).

Herpes Simplex 2 (HSV-2)

Maternal herpes simplex infection during pregnancy has been associated with microencephaly, hydrocephalus, mental retardation, eye defects, skin lesions, low birth weight and intracranial calcifications (Avgil and Ornoy 2006; Baldwin and Whitely 1989; Persaud 1985; South, Thompkins, Morris and Rawls 1969). It has also been associated with preterm birth and spontaneous abortion (Hanshaw and Dudgeon 1978).

The herpes simplex virus is able to cross the placental barrier and infect the fetus. The fetus may also become infected during its passage through the birth canal during delivery. A cesarean section is usually carried out to prevent such complications in mothers showing symptoms of the infection (Persaud 1985). Although the virus can cross the placental barrier during gestation, the primary period of transmission appears to be around the time of birth. Only approximately 8 percent of fetal infections are contracted prior to this period (Hutto, Willett, Yeager and Whitely 1985).

Recently, herpes simplex 2 infection has been associated with greater risk for development of schizophrenia in offspring. Buka, et al. (2001) utilized blood samples from the Providence cohort of the Collaborative Perinatal Project. These authors concluded that perinatal exposure to herpes simples-2 virus is associated with greater risk for the development of schizophrenia and other psychotic illness in offspring. In addition, Sever (1986) reports that the sequelae of children infected with herpes at birth include mental retardation, seizures and microecephaly. Sever (1986) also speculates that learning disabilities may be an outcome of more mildly affected children, but no study to date has tested this hypothesis. Several case reports provide evidence for a link between herpes simplex virus and autism (e.g., DeLong, Bean and Brown 1981; Gilberg 1986; Ghaziuddin, Tsai, Eilers and Ghaziuddin 1992; Greer, Lyons-Crews, Mauldin and Brown 1989). The combined sample size of these four case reports amounts to five participants, so any conclusion drawn regarding the link between HSV-2 and autism is tentative subject to further replication. For instance, Gilberg (1986) discussed the manifestation of autism in a 14 year-old-girl following herpes encephalitis. More recently, using a case-control design study of pregnant women born between 1959 and 1966, Yolken (2004) found an association between high levels of maternal antibody to HSV-2 and subsequent development of adult psychosis in 27 subjects who were later diagnosed with schizophrenia. However, Jorgensen, Goldschmidt and Vestergaard (1982) did not find an association between HSV-2 antibodies and later psychiatric outcomes. Thus, there appears to be inconsistent evidence regarding HSV2's association with later psychiatric outcomes.

Toxoplasmosis

Toxoplasmosis is an infection caused by a protozoan parasite. A pregnant mother may contract toxoplasmosis by ingesting uncooked meat, especially lamb or pork, or through exposure to cat feces containing toxoplasmosis parasites (Larsen 1986). There is no evidence that a woman infected prior to becoming pregnant can transmit the parasite to her developing fetus (Larsen 1986). However, once infection occurs during pregnancy, the parasite can cross the placental barrier and infect the developing fetus (Desmonts and Couvreur 1974). The incidence of fetal infection ranges from 0.25 to 8 per 1,000 in the newborn population (Larsen 1986)

Maternal toxoplasmosis infection during pregnancy has been shown to lead to hydrocephalus, blindness and mental retardation (Barron and Pass 1995; Hedrick 1996; Larsen 1986). The severity of this protozoan parasite infection appears to be related to the trimester of infection. The greatest teratogenic effects occur during the first trimester (Kumar and Prokay 1983; Larsen 1986). Recently, Brown, et al. (2005) found evidence that maternal exposure to toxoplasmosis may be a risk factor for the later development of schizophrenia. In particular, subjects with high maternal toxoplasmosis IgG antibody titers had a 161 percent increased risk of developing schizophrenia. This result is consistent with research by Torrey and Yolken (1995) who hypothesized that schizophrenia may be related to transmission from the feces of house cats.

Syphilis

Maternal syphilis infection during pregnancy, if left untreated, can cause abortion, stillbirth, abnormal bone and teeth development and mental retardation (Taber 1982). Early diagnosis and treatment before the 20th week of pregnancy is rarely associated with teratogenesis. Late treatment will prevent further damage, but will not reverse damage already imparted (Grossman 1986). Our review yielded only one citation on a possible linkage with psychological/behavioral outcomes. Lotspeich and Ciaranello (1993) describe a possible association between gestational syphilis infection and later onset of autistic spectrum disorders.

Summary

Each of the prenatal infections mentioned above are associated with physical teratogenesis. The exception is the influenza virus, which has been inconclusively linked with structural abnormalities observable at birth and extensively studied in relation to psychological and behavioral outcomes, with a number of associations reported for serious mental illness. The remaining prenatal infections deserve further study in this regard to determine any latent effects of prenatal exposure on the behavioral or psychological development of offspring.

For most prenatal infections the underlying pathogenic mechanism has not been well-elucidated, particularly in relation to behavioral teratology. It is often assumed that the direct effects of the virus or parasite which invaded the developing fetus contributed to the physical and neurological effects observed. However, there are a number of other processes related to infection (e.g., fever, inflammation, medication use) that could play a role. A neurodevelopmental hypothesis provides a general conceptual framework which is useful in understanding the role of prenatal infection in later psychological or behavioral outcomes. The forthcoming section will describe this hypothesis, followed by a detailed discussion of the postulated mechanisms of teratogenesis via the immune system response to infection.

Etiological Hypotheses

Neurodevelopmental Hypothesis

The association between influenza and schizophrenia has been explained as part of a neurodevelopmental hypothesis of brain perturbation. This hypothesis could plausibly be extended to other prenatal infections. The neurodevelopmental hypothesis posits that a disruption to brain development at an earlier stage creates a vulnerability to psychopathology in offspring at a later stage of life (Waddington, et al. 1999).

In the case of schizophrenia researchers have postulated that exposure during the second trimester may play a critical role in disrupting fetal neurodevelopment (Mednick, et al. 1988). The end of the second trimester of fetal development is marked by three important neurological events that, if perturbed, may be related to schizophrenic neuropathology: neural migration, an increase in brain growth and an increase in the risk of hemorrhage due to the dissolution of the germinal matrix (Barr, Mednick and Munk-Jorgensen 1990). Influenza exposure at this critical period of development may disrupt the process of neuronal migration from the periventricular area to a variety of sites on the cortex (Barr, et al. 1990). Akbarian, et al. (1993) suggest that second trimester disturbances can create cytoarchitectonic malformations and volume reductions in layers II and V of the cingulate and prefrontal cortex. In addition, Takei, et al. (1994) reports that influenza exposure may displace pre-alpha cells in the entorhinal cortex, and contribute to a lack of gliosis. Such neuronal disruption may produce decreased cell densities, cytoarchitectonic deviations and cell orientation disruptions, all of which are evident in histopathological studies of brains of schizophrenics (Barr, et al. 1990).

With influenza it is postulated that a symptom of influenza (e.g., fever) or a maternal or fetal immune response (e.g., circulating cytokines; maternal antibodies) contributes to a disruption or alteration of the developing central nervous system in a way that produces functional abnormalities (Wright and Murray 1996). The effects tend to alter development at the cellular level rather than at the structural level, and impart subtle damage in offspring that remains clinically latent until a later stage of development.

The Immune Response to Infection

Many of the commonly experienced prenatal infections discussed in this chapter– rubella, chicken pox, toxoplasmosis, cytomegalovirus, herpes simplex 2– have a profound impact on a child's physical development. These effects, as a result, often overshadow any associated neurobehavioral or psychiatric outcomes. These ill- nesses may be caused by viruses or parasites crossing the placental barrier and infecting the developing fetus. When viral trans-placental migration occurs, the virus is postulated to have a directly adverse impact on the developing brain. A second mechanism of teratogenesis is possible and has received increased research attention, particularly in relation to later psychopathology in offspring. In response to prenatal infection, the maternal immune system is mobilized and this immune response may play a role in central nervous system development.

Recent research has investigated the possible role of the immune system in disrupting fetal CNS development following gestational exposure to infection (Elbou, et al. 2004; Malek-Ahmadi 2001; Muller, Riedel, Ackenheil and Schwarz 1999; Patterson 2002). The immune system has evolved over time to protect the body from foreign organisms (e.g., viruses) or bodily trauma. Intricately balanced, the human immune system utilizes the mobilization of cellular, antibody and cytokine responses to foreign organisms. Aside from the deleterious impact of a direct viral infection, there are several immune system mechanisms that have been investigated for their possible role in contributing to psychological and behavioral outcomes following prenatal infection. These include circulating cytokines, maternal antibodies, fever, autoantibody response and heat shock proteins, each of which is described below.

Cytokine Effects

Cytokines are proteins produced by the immune system in response to infection, trauma or insult. There are dozens of cytokines in the body and their roles are extremely diverse (Benveniste 1992). Cytokines are important mediators of an individual's immunological defense (Benveniste 1992). Cytokines also have been studied for their role in promoting brain development.

Cytokines have been categorized into two groups. Type 1 cytokines (e.g., interleukin-2 (IL-2), interferon-lambda (IFN-λ) and tumor necrosis factor-α (TNF-α) are associated with the cellular immune system. Type 2 cytokines (e.g., IL-4, IL-5 and IL-10) are part of the humoral immune system. Type 1 cytokines are produced by various cells (e.g., macrophages) within the immune system. Type 2 cytokines are produced by the bone marrow and circulate within the bloodstream. Recent research has focused on the possible role of cytokines in producing adverse outcomes via either direct action or indirectly via their thermoregulatory properties. While cytokine activity has been extensively studied as it relates to respiratory infection and, to a lesser extent, brain development, only a few investigators have looked at how cytokines might disrupt the process of fetal CNS development (Gomez, et al. 1998; Patterson 2002).

An increasing body of evidence suggests that proinflammatory cytokines, such as IL-1, IL-2, IL-6 and TNF-α, generated by both the cellular and humoral immune system are important mediators in the relationship between maternal infection, abnormal fetal brain development and later psychiatric outcomes (Gilmore and Jarskog 1997; Malek-Ahmadi 2001; Nawa, Takahashi and Patterson 2000). Cytokines are thought to influence fetal brain development at the cellular level by disrupting important formative processes, either directly or indirectly. This association, however, is neither well-articulated nor fully understood. Much of the human research on the impact of cytokines during prenatal brain development has been conducted in the context of the schizophrenia-influenza association (Gilmore and Jarskog 1997; Patterson 2002).

Within the influenza-schizophrenia literature it is hypothesized that maternally generated cytokines cross the placenta and enter fetal circulation, although the precise mechanism by which cytokines enter fetal circulation remains largely unknown (Patterson 2002). Similarly, infections within the herpes virus family (e.g., HSV-2 or CMV) can induce a variety of proinflammatory cytokines and this mechanism is postulated to be linked to altered CNS development and subsequent psychopathology (Dalod, et al. 2002). Other researchers have discussed the possibility that cytokines generated by the fetus in response to prenatal infection may play an important role in altering fetal brain development (Gomez, et al.1998). Thus, both fetal and maternally generated cytokines may be responsible for adversely impacting the developing fetal brain.

Postmortem dissection studies have explored the possible role of cytokines in adversely affecting the brains of individuals with schizophrenia (Nawa, Takahashi and Patterson 2000). From this research it has been postulated that cytokines may play a role in the pathogenesis of schizophrenia, possibly exerting effects during gestational development. Both Type 1 and 2 cytokines have been observed in the CNS of individuals who developed psychiatric disorders during childhood (e.g., schizophrenia, OCD) (Mittleman 1997; Mittleman, et al. 1997). It is thought that cytokines, or some associated influence, were at least partially responsible for the genesis of these adverse behavioral and psychological outcomes.

The influence of cytokine activity on fetal CNS development seems plausible. Cytokines are known to regulate normal and abnormal brain development by playing an important stimulatory or inhibitory role in the development of neurons and glial cells (Mehler and Kessler 1999; Zhao and Schwartz 1998). Research has explored the influence of specific cytokines, particularly IL-1, IL-6, and TNF-α, on proliferation, survival, neurotransmitter expression and differentiation of neural cells during development (Rothwell and Hopkins 1995; Rothwell, Giamal and Toulmond 1996). Each of these cytokines is classified as proinflammatory and is reportedly toxic to a variety of developing cell structures in the brain (e.g., neurons and glia). Based on a rat model of brain perturbation, there is a hypothesis that developing neurons and glia in areas adjacent to the ventricles, including the germinal matrix, could be especially vulnerable to the direct effects of cytokines (Sarnat 1995). For example, IL-6 is known to directly impact neuron and glial proliferation, apoptosis and survival. Further, cytokines regulate neurotropic factor expression in glia (Hesse, Hock and Otten 1998). Other cytokines including IL-1β, IL-6 and tumor necrosis factor-alpha (TNF-α) may contribute to decreased survival of fetal dopaminergic and serotonergic neurons (Jarskog, Xiao, Wilkie, Lauder and Gilmore 1997). TNF-α may potentially lead to cell death by stimulating the release of excitatory (e.g., glutamate) amino acids which have been demonstrated to be neurotoxic (Chao and Hu 1994). IL-1β may contribute to alterations in neuron survival, particularly in the hippocampus. The plausibility of this association was demonstrated via experimental animal studies in which IL-1β contributed to reduced neuron survival in cultures of embryonic rat hippocampus cells (Arajujo and Cotman 1995). IL-1 has also been reported to modulate neuronal and glial cell survival and growth during development. IL-1 appears in the brain during prenatal development at about the same time that astrocytes appear (Giulian, Li, Li, George and Rutecki 1994). Recent research (e.g., Maier, Watkins and Nance 2001) suggests that IL-1 at low concentration could lead to inhibition of synaptic plasticity. Thus, IL-1 has been associated with alterations in synaptic plasticity, ultimately influencing learning and memory (Maier, Watkins and Nance 2001).

Based on the above research it is plausible that changes in the levels of cytokines in the fetal environment (in response to infection or trauma) may contribute to abnormal brain development. The ultimate impact on fetal brain development is likely to be dependent on both the timing and severity of prenatal insult in relation to critical periods. In turn, these factors probably interact with additional environmental and genetic risk factors to produce adverse outcomes (Urakubo, Jarskog, Lieberman and Gilmore 2001).

Indirect Effects via Hyperthermia

Research has pointed to a second mechanism by which circulating cytokines might disrupt fetal neurodevelopment. In response to trauma or infection, some cytokines (e.g., IL-1; TNF-α), called endogenous pyrogens, alter the set point of the hypothalamus to produce hyperthermia (e.g., fever) (Kluger, Wieslaw and Mayfield 2001).

There is a substantial body of research that demonstrates adverse fetal outcomes following first trimester hyperthermia exposure (Edwards 2006; Edwards, Walsh and Li 1997; Hunter 1984; Warkany 1986). An association has been found in human studies between maternal first trimester febrile episodes (e.g., fever) and later physical abnormalities including severe brain damage (Milunsky, et al.1992; Shiota 1982). This association can be demonstrated even more definitively in animal studies through the use of experimental control (Edwards, Walsh and Li 1997). In experimental animal studies with monkeys, sheep, guinea pigs, chickens, rats and mice, gestational first trimester hyperthermia exposure has a profoundly teratogenic impact on the developing embryo (Edwards, et al. 1997).

While these studies demonstrate first trimester teratogenic effects, there is some evidence that fever may have an adverse, yet less profound, effect if it occurs during the second trimester or third trimester of pregnancy. Dombrowski, Martin and Huttunen (2003) studied fever during each trimester of pregnancy and child outcomes in a birth cohort from Helsinki. In this study the authors reported a link between maternal report of fever during the second and third trimesters of pregnancy and later psychological and behavioral outcomes, including reduced academic performance, greater inhibition and reduced capacity to attend and remain on task. Researchers who have studied the association between influenza and schizophrenia have discussed the possible role of maternal fever as the mechanism through which influenza infections alter brain development (Barr, et al. 1990; Mehler and Kessler 1999; Patterson 2002).

The mechanism through which fever might perturb prenatal brain development is unclear. However, it is known that protein synthesis and enzyme production is sensitive to increases in temperature. Thus, it is possible that various cellular structures and formative processes (e.g., proliferation, migration, differentiation, myelination, apoptosis) during fetal development become altered or dysfunctional as a result of elevated body temperature. This raises the possibility that both endogenous (e.g., fever) and exogenous (e.g., sauna tub exposure; exercise-induced fever) hyperthermia can be teratogenic not only during the first trimester, but also during second and third trimesters of pregnancy. The possible relationship between maternal fever and adverse developmental outcomes for children deserves further study (Cordero 2003).

Autoimmune Response

Autoimmune mechanisms are another possible, but less researched, avenue of fetal brain perturbation (Kilidireas, et al. 1992; Strauss 1999). Typically, an individual's immune system has the capacity to differentiate the body's proteins and cells from foreign ones. The process is called tolerance (Strauss 1999). However, when there is a loss of self-tolerance, the immune system may target and attack the body's own tissues (Sinha, Lopez and McDevitt 1990). When this occurs the body's mechanism for attacking foreign organisms is mobilized against itself.

Environmental stressors (e.g., trauma, infection, toxins) are thought to trigger a breakdown in self-tolerance leading to autoimmunity (e.g., one's immune system attacking one's body) via molecular mimicry. This process occurs when antibodies raised against a foreign antigen (e.g., virus) mistakes the body's own proteins as foreign and attack those same proteins. If fetal neuronal structures are mistakenly attacked by the mother's or fetus's immune system, this could have devastating outcomes on fetal brain development.

While research has not, at this point, found a definitive link between autoimmune reaction during pregnancy and later psychiatric or behavioral outcomes in offspring, research has provided indirect support. Studies from the Collaborative Perinatal Project (CPP) have shown that elevated levels of total IgG and IgM immunoglublulins and antibodies are associated with increased risk for adverse psychological or behavioral outcomes. For instance, Buka, et al. (2001) used placental cord blood serum samples from the CPP and found that individuals with elevated levels of total IgG and IgM immunoglobulins and antibodies to herpes simplex virus type 2 at birth were at increased risk for the development of schizophrenia and other psychotic illnesses. Similarly, Yolken (2004) found a greater risk for autism in those with increased levels of total maternal IgG at birth. Using blood samples from the CPP, Yolken (2004) also described a 170 percent increased risk in developing cognitive impairments (e.g., low IQ) among children whose mothers reported increased influenza B antibodies at birth.

Further indirect evidence is based on research from two autoimmune diseases outside of pregnancy: Sydenham's chorea (Strauss 1999) and Rasmussen's Encephalitis (Rogers, Twyman and Gahring 1996). Individuals with Sydenham's chorea develop motor disturbances and psychiatric symptoms via an immune response to streptococcal infection in which an autoantibody cross-reacts with a neural antigen and attacks the body's nervous system (Bonthius and Karacay 2003). Rasmussen's encephalitis is a progressive disorder with childhood onset that includes seizures and dementia (Granata 2003). The purported mechanism of pathology is linked to direct autoantibody stimulation of CNS glutamate receptors (Rogers, et al. 1996).

The Heat Shock Response

The Heat Shock Response (Lindquist 1986) is produced when thermal stress (e.g., maternal fever) is encountered. This response is characterized by a decrease in normal cellular protein and RNA synthesis, and increased levels of production of heat shock proteins (HSPs). Heat Shock Proteins (HSPs) are a type of protein induced in response to infection, toxins and cytokine activation (Bates, Hawkins, Mahadik and McGrath 1996). Generally adaptive, heat shock proteins function to increase resistance to thermal stress at the cellular level (Lindquist 1986). Heat Shock Proteins also produce a variety of cellular effects which inhibit cellular growth, development and metabolism. Further, they cause a cessation of cell division and a reduction in mitochondrial activity (Petersen 1990). If any of the above noted cellular effects occurs during a critical stage of prenatal development, then important formative neurological processes may be disrupted.

Conclusion

The study of prenatal infection in relation to later psychological and behavioral outcomes has evolved from a focus on physical teratogenesis to behavioral teratogenesis. Given the latency with which many psychological and behavioral outcomes occur, there are many potential confounds to this research and many possible moderating relationships. Further, the current literature is hampered by inconsistent reports of adverse behavioral outcomes. Even in well-researched areas such as influenza-schizophrenia, there are studies which have not found an association. Finally, the precise mechanism of teratogenesis is difficult to uncover. With many infections it is unclear whether putative effect is the result of direct infection of the fetus or through some aspect of the immune response to the infectious agent. The immune response has many aspects. Potential mechanisms reviewed here include the cytokine response, hyperthermia due to fever, an autoimmune response or the heat shock response.

Chapter 6
Maternal Chronic Illness

There are a number of maternal conditions or diseases that place pregnancies and offspring at risk of mortality or morbidity. The United States government, through the Center for Disease Control, collects data on a selected number of these characteristics. Table 6.1 presents this listing and the rates of some of the most important maternal risk factors.

Data in Table 6.1 indicate that of those risk factors that are specifically tracked, anemia (low levels of iron in the blood), diabetes mellitus and risks related to hypertension have the highest rates of occurrence. These risk factors occur at a rate of more than 10 per 1,000, or in more than 1 percent of pregnancies ending in live births. The rates would be higher if calculated for pregnancies as opposed to live births, because it is known that many of these conditions increase risks of spontaneous abortions and stillbirth. There many other medical risks factors that do not occur at sufficient rates to be individually tracked. Categorized as Other Medical Risks, this group accounts for a larger rate of medical risks than all the individually tracked conditions combined.

One of the most striking aspects of the data in Table 6.1 is that the rate of most of the risks factors increased between 1992 and 2002. Further, the greatest increases have been in some of the maternal diseases that affect the largest number of pregnancies. For example, anemia has increased from 18.6 to 26.4 per 1,000 live births, and pregnancy-associated hypertension has increased from 29.3 to 39.3 per 1,000. Some of the risk factors listed have increased more than 30 percent during this 10-year period. Risks due to anemia will be discussed in Chapter 7, and risks due to genital herpes has been alluded to in Chapter 5. This chapter will focus on diabetes, hypertension and lung disease, as well as the role that obesity plays in many of these diseases.

Maternal Diabetes Mellitus

Diabetes Mellitus is a metabolic disease in which the pancreas does not produce sufficient insulin to combat the rise in glucose. The function of insulin is to facilitate the uptake of glucose into tissues. It can also occur when cells stop responding

R.P. Martin and S.C. Dombrowski, *Prenatal Exposures: Psychological and Educational Consequences for Children.*
© Springer 2008

Table 6.1 Medical Risk Factors of Mothers Per 1,000 Live Births: 1992, 2002

Risk Factor	1992		2002	
	Cases	Rate	Cases	Rate
Abruptio Placentae	23,075	5.9	21,409	5.4
Anemia	71,978	18.6	102,788	26.4
Cardiac Disease	15,551	3.9	20,308	5.1
Diabetes	102,285	26.6	131,027	33.9
Herpes, Genital	28,753	8.3	33,644	9.4
Hydramnios/Oligohydramnios	29,881	7.9	55,590	14.1
Hemoglobinopathy	2,161	0.6	3,150	0.8
Hypertension, Chronic	25,972	6.6	33,442	8.4
Pregnancy-Associated	112,467	29.3	150,854	39.3
Eclampsia	14,380	3.6	12,920	3.2
Incompetent Cervix	8,520	2.2	11,703	2.9
Lung Disease	16,596	4.2	49,263	12.5
Previous Preterm or SGA Infant	45,153	12.4	49,934	12.7
Renal Disease	8,936	2.3	12,185	3.1
Rh Sensitization	24,842	6.4	26,648	6.8
Uterine Bleeding	29,171	8.0	24,137	6.1
Other Medical Risks	458,652	131.6	765,468	237.1

to insulin resulting in an inability of cells to appropriately absorb glucose (American Diabetic Association [ADA] 2004).

Four types of diabetes are most prevalent. Type-1 diabetes, also known as insulin-dependent or juvenile diabetes, results from failure to produce a sufficient amount of insulin. Type-1 diabetes is an autoimmune disease in which the beta cell islets of the pancreas that produce insulin are destroyed by the immune processes of the body. There is a strong genetic component for this immune response, although environmental factors can play a role. It is typically diagnosed early in life. Type-2 diabetes, also known as non-insulin dependent diabetes, results from insulin resistance, a condition in which the body does not utilize insulin correctly. This insulin resistance is often combined with relative insulin deficiency. Risk factors for type-2 diabetes include age (older persons have a higher risk), obesity, physical inactivity and a family history of diabetes. A third type of diabetes is known as gestational diabetes. This type of diabetes occurs in pregnant women in whom the onset of diabetes or impaired glucose tolerance occurs during pregnancy. The predisposing factors are much the same as in the case of type-2 diabetes, although age does not play a major role. Finally, there is a prevalent condition known as prediabetes, in which a person's blood glucose levels are higher than normal, but not sufficiently high to signify type-2 diabetes (ADA 2004).

According to the ADA approximately 6 percent of the population has diagnosed diabetes. Of the 18 percent of the United States population with the disease, approximately 13 million have diagnosed type-1 or -2 diabetes. Of these, type-2 diabetes is the most common. There is an approximate 10 to 1 ratio of type-2 to type-1 diabetes (National Center for Chronic Disease Prevention and Health

Promotion of the Centers for Disease Control [CDC] 2005). Further, the prevalence rate of type-2 diabetes is probably significantly greater than the number of diagnosed cases. Some authorities suggest that perhaps only half of the cases of type-2 diabetes are diagnosed (Hampton 2004).

There are large ethnic differences with regard to the total prevalence of diabetes. Hispanic-Americans are given the diagnosis at a rate that is 1.5 times that of the non-Hispanic white population. African-Americans are diagnosed with diabetes at approximately 1.6 times the rate of non-Hispanic whites (ADA 2004).

Gestational diabetes occurs in 2 percent to 5 percent of all pregnancies. It is diagnosed in some women who probably have had diabetes prior to pregnancy, but have not received the diagnosis. For example, 5 percent to 10 percent of women with gestational diabetes are found to have type-2 diabetes after pregnancy, some of whom are believed to have been diabetic prior to pregnancy. Further, gestational diabetes seems to occur in women who have a predisposition toward the disease. Women who have had gestational diabetes have a 20 percent to 50 percent chance of developing the disease during the next five to 10 years (ADA 2004). Lauenborg, et al. (2004) found that of two samples of Danish women who had gestational diabetes 10 years previously, 27 percent and 40 percent of the samples had type-2 diabetes on follow-up.

Unfortunately, type-2 diabetes is on the increase across the globe. Based on current rates and recent increases, type-2 diabetes between 2000 and 2010 is expected to increase by 23 percent in the United States, 44 percent in South American, 33 percent in Australia, 50 percent in Africa and 57 percent in Asia (Zimmet, Alberti and Shaw 2001). It is now considered to be one of the main threats to human health in the 21st Century. In addition to genetic susceptibility, environmental and behavioral factors that lead to obesity such as sedentary lifestyle and overly rich nutrition also contribute to type-2 diabetes.

The effects of maternal diabetes that is poorly controlled during pregnancy, or of gestational diabetes, range from catastrophic to negligible. At the catastrophic extreme diabetes can result in the death of the fetus. Abnormal development early in pregnancy can also result in congenital malformations with serious effects. Malformations are most common in the heart and the neural tube, with the latter affecting development of the neurological tissues and related tissues in the spine. Diabetes can also reduce the growth of the fetus early in pregnancy (Pedersen and Molstead-Pedersen 1981). The mechanism through which diabetes produces malformations and early pregnancy growth retardation is not well understood. Studies in animals have shown that malformations can be reduced by injection of antioxidants (Al Ghafli, Padmanadhan, Kataya and Berg 2004). This kind of result points toward an overabundance of reactive oxygen species in mothers with diabetes.

On the other hand, the most common result of maternal diabetes on the fetus is a condition known as fetal macrosomia (unusually large fetuses). Diabetes results in an overabundance of glucose (e.g., hyperglycemia) which alters fetal insulin production and the action of the fetal insulin (Aerts, Pinjnenborg, Verhaeghe, Holemans and Assche 1996). As a result, during the last trimester the fetus abnormally gains weight. Unfortunately, fetal macrosomia can also predispose developing children to obesity, by increasing their risk of type-2 diabetes. These children are also susceptible to giving birth to their own diabetes-prone child (Hampton 2004).

Abnormally large fetuses are at risk for a variety of reasons. First, there may be difficulties in vaginal delivery related to asphyxia, subdural hemorrhage (hemorrhage within the brain), facial palsy and fracture of the clavical. However, modern fetal diagnostic tools typically can detect fetal macrosomia. When detected, the fetus is delivered via caesarian section, reducing these risks. However, biochemical abnormalities can occur in conjunction with macrosomia. One of these is that there is reduced production of surfactant in the lungs, a chemical that is necessary for the transport of oxygen into lung tissues from the inhaled air. This can result in respiratory distress syndrome, especially if the infant is delivered prematurely (see Chapter 4). Further, the infants of diabetic mothers are at higher risk of jaundice due to increased levels of bilirubin as a result of liver immaturity. Interestingly, the brain tissues of macrosomic fetuses seem to be unaffected by the disease. This results from uptake of glucose in brain cells that seems to be independent of insulin (Barrett 1987).

The most common biochemical abnormality afflicting infants of diabetic mothers is hypoglycemia (low levels of circulating glucose in the blood), affecting approximately 50 percent of infants of mothers whose diabetes was not or could not be controlled (Barrett 1987). Because the high levels of glucose available from the mother are stopped at the time of delivery, the infant can become hypoglycemic within the first few hours after birth.

It is instructive to determine the incidence rates of pregnancy complications and neonatal complications for each type of maternal diabetes. With regard to the most common form of maternal diabetes (type-2), a study carried out in Birmingham (England) is instructive. Dunne, Brydon, Smith and Gee (2003) studied 182 women with type-2 diabetes who delivered their babies between 1990 and 2002. Twelve percent of the pregnancies resulted in spontaneous abortions or stillbirths. An additional 2.7 percent of the births died within the first year of life. Twenty-eight percent of the babies were macrosomic. Congenital malformations occurred in 9.9 percent of the births. Fifty-three percent were delivered by caesarean section and 37 percent required admission to neonatal intensive care units. With regard to pregnancy complications for the mother, hypertension/pre-eclampsia was twice as common, polyhydramnios three times and postpartum hemorrhage six times more common than among non-diabetic women.

Women with gestational diabetes also tend to have higher rates of preterm births. Svare, Hansen and Molsted-Pedersen (2001) studied 327 women with gestational diabetes and 295 non-diabetic women. They found that gestational age was significantly lower for those with gestational diabetes, even when controls were instituted for induced deliveries.

Women who have type-1 diabetes have particularly complicated pregnancies. Evers, de Valk and Visser (2004) studied 323 women with type-1 diabetes who became pregnant between April 1999 and April 2000 in the Netherlands. Despite good control of blood sugar prior and during pregnancy, the rates of pregnancy complications were very high. For example, pre-eclampsia occurred in 12.7 percent of the sample, preterm delivery in 32.2 percent, caesarean section delivery in 44.3

percent and maternal mortality in 0.6 percent. Affects on the infants were also noted. These included 8.8 percent with congenital malformations, 2.8 percent with prenatal mortality and 45.1 percent with macrosomia. Of all infants delivered, 80.2 percent had some form of neonatal complication.

This brief review of the effects of maternal diabetes on mother and fetus reveals that diabetes, in all its forms, is associated with a substantial increase for abnormal pregnancies and abnormal outcomes. There is little direct evidence that maternal diabetes during pregnancy predisposes the child to learning and behavior problems. There are no long-term studies showing direct effects of maternal diabetes on child and adolescent behavior. However, diabetes is associated with prenatal and perinatal complications that are associated with long-term affects. These include preterm delivery and a variety of malformations that are known to result in learning and behavior problems (some neural tube anomalies).

Maternal Obesity

Women who are overweight or obese have many complications of pregnancy and delivery that can adversely affect fetal and newborn health, as well as long-term developmental outcomes. This is a problem of national consequence since an increasing number of women in the reproductive period are overweight or obese. An estimated 22 percent of nonpregnant women aged 18 to 49 in the United States are considered overweight, and an additional 22 percent are considered obese (Cogswell, Perry, Schieve and Dietz 2001). Overweight is typically determined in the medical research context by the use of the body mass index (BMI). It is calculated by dividing the body weight (in kilograms) by the woman's height (in meters) squared. A BMI of 19.8 to 26 is considered normal, while 26.1 to 29 is considered overweight, and over 29 is thought of as an index of obesity.

Obesity increases the chances of gestational diabetes, pregnancy-associated hypertension and preeclampsia, all of which have the potential for long-term negative effects on the child. For example, hypertension raises the risk of intrauterine growth retardation. Preeclampsia is a very dangerous complication to the mother and fetus that produces a combination of high blood pressure, swelling and protein in the urine of the mother. Untreated, it can cause the death of the mother and the unborn child. The only cure when preeclampsia develops is delivery of the baby. This often results in a premature delivery.

Problems of overweight or obese mothers can occur at the time of birth. Vahratian, Zhang, Troendle, Savitz and Siega-Riz (2004) have shown that these mothers often progress through labor more slowly than women with normal weight. Specifically, the time it took for the woman's cervix to dilate from four to 10 centimeters was used as the index of labor progression in this study. For obese women the median labor length was 7.9 hours, while for women of normal weight, median labor was 6.2 hours. The increased length of labor is often caused by babies that are too large to pass easily through the birth canal. Because of this longer labor there is increased risk to the infant, and obstetricians find themselves in the difficult position of deciding whether or not to reduce labor stress to the infant through a caesarian section delivery.

Weight gain during pregnancy is also a matter of considerable concern during pregnancy. There was a period when physicians recommended that women gain only 24 pounds during the nine months of pregnancy. However, some women seemed to overreact to this recommendation and reduced their food intake to the level that there was damage to the fetus. Many obstetricians now view weight gained in the range of 35 to 40 pounds as being within acceptable limits (Brody 2004). If an overweight woman is already pregnant, a weight loss program is not recommended. Thus, weight gain is calculated based on pre-pregnancy weight. However, weight gain recommendations are different for women who begin pregnancy at a normal weight than for those who begin pregnancy overweight. For example, the Institute of Medicine of the National Academy of Sciences recommends a gain of 25 to 35 pounds for women of normal weight, but not more than 15 pounds for women who are obese at the time of conception.

One of the most serious consequences of obesity on offspring is the increased risk of neural tube defects, including spina bifida (Hampton 2004). Anderson, Kim, Canfield, Shaw, Watkins and Werler (2005) investigated the link between obesity and nervous system birth defects, controlling for such factors as race, ethnicity, education level, alcohol use and periconceptional vitamin use. Also the presence of gestational diabetes was assessed. They found that obese women had increased risks of delivering offspring with anencephaly, spina bifida and hydrocephaly. The odds of these outcomes were higher if the mother was both obese and had gestational diabetes. The mechanism linking obesity to these congenital defects remains unclear.

This line of research makes it clear that obesity during pregnancy substantially increases the risk of central nervous system difficulties in offspring and, thus, can be linked directly to long-term behavior and learning problems of children. Further, research indicating that obesity increases the risks of prolonged and complicated deliveries raises concerns for long-term effects. Finally, obesity is related to type-2 and gestational diabetes, and to maternal hypertension. Given that there is a worldwide increase in obesity among women of childbearing age, increased risks to children are of considerable concern.

Circulatory Diseases Occurring During Pregnancy

Maternal Hypertension

Hypertension during pregnancy has been categorized into four different types: preeclampsia/eclampsia, gestational hypertension, the continued presence of chronic hypertension and the superimposition of preeclampsia on chronic hypertension.

In 2003 Roberts, Pearson, Cutler and Lindheimer summarized the results of a conference of the Heart, Lung and Blood Institute (NHLBI) of the National Institutes of Health in which the definitions of each of these types of hypertension in pregnancy were further delineated, and the epidemiological characteristics, pathophysiology and risks to the baby were described. Here we summarize this discussion with additional research findings also presented.

Preeclampsia is a pregnancy-specific syndrome that occurs after the midpoint of gestation. It is defined by the appearance of hypertention (systolic blood pressure of >= 140 mm Hg diastolic blood pressure of >= 90 mm Hg). It is accompanied by the onset of proteinuria (protein in the urine), usually albumin. The presence of albumin in the urine often indicates some level of kidney malfunction that can be brought on by hypertension. The definition of preeclampsia traditionally included the presence of edema (swelling due to poor circulation of bodily fluids) as a necessary condition, but this is not presently used as an indication of preeclampsia. The change was made because a portion of women have all the symptoms of preeclampsia without any indication of edema. Eclampsia occurs when preeclampsia progresses to a state in which the woman experiences life-threatening convulsions. Eclampsia usually occurs in the second half of gestation, but is most common at the time of delivery. One-third of eclampsias occur within 48 hours of delivery.

Gestational hypertension is defined by the appearance of hypertension in pregnant women who did not have clinical levels of hypertension before pregnancy. It is distinguished from preeclampsia by the absence of proteinuria. Typically the increases in blood pressure produce little harm to the mother, and blood pressure levels return to normal after pregnancy. It affects about 10 percent of pregnancies (Robillard and Hulsey 1994).

Chronic hypertension refers to high blood pressure that predates pregnancy. In these cases there is an increased risk of preeclampsia (occurs in about 25 percent of women with chronic hypertension). The outcomes for mother and baby in cases of preeclampsia occurring in the presence of chronic hypertension are worse than in cases of preeclampsia without hypertention prior to pregnancy.

Preeclampsia is the type of hypertension of most concern for offspring development. It occurs primarily in first pregnancies, but is also more common in women at the end of their childbearing years (Roberts 1998). The causes are unknown, but an immunological or infection-related etiology has been given some support. For example, Robillard and Hulsey (1994), and Li and Wi (2000) found that a change in sexual partners increased the risk of preeclampsia. Robillard and Hulsey found that in a sample of 1,011 women who had delivered babies in a five-month period, 11.9 percent of first-time mothers had pregnancy-induced hypertension. The rate for same paternity mothers with previous children was 4.7 percent, but for mothers with previous children who had a new sexual partner it was 24.0 percent.

Prior births or abortions confer a strong protective effect against preeclampsia. Saftlas, et al. (2003) examined whether nulliparous women with a prior abortion history who change partners also lose the protective effect of the prior pregnancy. They found that women with a history of abortion who conceived again with the same partner had nearly half the risk of preeclampsia as women who had no history of abortion. Further, women with no history of abortion who conceived with a new partner had the same risk of preeclampsia as women without a history of abortion. Thus, both prior pregnancies and exposure to the same sexual partner reduced the risk of preeclampsia. Interestingly, contraceptives that create a barrier between the seminal fluid of the father and the mother (condoms, diaphragms, spermicides) also create a higher risk of preeclampsia (Klonoff-Cohen, Havitz, Cefalo and McCann 1989).

Taken together, this and related evidence is interpreted by Roberts, et al. (2003) and others (Saftlas, et al. 2003) as an indication that immunological processes play a central role in preeclampsia. Apparently preeclampsia is the consequence of immunological intolerance between maternal and fetal tissues. This intolerance is lessened if the mother is exposed to the father's sperm, or has prolonged exposure to fetal antigens from a previous pregnancy.

Roberts, et al. (2003) provide a brief review of the evidence discussing preeclampsia's sizeable heritability. Daughters of preeclamptic women have more preeclampsia than daughters of mothers with no history of preeclampsia. Perhaps more interestingly, preeclampsia is more common in pregnancies fathered by sons of preeclamptic women.

In addition to genetic factors, a review of the pathophysiology of preeclampsia reveals that the placenta plays a central role in precipitating the symptoms associated with the disorder. This is due to a reduction of blood flow in the placenta. Roberts, et al. (2003) review a good deal of evidence showing that the chemical signals that guide the implantation of the placenta in the uterine wall do not perform properly in cases of preeclampsia. One of the primary errors that occur is that the spiral arteries that perfuse the placenta do not undergo the changes that occur in normal pregnancies. The arteries typically go from small muscular arteries to larger arteries, and the internal structures of the arteries also change. In cases of preeclampsia, these changes do not occur.

Hypertension and diabetes increase the risk of this kind of failure of arteries of the placenta and increase the risk of preeclampsia. In some cases the placental arteries give the appearance of rejected foreign tissue that occurs in transplant surgery. In support of prior findings implicating the immune system, the placental problems of preeclampsic women seem to indicate that the immune system inhibits the arterial adjustments that must be made for the placenta to be properly perfused. One theory is that the immune system particularly attacks endothelial cells of the arteries and other organs. The kidneys are often affected with hypertrophy (enlargement) of endothelial cells in offspring of preeclampsic women.

The risks to the fetus from maternal preeclampsia are well-known. In some cases the effects are profound, including growth retardation, hypoxia, preterm birth and death (Ananth, Peedicayil and Savitz 1995). The risks to the fetus are greatest for women who have severe preeclampsia, who do not have appropriate medical care and for those fetuses in which the preeclampsia episode occurred prior to 34 weeks gestation (Sibai 2006).

The less catastrophic outcomes of preeclampsia seem to be linked to the association with reduced vascular perfusion of the placenta. This relationship, however, is complex and not well understood. Preeclampsia is linked to preterm birth and small-for-gestational-age births. These perinatal conditions are known to have adverse effects on the long-term development of the child (see Chapter 3). However, a reduced blood flow in the placenta would be expected to greatly increase the risk of intrauterine growth restriction (IUGR). Only a small percentage of offspring of preeclampsic mothers have babies with IUGR. Further, the mothers of many IUGR babies did not experience preeclampsia. On the other hand, the failure to remodel blood vessels (arteries) to support vascular perfusion of the placenta that occurs in preeclampsia is observed in one-third of the pregnancies ending in spontaneous preterm birth (Roberts, et al. 2003).

In summary, severe and untreated preeclampsia is known to have significant long-term effects on offspring. These effects are so well understood that there is little need for further research. However, the consequences of more moderate preeclampsic episodes of pregnant women are less clear. Further, the mechanisms by which preeclampsia produces long-term neurological effects are not well understood. Failures in vascular placental perfusion seem to be one of the pathways to fetal developmental anomalies.

Maternal Heart Disease

Approximately 1 percent of all pregnancies are affected by heart disease of the mother (Thilen and Olsson 1997). Heart disease is of particular concern to obstetricians and specialized pediatricians who monitor the progress of fetal growth throughout pregnancy. This concern is based on the central role played by the circulating blood levels in fetal growth and development. This concern is also based on the circulatory challenges of pregnancy. These challenges include increased blood volume, increased red cell mass and increased heart rate. Due to these factors, cardiac output during pregnancy increases by 30 to 50 percent. This is achieved through increases in stroke volume and heart rate. Stroke volume increases until the second trimester, then remains constant until term (Lupton, Oteng-Ntim, Ayida and Steer 2002; Siu and Coleman 2001; Thilen and Olsson 1997). Heart rate continuously increases to 15 to 30 percent above pre-pregnant levels during pregnancy (Thilen and Olsson 1997). Despite these changes in blood volume, heart rate and stroke volume, there is a small decrease in vascular resistance during pregnancy due to the incorporation of low resistant circulation of the placenta. This small fall in blood pressure reaches its lowest point at the end of the second trimester (Thilen and Olsson 1997). In cases of twins the increase in heart rate and stroke volume is further increased. At the time of delivery, contractions further increase cardiac output, sometimes by 60 percent (Thilen and Olsson 1997).

Historically, most cardiac problems in women of childbearing age were the result of congenital malformations due to effects of rheumatic fever. Following the introduction of penicillin, the rate of congenital malformations decreased from approximately 3 percent to 1 percent of pregnant women. Many female infants and children who had other forms of congenital heart defects perished prior to their reproductive years. During the past 20 years a much higher percentage of these women survive to participate in reproduction, and thus the rate of heart disease in pregnancy has not continued to fall. In fact there is some indication of modest increases (Lupton et al. 2002). Thus, the prevalence of heart disease in pregnant women is sufficiently high to cause concern for both the welfare of the mother and the development of offspring.

Siu et al. (2001) point out that much of the available research evidence on the effects of heart disease come from old, small sample studies, with most information obtained from retrospective reports. Recently, these researchers as part of the Cardiac Disease in Pregnancy investigation team, studied 596 consecutive pregnancies of 532 women with heart disease in 13 Canadian hospitals. The pregnancies of 23 women were terminated due to life-threatening heart disease. Of the remaining women, the principle cardiac problems were congenital malformations (455 pregnancies), acquired lesions (127 pregnancies) and arrhythimia (27 pregnancies). A primary cardiac event (a clinically significant change in heart functioning requiring medical intervention) occurred in 80 of the pregnancies. In almost all cases this was due to pulmonary adema (access fluid in the lungs caused by cardiac insufficiency) or arrhythmia. Strokes occurred in four pregnancies due to embolisms (obstruction of a blood vessel due to a blood clot or other foreign object). In 37 pregnancies secondary cardiac events occurred that worsened the cardiac functioning of the mother. Pregnancy-initiated hypertension complicated 4 percent of the pregnancies.

With regard to outcomes for the fetus, 105 pregnancies (18 percent) resulted in preterm births, a rate that is much higher than in the general population in Canada. In 22 pregnancies the fetus was small-for-gestational-age (3.7 percent). About 1 percent of the fetuses died prior to birth, and 1 percent died within the first three months of life. Among the 432 women with congenital heart disease, 7 percent had infants with congenital heart disease (Siu, Sermer et al. 2001).

There is some evidence that heart defects of pregnant women that involve diseases of the valves of the heart (e.g., mitral stenosis) are particular troubling. With regard to the effect on the fetus, Hameed, et al. (2001) found that valvular disease resulted in increased preterm deliveries, intrauterine growth retardation and reduced birth weight. These negative outcomes were observed mostly for women who had moderate to severe mitral stenosis and aortic stenosis.

In summary, heart disease affects about 1 percent of all pregnant women. Because of the central role played by the cardiovascular system in fetal development, there is great concern by attending physicians in the welfare of the fetus of women with heart disease. Data collected over the past three decades makes it clear that moderate to severe heart disease is associated with increased risks of preterm deliveries, IUGR and low birth weight. It is also associated with increased rates of heart disease of offspring. While there have been no long-term follow-up studies of the developmental outcomes of these offspring during childhood and adolescents, the literature on IUGR, preterm deliveries and low birth weight provide a clear pathway from maternal heart disease to developmental problems during childhood.

Pulmonary Diseases: Asthma

Asthma is a chronic disease of the lungs which in characterized by recurring episodes of breathing problems, including coughing, wheezing, chest tightness and shortness of breath. There is no cure, but progress has been made in controlling the symptoms.

There is considerable evidence that the rates of asthma are increasing in all western affluent countries (von Mutius 2001). Peat, Gray, Mellis, Leeder and Woolcock (1994) reported that in one state in Australia (New South Wales), there was a near doubling of prevalence of wheeze and airway hyper-responsiveness in children between 1982 and 1992. Similar data have been reported in the United States. The Epidemiology and Statistical Unit of the CDC (2001) reported that, for persons less than 18 years of age, the attack prevalence rate per 1,000 persons in 1982 was 40.1; in 1996 the prevalence rate was 74.9 per 1,000. For persons between 18 and 44 the rate in 1982 was 29.0 and in 1996 was 56.9. Trends are less clear when hospitalization discharge records are used, but the body of evidence indicates an increase in asthma in children and young adults. The prevalence rates for adults in industrialized countries are in the range of 5 to 6 percent of the population (Peat, et al. 1994).

Asthma is strongly associated with gender; it is more prevalent in women, and the rate of increases in prevalence is higher in women than in men. For example, the CDC (2001) reports that the increase in death from 1979 to 1998 from asthma was from .9 to 1.2 per 100,000 (a 33 percent increase), but for women this increase was from .9 to 1.5 per 100,000, a 67 percent increase. Asthma is also related to ethnic/race and socioeconomic status. The death rate due to asthma for the black population is more than three times the death rate for the white population. Deaths due to asthma are rare (3.7 per 100,000 for blacks, 1.1 per 100,000 for whites), but death rates provide one indication of the relative prevalence of the disease in various subgroups in the population. Death rates are also age-related and are highest in the elderly.

About 6 percent of women of childbearing age suffer from asthma (Dombrowski, et al. 2004). Women who have asthma and are pregnant have been found to have increased incidence of hyperemisis gravidarum (e.g., extreme pregnancy-related nausea), vaginal bleeding, pregnancy-induced hypertension, toxemia (e.g., generalized infections in which poisonous production of bacterial infection are transmitted throughout the body in the circulating blood supply), preeclampsia, instrument deliveries, cesarean section deliveries and gestional diabetes (Kallen, Rydhstroem and Aberg 2000; Mineribi-Codish, Fraser, Avnun, Glezerman and Heimer 1998; Perlow, Montgomery, Morgan, Towers and Porto 1992). With regard to neonatal outcomes, asthma during pregnancy has been associated in some studies with increased incidence of hypoxia, perinatal and neonatal death, preterm delivery, low birth weight and intrauterine growth retardation (Kallen, et al. 2000; Minerbi-Codish, et al. 1998).

The good news for mothers with asthma is that these negative outcomes are rare if asthma is controlled during pregnancy. Dombrowski, et al. (2004) conducted one of the largest and best controlled studies of the perinatal effects of maternal asthma during pregnancy. They collected data from 16 university hospital centers resulting in 881 nonasthmatic controls, 873 patients with mild asthma, 814 with moderate asthma and 52 with asthma that was classified as severe. In comparisons of neonatal and maternal outcomes of the asthmatic groups with controls, it was determined there were two primary adverse outcomes. There were more cesarean deliveries among the moderate and severe asthma groups. Also, the mild asthma group had neonates with a higher rate of sepsis (a generalized infection). The connection between asthma and neonatal infections has been established in other studies (Minerbi-Codish, et al. 1998).

Two main potential mechanisms have been hypothesized to explain the findings that asthma is associated with perinatal difficulties of mothers and neonates. The first implicates a lack of appropriate asthma control during pregnancy which then leads to fetal hypoxia during critical stages of development. The second hypothesis is that the medications used to manage asthma in pregnant women damage the fetus. In an attempt to address these issues Schatz, et al. (2004) studied the effects of asthma medications on perinatal outcomes of pregnancy. This large sample (n = 2,123) analysis of medical charts of pregnancies of women with asthma revealed that of the four types of medications most often used to control maternal asthma, negative affects were found for only one. Specifically, no significant relationship was found between use of inhaled beta-agonists (n = 1828), inhaled corticosteroids (n = 722) or theophyline (n = 273) and negative outcomes. However, even after adjusting the data for demographic and asthma severity covariates, oral corticosteroid use was found to be associated with both preterm birth (< 37 weeks) and low birth weight (< 2,500 grams). Similar results were reported by Bracken, et al. (2003).

Summary and Conclusions

Medical conditions of the mother constitute a risk of about 5 percent of all pregnancies. Maternal diabetes, obesity, maternal heart disease and maternal pulmonary disease are among the most common maternal illnesses that have been linked to adverse outcomes for the fetus. Diabetes presents problems for the fetus primarily at the time of delivery, particularly when the disease produces macrosomic infants. However, at lower levels it is associated with a wide range of congenital malformation and complications. Maternal heart disease and pulmonary disease place the infant at risk of hypoxia/anoxia, IUGR and preterm birth, in addition to a range of other factors. Maternal obesity is associated with all of these risks, particularly diabetes, and thus is associated with many of the negative outcomes associated with these other maternal diseases. These relatively common maternal diseases are of particular concern to public health officials and others because the rates of diabetes, obesity and maternal pulmonary disease are increasing among women of childbearing age.

Chapter 7
Nutrition

Our bodies are, for the most part, a direct reflection of what we eat and how our genetic makeup sets up physiological processes to utilize what we eat. Therefore, it is not surprising that the construction of the body of the fetus is strongly influenced by what food the mother ingests. The fetus can utilize food stuffs carried by the mother in the form of fat, and can obtain some minerals, such as calcium, from other stored resources that the mother has retained in her body. However, how much and what the mother eats plays a critical role in the development of her baby.

Poor nutrition is known to have a significant impact on the development of the CNS of the fetus. Nutritional inadequacies that are of physiological significance can affect brain development in the prenatal period through effects on neuroanatomy, neurochemistry, or both. The structural effects are primarily due to the influence of nutrients on cell division and growth (Rao and Georgieff 2000). These effects could result in fewer neurons being developed. It could also result in adverse effects on non-neuronal supporting structures in the brain, such as oligodendrocytes that play a critical role in the myelination of neurons. Without appropriate myelination, nerve conductance is slowed and cognitive performance is hampered. The effects of nutritional inadequacies on the neurochemistry of the brain are most easily seen in effects on neurotransmitters. This effect can be through the alteration of levels of neurotransmitters, on the release and uptake of the neurotransmitters or on the sensitivity of the receptors.

Nutritional changes, like many other perturbations of fetal development, vary in their effect based on the timing of change. In research with rats it is known that iron deficiency around the time of birth results in smaller brain size (Rao, et al. 1999), and permanent negative effects on learning and behavior (Felt and Lozoff 1996). However, iron deficiency occurring after the rat pup has been weaned has minimal effects (Chen, Conner and Beard 1995).

An additional factor that is observed throughout the nutritional literature is that a nutrient can negatively affect brain development by being in short supply or by being overabundant. Stated another way, many nutrients are regulated within narrow therapeutic ranges (Rao and Georgieff 2000). For example, Vitamin A is a nutritional component that is necessary in normal brain development. However, if this component is ingested or absorbed through the skin by pregnant women in high levels, it is associated with microcephaly and mental retardation (Willhite, Hill and Irving 1986).

Inadequate nutrition can be general, or it can be specific to one or more nutrient compounds. Our review of the effects of nutrition during pregnancy on child outcomes will begin with a discussion of general nutritional deficiencies and then consider a number of specific nutrients that have been linked to poor child outcomes.

Protein-Energy Malnutrition

Generalized malnutrition in the form of insufficient food supply is the most common and most studied form of nutritional perturbation during fetal development. Referred to more accurately as protein-energy malnutrition (PEM), this condition is most often observed in those human populations that are economically disadvantaged. It is also observed in populations in periods of extreme distress due to famine that results from war or natural disasters. Research on PEM is difficult to interpret in human populations, however, since those affected are generally affected by a variety of other factors such as low education level, social isolation, mental illness, teenage pregnancy or high levels of stress.

Classic studies of famine during pregnancy have demonstrated that offspring have higher rates of neurological and psychiatric disease at some point in development. For example, Susser and Lin (1992) studied the Dutch Hunger Winter of 1944-1945. During this period the Nazis blockaded western Holland. Individuals who were conceived during this period were found to have a two-fold increase in risk of schizophrenia. Schizophrenia has a multifactor etiology; however it is now generally considered to be a neurodevelopmental disease in which environmental factors increase the morbidity risk of persons who are genetically predisposed (Cannon, Kendell, Susser and Jones 2003). Unfortunately, the interpretation of the results of the Dutch famine is clouded by the small number of subjects that were conceived during this period (famine decreases reproductive activity and fecundity), and by the presence of a variety of other stressors (war) during the period. Further, the result could be due to PEM malnutrition, to the lack of some trace element or to the presence of neurotoxins in the environment. Many Dutch citizens, for example, had to eat plants (e.g., tulip bulbs) not generally considered edible because of the lack of other food sources. It is possible that some of the food that was eaten, including tulip bulbs, contained toxins that had an adverse affect on the developing fetus.

A more recent study has investigated a Chinese famine (St Clair, et al. 2005), that was inaugurated by an abrupt change in agricultural practices instituted by the Communist Government during the period 1959-1961. The study investigated birth patterns and the risk of schizophrenia in the Wuhu region of Anhui, one of the provinces that was most affected by this famine. During the famine, birth rates per 1,000 decreased approximately 80 percent, from 28.28 in 1958 to 8.61 in 1960. Of the births that did occur during these years, the risk for developing schizophrenia in later life closely approximated that found for the Dutch study. Persons born at the height of the famine in 1960 had twice the rate of schizophrenia as those born in non-famine years. It is noteworthy that the Chinese famine did not occur during a period of extreme stress (other than the stress of the famine) and a far larger sample was available for study than in the Dutch famine.

All natural experiments like famines have a number of confounding factors that remain uncontrolled. From a research point of view, interuterine growth retardation (IUGR) due to placental insufficiency (disruption of adequate blood supply to the fetus via the placenta) is a good model for evaluating the effects of PEM on brain development and behavior (Rao and Georgieff 2000). IUGR has been found to result in structural abnormalities, as well as decreased neurotransmitter production (see Rao and Georgieff 2000 for a brief review). Cognitive impairments due to IUGR have been widely documented (Gottleib, Biasini and Bray 1988; Strauss and Dietz 1998).

One of the strongest investigations in this area has been that of Strauss and Dietz (1998). They studied 2,719 infants that were small-for-gestational-age (SGA) due to IUGR as part of the National Collaborative Perinatal Project. The development of these children was compared to that of 43,104 appropriate-for-gestational-age infants (AGA). A smaller sample (n=220) of SGA infants were also studied, compared to AGA siblings. Assessments at age 7 included the Wechsler Intelligence Scale for Children (WISC) and the Bender-Gestalt Test.

Children with IUGR had lower WISC full-scale IQs than the AGA control group (90.6 vs. 96.8), and lower scores on the Bender Gestalt Test (57.3 vs. 62.3). However, in comparison to AGA siblings, the differences were much smaller (IQ; 91.0 vs. 92.4). Only those children whose head circumference was more than two standard deviations below the mean had IQ and Bender Gestalt scores that were lower than the control AGA group and the sibling group. One criticism of this study is that the measures used were broad screening devises used to assess general cognitive and visual-motor development. It is possible that more specific measures of visual-motor integration, memory, attention, word recognition or motor coordination or strength could have produced results showing specific deficits related to IUGR.

Premature birth presents a special set of problems from the point of view of nutrition. Delivery of nutrients from the mother to the fetus is at maximal levels during the third trimester (Rao and Georgieff 2000). Infants who are born prematurely do not have access to this nutrition for some portion of the third trimester. In addition, because the premature infant's digestive and metabolic processes have not fully developed, these systems can be overwhelmed by high levels of nutritional supplementation. Often the premature infant also has a variety of other physiological challenges (e.g., infectious disease) that can further complicate obtaining appropriate nutritional levels. About one-quarter of all infants with birth weight less than 1,500 grams (all of whom are born premature) have head circumferences less than the fifth percentile (Hack, et al. 1991). Some portion of this problem may be due to prenatal nutritional insufficiency, but a sizeable portion may be due to difficulties of obtaining sufficient nutrition during the first weeks after birth.

In summary PEM is known to adversely affect cognitive and behavioral development of children. However, the extent of the damage and the specific neuropsychological functions that are affected remain unclear. PEM is primarily a problem for those at the lowest levels of the socioeconomic ladder and for those whose prenatal development occurred at a time of severe societal disintegration (as in war). PEM remains a major problem in many parts of the Third World. However, in industrialized countries, infants that were born prematurely may suffer some of the effects of PEM due to inadequacies of their digestive systems and the impact of other problems related to premature birth (e.g., pulmonary insufficiency) that impact the infant's general ability to metabolize food. These problems are particularly acute if the premature neonate does not receive specialized care.

Iron Deficiency

Iron deficiency is the most common single nutrient deficiency in the world. It occurs in less than 1 percent of pregnancies in the United States, but at much higher rates in developing countries. DeMaeyer and Adiels-Tegman (1985) estimated that iron deficiency anemia affects 20 percent to 25 percent of the world's infants. In the United States anemia is much more common in low-income and minority infants than among the middle-class (Yip, et al. 1992)

In addition to low-income minority women, several other groups of women are at high risk for iron deficiency that could adversely affect fetal development. One such group is teenage girls. National nutritional surveys suggest that approximately 10 percent of adolescent girls of childbearing age are iron deficient (Looker, Dallman, Carroll, Gunter and Johnson 1997). Low iron levels in this group are due to high levels of menstrual blood loss, and to inadequate levels of iron in the diet. There is also evidence that pregnancy during the teenage years increases the risk of iron deficiency (Groner, Holtzman, Charney and Millitts 1986).

Two other groups of women who have higher risks of iron deficiency are those with maternal diabetes mellitus or women who have hypertension. From 5 percent to 10 percent of pregnancies are complicated by maternal diabetes mellitus (see Chapter 6). More than half of the infants born to mothers with diabetes have low iron levels (approximately 150,000 infants annually; Georgieff, et al.1990). IUGR that results from maternal hypertension occurs in approximately 3 percent of pregnancies in the United States. Decreased iron levels occur in about half of the infants delivered with this complication (Rao and Georgieff 2000).

Rao and Georgieff (2000) provide a summary of findings on the cognitive effects of iron deficiency in infants. In general, infants and toddlers with iron deficiency anemia have mental development scores on the Bayley Scales that are 10 and 12 points lower than control groups (Lozoff 1990).

Lozoff and colleagues (Lozoff, et al. 1998) have described a range of behavior abnormalities among iron deficient infants. They studied the behavior of 52 Costa Rican children, ages 12 through 23 months, who had been diagnosed with iron deficiency anemia. The behavior of a similar group of children known to have better iron status was observed. Behaviors were videotaped and coded while the children were being assessed using the Bayley Scales of Infant Development. They were assessed again after three months of nutritional therapy. The toddlers with iron deficiency anemia spent more time in close contact with their mothers, showed less pleasure, were less playful, more wary or hesitant and were easily fatigued. The toddlers who were anemic also paid less attention in the assessment to instructions or demonstrations of items. It should be noted that assessments in this study and many similar studies have often been done between six and 24 months of age. Thus, the observed difficulties could be related to post natal iron deficiency.

Rao and Georgieff (2000) report that attempts to reverse cognitive impairments due to iron deficiency anemia through supplementation have generally failed. This finding is often interpreted to indicate that the effects of iron deficiency on the developing brain are specific to one time period in brain development, and that supplementation after that time period cannot alter the permanent damage that has been done. An alternative explanation is that iron deficiency is associated with a range of sociocultural factors which adversely affect cognitive performance. These factors would continue to have an effect on the child after iron supplementation.

The mechanisms for effects of severe pre- and perinatal iron deficiency are numerous. One clear effect demonstrated in animal models is a decrease in myelination. Iron is essential for lipid metabolism in the nervous system (Rao and Georgieff 2000). Myelination is a 'once and for all' process; it occurs only during specific stages of brain development. Thus, factors that disrupt myelination result in irreversible impairment. There is also evidence that iron deficiency decreases the activity of some dopamine receptors in the brain (particularly D2 receptors). This effect is thought to be responsible for some of the behavioral changes observed in iron deficient infants (see Lazoff, et al. 1998 above).

This brief review indicates that there is sufficient evidence to suspect that iron deficiency anemia during prenatal development is a significant concern for the subsequent development of the child. For this reason women in industrialized countries are prescribed iron supplementation as soon as they are known to be pregnant. The need for this supplementation is just one additional support for the importance of adequate prenatal care.

Vitamin Deficiences

Vitamin A

Vitamin A is a necessary nutritional constituent. It is particularly important for the health of skin, eyes, bones, teeth and the immune system. It also plays a role in human physiologic processes such as growth, reproduction and immunity. It is essential throughout the lifespan, but is particularly critical during periods of cell proliferation, differentiation and, in general, organogenesis. One metabolite is retinaldehyde, which plays a critical role in signal transmission to neurons of the optical nerves. A second metabolite is retinoic acid. It is a lipid-soluble hormone that controls gene expression. It is this relation to gene expression that seems to play an important role in organogenesis (Azaois-Braesco and Pascal 2000).

Vitamin A is accessible to humans in two types of food sources. The first source is through the antioxidant compound beta-carotene which is obtained from carrots, sweet potatoes, cantaloupe and green leafy vegetables. The second source is through the retinol or preformed vitamin A. Retinol is obtained in the human diet through animal products such as liver, egg yolks, cheese and milk. It is stored primarily in the liver, with smaller amounts stored in the lungs, kidneys and fat cells.

While vitamin A is necessary for human health, it was the first vitamin to be shown to have teratogenic effects if ingested at high doses. More specifically, it was shown in animal models that retinol was toxic in high doses to the developing fetus during the first trimester. Vitamin A obtained from beta-carotene (carotenoids, a vitamin A precursor) is not toxic to the fetus (Smithells 1996). Thus, some Vitamin A is healthy, while a lot is toxic. But, how much is too much?

An indirect answer to this question came from research on cosmetics. In the early 1980s it was discovered that retinol had positive effects on the skin if applied directly to the skin. Pharmaceutical and cosmetic companies began to put synthetic retinol (isotretinoin and etretinate) in skin creams and acne medications. Some of these preparations contained very high levels of these compounds. It was determined that retinol could enter the blood stream through the skin. High doses that fostered healthier skin turned out to have deleterious effects on the developing fetus if the medications were administered during the first trimester of pregnancy, particularly during the first eight weeks. When maternal intake of vitamin A exceeded 10,000 international units per day, the risks of malformations of the fetus increased significantly. Malformations included hydrocephaly, microcephaly, mental retardation, craniofacial abnormalities, cleft lip/palate and heart defects. The rate of psychiatric disorders during development also increased.

One of the foundation studies in this area was conducted by Rothman, et al. (1995). They studied birth defects of the offspring of 23,000 mothers for whom vitamin A intake prior to and during early pregnancy was known. If the intake was greater than 15,000 international units (IU) birth defects were observed in significantly greater numbers than in controls. This level of intake was associated with craniofacial abnormalities, central nervous system abnormalities and heart defects. Very few of the mothers with intakes greater than 10,000 IU obtained this level of vitamin A from food alone. Most had been exposed to synthetic vitamin A in skin preparations.

It has been determined that there is a classic dose-response relationship between vitamin A exposure during the first trimester and risk of some type of malformation. For example, simply taking too many vitamin A supplements could double the risk of malformation. Eating too much liver (more than 50 grams per week) can increase the risk of miscarriage and malformation. At the highest risk levels exposure to more than 20,000 international units of vitamin A increases the risk of miscarriage by 25 percent.

Because these dangers are well-known, women who receive adequate prenatal care are prescribed vitamin supplements with appropriate quantities of vitamin A, and are instructed to limit some foods (such as liver) during pregnancy. They are also strongly cautioned to avoid use of skin creams and acne medication that contain synthetic retinol.

At the other end of the continuum inadequate supplies of vitamin A create significant risks for the developing fetus. Ramakrishnan, Manjrekar, Rivera, Gonzales-Cossio and Martorell (1999), in an extensive review, report on a number of studies in which vitamin A status of the infant was associated with premature birth or IUGR. Most of these studies were done in the developing world with samples that included mothers and infants with clear vitamin A deficiencies. Similar studies in the United States have not found links to premature birth or IUGR, perhaps because the samples contained few women or infants with significant vitamin A deficiencies.

There is compelling evidence that levels that are too low also negatively affect the immune system of the newborn. The lowered immune status of the infant leaves them susceptible to upper respiratory infections, diarrhea and diseases such as measles. These infections can have profound effects on infants, particularly in areas of the world where adequate health care is unavailable or too expensive to be utilized by many parents. Azais-Braesco and Pascal (2000) present a persuasive case in arguing that the effects of too little vitamin A are far more wide ranging (affecting millions of infants worldwide) than are the effects of too much for which there have been less than 20 documented cases. Still, these authors strongly suggest that vitamin A intake during pregnancy should not exceed 10,000 IU per day.

Vitamin B Complex

Relatively little is known about the effects of vitamin B complex on pregnancy outcomes, particularly long-term outcomes (Ramakrishnan, et al. 1999). Thiamine (vitamin B_1) deficiency in pregnant rats has been shown to result in IUGR in the offspring. Further, thiamine deficiency could play a negative role in brain development, since enzymes that depend on the presence of thiamine are essential for the energy metabolism necessary for lipid and nucleotide synthesis in the developing brain (Butterworth 1990).

Vitamin B_6 also plays an important role in the development of the central nervous system because of its involvement with protein metabolism. Ramakrishnan and colleagues (1999) review a number of studies that show that Apgar scores of infants born to women with low dietary intake and low serum levels of vitamin B_6 were lower than those born to controls.

Folic acid is a member of the vitamin B group. It is found naturally in green plants, animal livers and yeast. It is required for the synthesis of DNA. In rapidly dividing cells, folic acid deficiency can result in chromosomal abnormalities (Ramakrishnan, et al. 1999). Since the mid 1990s there has been unimpeachable evidence that mothers who ingest inappropriately low levels of folic acid prior to and during the first trimester of pregnancy have babies that are at higher risk of neural tube defects (Smithells 1996). Neural tube defects include hair lip, cleft palate, spina bifida and a variety of other structural defects. Folic acid deficiencies are also associated with a variety of pregnancy complications such as bleeding, abruption placenta and preeclampsia, all of which are known to be related to negative outcomes for offspring (Ramakrishnan, et al. 1999).

While low levels of folic acid in the first trimester are known to cause neural tube defects, inadequate levels occurring later in pregnancy also have a variety of negative consequences for the developing fetus. These include low birth weight and preterm delivery. For example, Goldenberg, et al. (1992) studied 295 African-American women. They found that infants born to mothers in the upper two quartiles of serum folate levels assessed at 30 weeks gestation had higher birth weights and lower rates of IUGR.

In 1998 the Food and Drug Administration mandated that United States manufacturers fortify grain-based foods such as cereals and breads with folic acid. This policy initiative significantly altered the rate of neural tube defects in children, decreasing occurrence by approximately 25 percent. Unfortunately, this and related public health initiatives have not reached the majority of pregnant women. More than 3,000 children are born in the United States each year with neural tube defects (Smithells 1996). Currently, pregnant women are advised to take 0.4 mg of folic acid daily, starting before or soon after conception.

Vitamin C

In their extensive review of micronutrients and pregnancy, Ramakrishnan, et al. (1999) report that there is some evidence linking vitamin C (ascorbic acid) deficiency to premature rupture of membranes. The chorioamnion membrane gains much of its elastic strength from collagen, and free radicals can weaken the structure of collagen. Vitamin C helps control the activity of free radicals, so this may be the mechanism through which vitamin C is related to premature membrane rupture. Premature membrane rupture can negatively affect pregnancies and pregnancy outcomes through premature delivery or increased risks of infection.

Vitamin D

Vitamin D is a fat-soluble vitamin that is produced in the skin in response to solar radiation. The active form of vitamin D is technically referred to as 1,25 hydroxyvitamin D_3 (sometimes as calcitriol or cholecalciferol). Sunlight interacts with 7-dehydrocholesterol, which is hydroxylated first in the kidney and then in the liver to produce 1,25 hydroxyvitamin D3. (From this point on, vitamin D will be used to denote this compound.) Vitamin D is also obtained from some foods, including oily fish, eggs, liver, milk and margarine. Milk is the primary food in United States diets that contains vitamin D. It is typically fortified with 400 I.U. of vitamin D per quart. However, exposure to sunlight is considered the primary source of vitamin D for women, since the quantities of milk consumed by women in the United States is quite small. One survey indicates that only 4.1 percent of white women in the United States ages 18 to 44 drink sufficient milk to provide the amount of vitamin D that is recommended for adults (United States National Center for Health Statistics 1979).

Only light in the ultraviolet (UV) wavelength stimulates the synthesis of vitamin D. Within this range three types of UV light have been identified: types UVA, UVB and UVC. Of these types UVB is primarily responsible for the stimulation of vitamin D synthesis in the skin. Many studies have shown that vitamin D concentrations reach their zenith concentration in the blood in summer and the nadir in winter (Need, Morris, Horowitz and Nordin 1993; Nakamura, Nashimoto and Yamamoto 2000).

The primary function of vitamin D is to facilitate the absorption of calcium and phosphate by the intestines. Thus, during the winter months when UV exposure is low, there is a decrease in the plasma level of ionized calcium, and an increase in plasma parathyroid hormone which is a sensitive indicator of calcium levels (Cheng, et al. 2003).

Low levels of vitamin D have been frequently reported in both developed and developing countries. For example, Thomas, et al. (1998) report that 58 percent of persons admitted to general medical wards in Boston were vitamin D deficient. Due to relatively high latitude and the resulting long winter period, vitamin D deficiencies in New England, including the Boston area, should be higher than in more southern parts of the country. In a broader study of a large community-based sample of non-institutionalized adults in the United States (n = 15,778), 9 percent of the population were found to be vitamin D deficient (Looker et al. 1997).

Vitamin D binds to many proteins that are expressed in the brain. Thus, it is assumed to play a role in fetal brain development. Vitamin D receptors (VDR) are widely distributed throughout the embryonic brain, prominently in the neuroepithelium and proliferating zones. VDR is also expressed widely in the adult brain in the temporal, orbital and cingulate cortex, in the thalamus, in the accumbens nuclei, parts of the stria terminalis and amygdala, and widely throughout the olfactory system.

McGrath (2001) has recently hypothesized that low prenatal levels of vitamin D may leave the individual at risk for a number of diseases, including neurological and psychiatric disease. For pre- and perinatal vitamin D hypothesis to be viable, it would first have to be demonstrated that pregnant women are at risk of vitamin D deficiencies. There is such support. A United States survey of women aged 20 to 29 (the peak years for childbearing) reported that 12 percent had serum 1,25 hydroxyvitamin D3 levels below the generally accepted threshold for deficiency

(Looker and Gunter 1998). Further, several research teams have commented on the fact that increased needs of the fetus for vitamin D (particularly during periods of rapid bone development) place pregnant women at risk of greater levels of deficiency than would be observed in the general population. Further, the behavior of pregnant women may change in such a way as to reduce outdoor activity and, therefore, UV exposure (Hilman and Haddad 1976).

Also, if the prenatal vitamin D hypothesis is true, then exposure to solar radiation, particularly the UVB component, should be shown to be related to developmental indices that are apparent early in life. One such indicator is body size. Wohlfahrt, Melbye, Christens, Anderson and Hjalgrim (1998) demonstrated that there were seasonal variations in length and weight at birth. Waldie, Paulton, Kirk and Silva (2000) directly studied the effects of pre- and perinatal exposure to sunlight on body size at birth and at regular intervals up to age 26. They studied data on 20,021 infants born in Dunedin, New Zealand, between the first day of August 1976 and the last day of July 1978. Spectral analyses revealed that monthly means for neonate height and weight varied in a cyclical pattern at the same frequency as that for monthly variation in hours of bright sunlight. The period of greatest sunlight peaked six to nine months prior to the period of greatest body size, indicating that sunlight was most associated with birth height and weight if it occurred during the early months of pregnancy. These same researchers found that height at age 11 was significantly related to sunlight hours experienced during the prenatal period. Thus, the effect of prenatal sunshine is not only pertinent to birth weight and height, but the effect continued throughout the first 11 years of development. However, paradoxically, it was last trimester sunlight that was most related to height at age 11. At birth it was first trimester sunlight that was most influential.

Persons who get little sun exposure due to clothing customs (e.g., some Muslim women), should demonstrate high rates of vitamin D deficiency and should have a higher prevalence of the diseases outline by McGrath than other populations. A similar pattern should occur for persons with darkly pigmented skin because pigmentation slows the synthesis of vitamin D. This hypothesis has been investigated by Grover and Morley (2001). They found that 100 percent of their sample who were very dark skinned and were consistently covered (face, limbs, body) when outside the home were vitamin D deficient. Both bodily covering and pigmentation seemed to play a role. Pigmentation has been shown by other researchers to reduce serum vitamin D levels (Norman 1998; Feleke, et al.1999).

The angle of the sun as it strikes the earth greatly affects the amount of ultraviolet light that reaches the earth. That is, as the latitude gets higher (further north in the northern hemisphere or south in the southern hemisphere) the quantity of UV light that is available is reduced. If there is a relationship between UV light and, thus, vitamin D during prenatal development, there should be a higher prevalence of neuropsychiatric disease at higher latitudes. Davies, Welham, Torrey and McGrath (2000) have analyzed the available literature on seasonality of schizophrenia in the northern hemisphere. Data were included if the article indicated the prevalence of schizophrenia for persons born in the winter/spring and in the summer/fall. Data from 62,934 subjects drawn from 20 sites were available. A significant positive relationship was obtained between the size of the difference in schizo-phrenic birthrates (controlling for population birthrates) and latitude ($r = .48$).

Is there any direct evidence in animals or humans that UV exposure of women prior to and during pregnancy affects the neurological development of the fetus? The answer is that this hypothesis has only recently been advanced so there is very little published data. However, in animal models it has been observed that rat dames that were deprived of vitamin D and UVB gave birth to pups with abnormal brain development (Eyles, Brown, Mackay-Sim, McGrath and Feron 2003).

Inadequate vitamin D may directly alter fetal development through some of the mechanisms pointed out above. However, it is possible that vitamin D deficiency is one part of a multistage process in which the deficiency creates conditions under which other processes occur that may alter fetal development. One candidate for the mediating role is the effect of vitamin D on the immune system. The immune system provides a rapid response to cope with assaults from a variety of infectious agents including bacteria, viruses, fungi and parasites. One component of this system is a group of antimicrobial peptides that includes cathelicidins. In a recent study Gombart, Borregaard and Koeffler (2005) found that the active from of vitamin D induced expression of the gene that produces this peptide. A chemical precursor to this peptide is stored in neutrophils and in various white blood cell populations, including natural killer cells, monocytes and mast cells. The human cathelicidin antimicrobial peptide is synthesized and secreted by tissues that are exposed to infectious agents, including the squamous epithelia of the mouth, tongue, esopha-gus, lungs, intestine, cervix and vagina.

The finding that this important antimicrobial peptide is strongly influenced by vitamin D helps explain a variety of disparate clinical and epidemiological findings. For example, it has been found that persons with rickets (a bone disease brought about by vitamin D deficiency) suffer from an increase rate of dental abscesses and other infections (Seouw 2003). Persons with atopic dermatitis have an increased susceptibility to skin infection and have decreased levels of cathelicidin (Ong, et al. 2002). Cannell (Raloff 2006), a prison psychiatrist, reports that in a large state prison in which he worked, during a major influenza epidemic in the prison, per-sons in one wing of the facility did not report any influenza symptoms. This was the wing in which Cannell had prescribed high doses of vitamin D because the prisoners were found at an earlier date to be vitamin D deficient. Finally, the com-monly observed increase in upper respiratory infections during the winter may, in part, be a function of decreased vitamin D levels due to decreased sun exposure, which reduces activation of the genes that produce cathelicidin.

Research on vitamin D deficiencies has produced results that are provocative for considering perturbations during the prenatal period. First, infection is one of the primary causes of pregnancy complications leading to low birth weight babies, babies born prematurely and other complications (see Chapter 5). For women who are pregnant during the winter, the risk of infection may rise due to the lack of suf-ficient sunlight exposure. This would lead to the hypothesis that children born in the late winter through late spring/early summer are at greater risk of the develop-mental anomalies brought on by infection during critical periods of fetal development, particularly of neurological development. Indeed, Martin and colleagues (Martin, Clanton, Foels and Moon 2004; Polizzi, Martin and Dombrowski 2007) have shown that children receiving special education services in public schools are more likely to have been born during the spring months. Further, since African-American and other women with darkly pigmented skin have higher rates of pregnancy complications than women with lightly pigmented skin, the vitamin D/infection hypothesis may help explain some of these differences. Finally, maternal insufficiency of vitamin D during pregnancy has been linked to multiple sclerosis in their children. Viral infection is a presumed risk factor for MS, and adequate serum vitamin D levels during pregnancy appear to reduce the risk of MS. It is known, for example, that the risk of developing MS is higher for person born during the spring than for others (Willer, et al. 2005).

In summary, there is strong circumstantial evidence that prenatal vitamin D levels are related to a variety of human health outcomes, including psychiatric disease. There is also strong evidence that vitamin D deficiencies are not uncommon, even in the United States. Among women of childbearing age probably 10 percent of the population is deficient during the winter months. Further, women with darker pigmentation have higher rates of vitamin D deficiency. Finally, in animal models, vitamin D deficiencies result in abnormal brain development. For all these reasons, much more research is need on the connection between vitamin D levels in pregnant women, and the health and behavior of their offspring.

Vitamin E

There is no known literature on cognitive or behavioral effects of prenatal vitamin E intake by pregnant women. However, there are animal studies that demonstrate that vitamin E deficiency can result in neurological abnormalities (Ramakrishnan, et al. 1999). Several groups of researchers have found associations between childhood asthma and reduced intake of antioxidant vitamins (vitamins C, E and Beta-carotene) (Harik-Khan, Muller and Wise 2004; Gilliland, et al. 2003). Reduced intake of the trace elements selenium, zinc, cooper, iron, manganese and magnesium have also been associated with increases in asthma symptoms among children (Schwartz and Weiss 1990). Interestingly, some of these trace elements also have antioxidant properties. In these studies, it is unclear whether deficits in vitamin E and other antioxidants had been present since prenatal development or was the result of childhood nutritional intake.

A recent study by Devereaux, et al. (2006) attempted to clarify this issue. These researchers obtained surveys of eating habits of women during pregnancy. Further, food preference surveys about their child's eating habits were obtained from mothers when the children were five years of age. Also, symptoms related to asthma were assessed at five years and parents reported if the child had received a medical diagnosis of asthma. These researchers found that vitamin E intake during pregnancy was negatively associated with the occurrence of wheeze (the predominant symptom of asthma), and was also associated with a diagnosis of asthma. Beta-carotene and vitamin C intake during pregnancy were not related to the asthma diagnosis or symptoms. However, maternal intake of zinc during pregnancy was also associated with whether or not asthma had been diagnosed in offspring.

Summary and Conclusion

With the exception of general protein-energy malnutrition and iron deficiency, there have been very few long-term studies of the effects of vitamin or trace mineral deficiencies on academic or behavioral outcomes of children or adolescents. The vast majority of the research has been concerned with outcomes that could be observed at birth (e.g., malformations, low birth weight, premature birth). However, many of the nutrients reviewed are known to play a role in the health and development of the central nervous system. The current research activity on vitamin D is particularly provocative. Thus, there is a critical need for more long-term follow-up studies of children who were at risk during the prenatal period due to inadequate nutrition.

Chapter 8
Maternal Stress

In Act IV of King Henry VI a pregnant Queen Elizabeth, on learning of the imprisonment of her husband, says that she must stop her tears so that she doesn't damage the heir to the English crown (Shakespeare, King Henry VI, Part 3, Act IV, Scene IV). Ancient Finnish folklore provides several proverbs about the effects of maternal trauma on the temperament and behavior of the offspring. These proverbs typically indicate that when pregnant women are stressed they will give birth to a shy and frightened child. In these proverbs the offspring of stressed mothers are compared to the shy and sensitive rabbit (Huttunen, personal communication).

Based on research findings and general medical opinion, the March of Dimes recommends that stress during pregnancy should be reduced *(http://www.marchofdimes. com/professionals/681_1158.asp)*. This might be accomplished by having the mom-to-be devise a coping plan to deal with expected stresses, getting the proper amount of sleep, exercising, having a good social support network in place and practicing stress reduction techniques such as biofeedback, meditation, yoga or guided mental imagery.

On what research does the March of Dimes base this recommendation? Does ancient wisdom as represented by Shakespeare or Finnish folk wisdom hold up under the scrutiny of modern empirical and scientific methods? What is the quality of the research in this area? These are some of the questions that will be addressed in Chapter 8.

Definition

While environmental stress has a central place in psychology, it is an illusive and often vaguely defined construct. Some use the term to indicate a stimulus, others a response to the stimulus, and others the psychological consequences of that response. Most definitions mention two aspects. First, an unexpected, threatening, and/or potentially damaging environmental stimulus is experienced. Thus, we say that a gardener who stumbles upon a rattlesnake is said to experience the stressor of the snake due to the potential for bodily harm. We also say that the CEO of a corporation who might be demoted due to falling profits also is experiencing stress. In the latter case there is no threat of bodily harm, but perhaps a psychological threat of loss of status.

R.P. Martin and S.C. Dombrowski, *Prenatal Exposures: Psychological and Educational Consequences for Children.*
© Springer 2008

Second, the interpretation of the stimulus depends on characteristics of the individual experiencing the stimulus. Some people who ride a motorcycle for the first time experience the event as highly stressful, while others find the experience more pleasant than stressful.

Grant, et al. (2003) have reviewed the literature on stress and child psychopathology, and have defined stressors as "environmental events or chronic conditions that objectively threaten the physical and/or psychological health or well-being of individuals of a particular age in a particular society" (pg. 449). Lazarus and Folkman (1984) define a stressor more broadly as a circumstance that threatens a major goal, including the maintenance of one's physical integrity or one's psychological well-being. Distress is a negative psychological response to such threats and can include a variety of affective and cognitive states, such as anxiety, depression, frustration, the sense of being overwhelmed or helplessness (Kemeny 2003).

Some stress (at low levels) has a positive effect on the coping mechanisms of most people. Lederman (1995) refers to this type of stress as eustress. Like Kemeny (2003), Lederman labels severe and prolonged stress as 'distress,' and points out that it is this type of stress that has a negative effect on performance, relationships and the biological functioning of the individual.

The Psychobiology of Stress: A Brief Overview

In order to understand the research on the effects of antenatal stress on offspring behavior, it is important to understand some of the biological responses made in response to a stressor. There are two psychobiological pathways for the stress response to influence the central nervous system and the immune system (Kemeny 2003). The first is the hormonal pathway known as the Hypothalamic-Pituitary-Adrenal axis (HPA). When a stressor is perceived by the central nervous system the organism initiates a cascade of effects that involve the hypothalamus, the anterior pituitary gland, and the adrenal cortex. In response to a real or perceived stress, the hypothalamus produces corticotrophin releasing hormone (CRH), which stimulates the anterior pituitary gland. This gland, in turn, produces adrenocorticotropic hormone (ACTH) that subsequently stimulates the adrenal cortex (outer layer of cells of the adrenal gland). In turn, the adrenal gland then produces cortisol, which has a number of biological effects that prepare the individual for 'flight' or 'fight.'

At the biological level, in addition to the hormonal pathway, stress produces an effect on the autonomic nervous system (ANS) via the action of norepinephrine (a neurotransmitter) on the adrenal medulla (central portion of the adrenal gland). This gland produces epinephrine that also has a variety of effects on the body that prepare the individual for actions to limit the damage due to the perceived stressor.

Researchers who study stress reactions often assess the hormonal or neurotransmitter changes following presentation of the stressor stimulus. For example, increases in CRH, ACTH or cortisol levels in blood samples are often taken as a biological marker of the organism's response to a stressor.

The Sociology of Stress

Socioeconomic status (SES) is strongly related to stress proneness. This is true for a wide range of reasons. SES is a reflection of social position (Adler and Snibbe 2002) and is commonly assessed using measures of education, occupation or income (personal or family). Each index indicates the amount of resources an individual or family has to cope with stressors. Also, low SES can be a source of distress in itself and individuals may perceive themselves as being lower than others on some social hierarchy. This problem is exacerbated by minority social status.

Adler and Snibbe (2002) point out that when there is a decline in SES, environmental demands increase and resources for dealing with these demands decrease. Thus, across many domains of life, individuals with lower SES are exposed to a larger number of stressors than their high SES peers. Further, at any given level of the stressor, they experience a larger psychological response.

Pregnancy is a biologically, and sometimes psychologically, stressful event. Pregnant women of low SES experience a higher rate of physical problems associated with pregnancy (sometimes due to poor prenatal care), have fewer social supports for pregnancy and less education on average to help them understand all the health and social consequences of pregnancy. Further, the pregnancy may take place in an environment that exposes the woman and fetus to more levels of toxins, bacterial or viral pathogens, and noise. Low SES women may have jobs that present more physical risks. They may live in social circumstances with higher risks of crime, social conflict and crowding.

All these factors increase the likelihood of negative consequences for offspring. One of the clearest socioeconomic gradients in health is for fetal and infant mortality. That is, the lowest SES groups have a higher infant mortality than the lower-middle-class, and the lower-middle-class has a higher infant mortality than the middle-class, etc. All these effects are not attributable to specific stressors or the stress responses. However, the role of SES in increasing the stresses on pregnant women is a major theme that is clear in much of the research and thinking about prenatal stressor effects on offspring.

Prevalence of Stress or Distress Occurring During Pregnancy

The prevalence of environmental stresses during pregnancy is difficult to determine because environmental stressors are often unexpected and random (e.g., accidents). Further, the prevalence of some events can be calculated, but due to the subjective evaluative nature of perception of the event as stressful, it is difficult to know how many persons might be affected by the event.

It is somewhat easier to determine the number of pregnant women who state that they experience distress; that is, they experience adverse responses to stressors (e.g., anxiety or depression). The evidence that is available indicates that a large percentage of pregnant women describe some symptoms of distress. For example,

Jarrah-Zedeh, Kane, Van be Castle, Lachenbruch and Ewing (1969) reported that 50 percent of the average obstetric population complained of lability of mood, insomnia, increased tendency to worry, anxiety or depression. Luoma, et al. (2001) found that 11 percent of their large sample of Finnish women scored in the high range for symptoms of depression on the Edinburgh Postnatal Depression Scale (the measure was used for pre- and postnatal measurements) when assessed during the last trimester of pregnancy.

In addition to external stressors that are unrelated to pregnancy, pregnancy itself often is perceived as stressful. Rofe, Blittner and Lewin (1993) asked 282 women who had just given birth with what frequency they had experienced various symptoms during each trimester of pregnancy. They found that symptoms related to physiological changes were common during the first trimester. These included nausea, vomiting and dizziness. By the time of the third trimester anxiety and emotional distress became the most significant symptoms. These investigators also found that the experience of these symptoms was significantly related to the women's socioeconomic level, number of previous births and her personality. Across all three trimesters primiparae (first-time mothers) and women of higher socioeconomic levels reported less emotional stress than multiparae and women of lower socioeconomic status. Also, women who were characterized as repressors (versus sensitizers) reported less emotional stress. While not all researchers have found that anxiety and distress during the third trimester is typically greater than during the first or second trimester (see Lubin, Gardener and Roth 1975), the results of this research make two important points that have been often affirmed. Pregnancy is inherently stressful for many women. The experience of distress depends on a variety of other factors, including previous experience with pregnancy, general life circumstances and the personality of the mother (Carlson and LaBarba 1979; Leifer 1980; Lips 1985; Spielberger and Jacobs 1979).

Effects of Pregnancy Distress on Offspring: Introduction

During the second half of the 20th Century, a rapidly maturing psychological science began to consider the effects of maternal anxiety, depression and stress as an etiological factor contributing to behavioral, emotional and learning problems (Montagu 1962; Sontag 1941). Because distress cannot be ethically induced in pregnant women, experimental research on the effects of stress during pregnancy has been limited to animal models. Typical stressors used in this research included removal from the home cage or random noise. This research has been buttressed by a growing number of studies in which researchers studying humans looked for natural 'experiments' in which an event thought to be a stressor was studied, or pregnant women who were experiencing distress were studied. This research has often included one of the following elements: (a) an identifiable general stressor (e.g., war) on the population of which the mother was a member, (b) an identifiable group of women who were known to have experienced stressful events (e.g., death of husband) and (c) women who reported high levels of anxiety or depression during pregnancy.

Animal Studies

Schneider (1992) conducted a study of rhesus monkey infants whose mothers had been presented with a mild stressor during pregnancy. The stressor consisted of being removed from the home cage daily during pregnancy for 10 minutes and being exposed to three unpredictable noise stimuli. A matched set of infants whose mothers had not undergone this procedure were tested. It was determined that the infants whose mothers had been stressed during pregnancy had lower birth weights, were delayed in self-feeding, were more distractible and had lower motor maturity scores than those infants from undisturbed pregnancies. In a similar study Fride and Weinstock (1984) found that, for rodent offspring of dames that had been randomly stressed throughout gestation, motor development was delayed.

Clarke, Soto, Bergholz and Schneider (1996) studied the effects of maternal prenatal stress on adolescent monkey behavior during a mildly challenging condition. Removal from the home cage and presentation of short bursts of noise were used as the stressor. Offspring were removed from mothers on the day after birth to control for maternal rearing effects. Monkeys were reared in standard nursery conditions, then with a peer group. At age three or four (rhesus monkey adolescence), each animal was housed alone for three weeks, then housed in a new social group. Animals stressed during the prenatal period showed more locomotion and higher rates of abnormal and disturbed behavior than controls when housed with the new social group. Controls showed approximately six times more play than animals that experienced prenatal stress. The stressed male animals showed more clinging to others than controls. In free play situations, the control animals showed more exploratory behavior and the stressed animals showed more inactivity. Finally, in a playroom control animals decreased in their distress vocalization over time, while animals stressed during the prenatal period showed increasing levels of distress vocalization. Taken together, the results indicate that the animals whose mothers were stressed during pregnancy showed more distress in adolescence when placed in a novel situation and were less able to adapt to new social circumstances.

Schneider and colleagues (Schneider, Roughton and Lubach 1997) also provided data on the interaction of stress with another factor known to have detrimental effects on offspring development-alcohol use during pregnancy. They studied 33 rhesus monkey infants from females that had been given one of three treatments during pregnancy: (a) alcohol daily throughout gestation (equivalent to one to two drinks), (b) daily alcohol consumption, but also exposure to a mild set of psychological stresses (removal from cage and three random noise bursts) and (c) sucrose solution consumed daily that had the same volume and the same calories as the alcohol consumed in treatment 'a.' Infants from the moderate alcohol-consuming group had deficits in attention and neuromotor functioning, despite being normal in gestational length, birth weight and facial structure. These effects were exacerbated by maternal exposure to psychological stress, particularly the neuromotor impairments. Further, males from the alcohol/stress condition had lower birth weights than those from other conditions. Some of the most profound effects of the stress were observed when fetal loss was considered. Alcohol, accompanied by stress during fetal development, resulted in 23 percent fetal losses (spontaneous abortions and stillbirths), while there was no fetal loss for the group exposed only to alcohol.

This research increases understanding of the common human circumstance in which stress and other detrimental factors co-occur. The research of Schneider and colleagues seems to indicate that there is an additive or perhaps multiplicative effect of stress and other factors (e.g., maternal alcohol use) that is detrimental to fetal development.

Most research on stress posits that mild forms of stress have a positive effect on the ability of the organism to respond to stress in the future. Exercise programs are designed based on this idea. One animal study (Fujioka, et al. 2001) was found that seemed to support this idea. In this research a mild stress was applied to pregnant rats and was shown to actually enhance the ability of the offspring to learn more quickly in standard laboratory procedures.

Human Research: Effects Observed During the Prenatal Period

If maternal distress has an effect on the development of the nervous system during prenatal development, it seems likely that behavioral responses of the developing fetus to specific stressors might be observed. In fact there have been anecdotal reports from mothers for many years, in addition to single case studies, that have documented that stressful events increase the movement of the fetus (Hepper and Shahidullah 1990). Since the 1940s, a small body of research has documented that the fetus moves in utero in response to stress (Sontag 1941). In more fine-grained analyses, DiPietro, Hodgson, Costigan, Hilton and Johnson (1996a) found that maternal stress is associated with reduced fetal heart rate. This same research group also reported that fetal heart rate is associated with fetal movement (DiPietro, Hodgson, Costigan, Hilton and Johnson 1996b) beginning at 20 weeks gestation. Attempts to experimentally induce mild stress and then find increases in fetal heart rate have met with mixed results (Van den Bergh, et al. 1989).

One of the strongest studies of stress responses during the fetal period was provided by DiPietro and colleagues (DiPietro, Hilton, Hawkins, Costigan and Pressman 2002). They studied 51 mothers and their fetuses at 24, 30 and 36 weeks gestation. Women who rated themselves as more affectively intense, appraised their lives as more stressful (using the Daily Stress Inventory) during pregnancy and reported more hassles related to pregnancy. These mothers had fetuses that were more active from 24 weeks through 36 weeks gestation. Women who perceived their pregnancies to be more positive and uplifting had less active fetuses. Activity was associated with fetal heart rate at the 36 weeks assessment.

One of the most consistently reported adverse effects of maternal prenatal stress has been increased irritability or negative emotionality of offspring during the neonatal and infancy periods. In a large study Zuckerman, Bauchner, Parker and Cabral (1990) studied 1,123 mothers and their term infants (>36 weeks gestation). The mothers were most often unmarried (63 percent), had low incomes and were members of ethnic minority groups. Maternal depressive symptoms during pregnancy were measured by the Center for Epidemiologic Studies-Depression Scale during a prenatal interview (timing during gestation was not specified). Infants were evaluated by pediatricians who were unaware of the mothers' prenatal or intrapartum history using a structured neurobehavioral examination. Infant consolability was evaluated by a trained examiner during the first 15 second crying episode that was encountered during the examination. No relationship was found between maternal depression scores and the pediatric neurobehavioral examination. However, maternal depression was associated with poor consolability and excessive crying of the infants. Women at the 90th percentile on depression were 2.6 times more likely to have an unconsolable newborn than women at the 10th percentile. The findings were unchanged when the researchers controlled for smoking, alcohol, cocaine, marijuana, opiate and other drug use, poor weight gain, income and birth weight. This result is consistent with earlier research by Ottinger and Simmons (1964) who found that, two to four days postpartum, infants of high anxious mothers cried significantly more than infants of low anxious mothers.

Vaughn, Bradley, Joffe, Seifer and Barglow (1987) found that infants of high anxious mothers were perceived by their parents as having a more difficult temperament, defined primarily as negative emotionality. In addition Abrams, Field, Scafidi and Prodromidis (1995) found that newborns of depressed mothers showed more irritability and distress during the Brazelton Neonatal Assessment than newborns of non-depressed mothers. These infants also had increased levels of norepinephrine and disturbed sleep patterns, when compared to infants of non-depressed mothers. Niederhofer and Reiter (2000) reported that negative psychological circumstances during pregnancy were associated with maternal ratings of difficult infant temperament (primarily negative emotionality) at age six months. Huizink, et al. (2002, 2003) also found significant effects during the first year of life for maternal anxiety on infant temperament. Maternal anxiety at 15 to 17 weeks and 27 to 28 weeks gestation showed the strongest effect on infants' difficult temperament assessed at three months.

Among the strongest research of this type is that of Van den Bergh and colleagues. Van den Bergh, Vandenberghe, Daniels, Casaer and Marcoen (1989) found that antenatal anxiety explained 10 percent to 25 percent of the variance in behavioral states including hyperactivity, frequent crying, sleeping and feeding difficulties and difficult temperament during the first seven months of life. Associations were strongest for anxiety between 12 and 22 weeks gestation.

In addition to adverse affects on infant emotionality, some researchers have found that antenatal maternal stress relates to general development and attention. Huizink et al. (2002, 2003, 2004), in a series of studies, found that prenatal maternal anxiety is negatively related to attention regulation and mental/motor development observed at three and eight months of age. These studies were noteworthy for their rigor. Data were reported on a large sample (n = 170 pregnant women), and links between daily hassles and salivary cortisol levels were established, as well as between cortisol levels and lower mental/motor development.

Attention effects were observed by Brouwer, van Baar and Pop (2001). They found maternal anxiety was negatively correlated with measures of attention at three weeks and 12 months of age, but it was maternal anxiety assessed at 32 weeks gestation that had the strongest negative association with infant outcomes. Standley, Soule and Copans (1979) found anxiety specific to the prenatal period was associated with poor motor maturity. Oyemade, et al. (1994) found prenatal stressful life events and maternal anxiety were associated with poorer neonatal habituation on the Brazelton Neonatal Behavioral Assessment Scale.

In addition to studies of infant behavior, several studies have noted relationships between structural anomalies observed during the newborn period and stressful events in the mother's life. For example, Hansen, Lou and Olsen (2000) found that facial malformations such as cleft lip and cleft palate have a typical prevalence rate of 0.65 percent. However, for mothers under extreme stress (death or illness of the woman's spouse or older child) the prevalence of malformations increases to 1.18 percent. More specifically, if the stress was the death of an older child, there was a five-fold increase in facial malformations, as compared to the average level. Further, if the death of the older child was unexpected, the risk of facial malformations was almost eight times the normal rate.

Other researchers have found relationships between antenatal stress, and birthweight and prematurity. For example Rondo, Ferreira, Nogueira, Ribeiro, Lobert and Artes (2003) assessed prenatal stress and maternal distress of 865 pregnant women. Maternal distress was associated with low birth weight (RR = 1.97) and prematurity (RR = 2.32). (The relative risk index indicates that when maternal distress was high, the infants had approximately twice the probability of being low in birth weight, and 2.3 times the rate of prematurity.) In a similar study Hobel, Dunkel-Schetter, Roesch, Castro and Arora (1999) found that the maternal plasma corticotropin-releasing hormone was associated with stress at 20 weeks gestation in pregnancies ending in preterm delivery.

One potential pathway for stress to contribute to low birth weight is through affects on blood pressure and other circulatory processes of the mother. In support of this link Kurki, Hiilesmaa, Raitasalo, Mattila and Ylikorkala (2000) have shown that high levels of depression and anxiety are associated with the risk for pregnancy complications, specifically maternal preeclampsia. Maternal preeclampsia, in turn, is related to early labor and low birth weight.

There have been few long-term studies of maternal stress during pregnancy. In one such study Martin, Noyes, Wisenbaker and Huttunen (1999) followed a cohort of children born in Helsinki between July 1, 1975 and June 30, 1976. The mothers of these children had completed a questionnaire at each prenatal visit designed to assess somatic and mental health problems during the past month. Also, the mothers again provided temperament ratings of their children at age five. First trimester self-ratings of anxiety/depression and first trimester mood lability scores were significantly and positively related to maternal rating at age five of inhibition, biological irregularity, negative emotionality, emotionality intensity and the tendency to be unhappy/nonadaptive. In all cases the correlations were stronger for male offspring than for female offspring. Some significant correlations were reported for second and third trimester maternal anxiety/depression and mood lability, but in all cases the correlations were stronger for first trimester scores.

Research by O'Connor, Heron, Golding, Beveridge and Glover (2002) in England found that prenatal maternal anxiety was positively associated with emotional problems in both sexes. It was associated with conduct disorder in girls and hyperactivity in boys at age four.

Van den Bergh and Marcoen (2004) conducted a follow-up of their original sample which reported effects of maternal anxiety during the infancy period. At follow-up the sample consisted of 71 women and their eight- and nine-year-old firstborn children. Women had completed the State-Trait Anxiety Inventory (STAI) at 12 to 22, 23 to 31 and 32 to 40 weeks gestation. Child behavior was assessed using a Dutch language version of the Child Behavior Checklist with maternal and teacher reports. During a home visit, the child's behavior was observed and the child completed the State-Trait Anxiety Scale for Children. Child gender, maternal educational level, prenatal smoking behavior of the mother, birth weight and postnatal maternal trait anxiety were used as covariates. The results showed that prenatal maternal anxiety was significantly associated with ADHD symptoms, externalizing problems and self-reported anxiety of the children. Anxiety assessed at 12 to 22 weeks gestation was the best predictor.

A similar finding was obtained by Luoma, et al. (2001). They studied 270 mother-child pairs. Measures of maternal depression were obtained during the last trimester of pregnancy (prenatal assessment), three times during infancy and once when the child was eight to nine years of age. Measures of child behavior problems were obtained at age four to five and eight to nine using the parent and teacher forms of the Achenbach Child Behavior Checklist. Maternal prenatal depression was a strong predictor of the child's total number of behavior problems (odds ratio 8.5), as well as externalizing scores (odds ratio 3.1). However, the most adverse effect was for women who exhibited prenatal depression and had high levels of depressive symptoms at the time of the behavior problem assessment (concurrent depression).

Not all studies of prenatal stress have resulted in negative outcomes for offspring. In a research report by DiPietro (2004), high levels of anxiety during the second trimester of pregnancy were associated with higher scores on the Bayley Scales of Infant Development (primarily a measure of motor maturity and visual/motor integration at this age). The effect remained even when statistical controls were applied for maternal education level, and stress and anxiety during the postnatal period.

Leckman, et al. (1990) studied a small sample (31) of children with Gilles de la Tourette's syndrome (TS), most of whom were adolescents. These subjects were rated independently on the severity of their tic behaviors (involuntary motor movements). The researchers found that severity of maternal life stress during pregnancy was a significant predictor of tic severity. This occurred even though the mothers of TS patients had experiences during the perinatal period that were within normal limits (e.g., Apgar scores were normal), as was gestational age. The only other symptom that was related to severity of tic behavior was nausea and vomiting during the first trimester.

Van Os and Selton (1998), using the Netherlands National Psychiatric Case register, tracked the mental health hospitalization histories of more than 100,000 men and women born during the German invasion of the Netherlands in 1940. They compared the prevalence of hospitalization for mental disorders of this group to those born in the prior and subsequent year. They found a small (0.5 percent), but statistically significant, higher rate of hospitalizations for schizophrenia for those persons born during the invasion than those born during the comparison years. There were no effects for affective disorders. The effect was larger for those persons exposed to the stressor (the invasion) when their mother was in the first trimester of gestation.

The studies by Leckman, et al. on Tourette's syndrome and of Van Os on schizophrenia point to an important issue in the etiology of these syndromes. Both Tourette's syndrome and schizophrenia are chronic neuropsychiatric conditions that are known to be genetically mediated. These studies support the notion that the severity of the expression of the genetic diathesis is associated with effects of non-genetic factors. Such studies point out the potential interaction of genetic and prenatal effects in the etiology of many psychopathologies.

Huttunen and Niskanen (1978) provided one of the clearest examples of a natural experimental study of prenatal stress. Utilizing population registers kept by the Finnish government, they found mental health records of 167 adults whose mothers had lost a husband during their prenatal development. These adults were then matched with a group who had lost their fathers during their first year of life. The adults who had lost a father during prenatal development had a significantly higher incidence of adult psychiatric disorders. Additionally, the time of the father's death seemed to be important. A greater number of the adults with psychiatric disorders had fathers who died between the third and fifth months of gestation.

Etiological Mechanism

Five mechanisms have been described most often by researchers as having the potential to explain the relationship between maternal psychological distress during pregnancy and child behavioral or learning outcomes (DePietro 2004). The first hypothesized mechanism is that stressed, anxious and depressed mothers behave differently from happy, contented mothers. One set of behaviors that might be important for fetal neurological development is increased smoking, use of alcohol or use of other substances by those that are stressed. It is known that these substances have a deleterious effect on the developing fetus if used in sufficient quantities, and it is known that persons who are anxious or depressed have a higher rate of self-medication with these substances.

A second mechanism involves the effect of the stress reaction on blood flow. Stress sets up a persistent fright/flight response. This response, in part, involves the diversion of blood flow from 'maintainence' functions (e.g., digestion) to functions related to movement (muscles and heart). Placental blood flow is similarly affected. This effect has been demonstrated by Sjostrom, Valentin, Thelin and Marsal (1997) who reported a significant negative relationship between maternal anxiety and blood flow to the fetus. Thus, the fetus may be deprived of oxygen and nutrients by this reduced blood flow, resulting in a broad range of developmental difficulties. The developing neurological system may be particularly sensitive to reduced blood flow during critical periods of rapid development.

A third mechanism involves the transport of neurohormones to the fetus through the placenta. Neurohormones released in response to stress (e.g., cortisol) are necessary for normal fetal development. Thus, they easily cross the placental barrier. This has been demonstrated by Gitau, Cameron, Fisk and Glover (1998) who found that maternal and fetal levels of stress hormones are closely linked. Van den Bergh and colleagues have posited that high levels of these neurohormones alter neurological development by 'programming' neurological structures in a way that is maladaptive. This hypothesis is based on the influence work of D. J. Barker (Barker 1998), the central tenants of which is that when "disturbing factors act during specific sensitive periods of development, they exercise organizational effects—or program some set points—in a variety of systems." (van den Bergh and Marcoen 2004, pg. 1087). This hypothesis posits that if these set points were programmed to fit environmental circumstances different from those faced by the organism later in life, the organism is then hampered because the programmed set points do not easily adapt to this new environment. These maladapted set points constrain the flexibility of biological systems to adjust to altered environments, and can result in poorly adapted physiology and disease. For example, if a person's physiological ability to metabolize glucose was set in a nutritionally deprived environment during the prenatal period, and they then encounter an enriched glucose environment after birth, diabetes mellitus can result due to the inability of the body to cope with the higher glucose environment.

Van den Bergh and Marcoen (2004) and others posit that the hypothalamic-pituitary-adrenocortical (HPA) axis is particularly susceptible to prenatal programming by glucocorticoids, as has been demonstrated in animal studies. Prenatally stressed animals that are stressed during the postnatal period show pronounced and prolonged stress responses. These animals also have associated neurochemical changes in various brain areas, including glucocorticoid receptor expression in the hippocampus and elevated corticotropin-releasing hormone response in the amygdala (Weinstock 2001; Welbert and Seckl 2001).

Two other explanations for connections between stress and pregnancy outcomes implicate the HPA responses described above. One such hypothesis relates stress to increased risks of premature birth. When a person is under stress, the level of corticotropin-releasing hormone increases. This hormone is closely tied to the initiation of labor. Thus, increased CRH levels may set the placental clock for early delivery because CRH prompts the body to release prostaglandins which trigger uterine contractions.

The responses of the HPA have a variety of other effects, including a suppression of immune system functioning. Suppression of immune system functioning during pregnancy may be particularly detrimental to maternal and fetal health because the immune system is already suppressed as a normal part of pregnancy. Normal suppression of immune functioning during pregnancy occurs because one of the functions of this system is to identify 'self' and 'non-self' cells, and then to kill 'non-self' cells. Through this method the immune system kills its own cells that have undergone alternations associated with malignancy and kills foreign cells (antigens) such as viruses or bacteria (also fungi and protozoa). The immune system carries out these functions using white blood cells (leukocytes) and the complement system, a complex series of more than 20 proteins that initiate and promote leukocyte activity as well as other functions. One of the negative side effects of this process is that it impedes medical transplantation. The immune system defines the transplanted organ (e.g., kidney) as 'non-self' or attacks these cells, so transplant patients have to have their immune system suppressed to help preserve the transplanted organ.

A similar process takes place during pregnancy. The developing fetus is defined by the immune system as 'non-self.' It is what physicians refer to as an allogeneic graft, having many characteristics of a transplanted organ. The fetus is not destroyed by the mother's immune system because the uterus has protective features rendering it a privileged site for implantation. The mother and the fetus also have separate circulation systems and some subsets of maternal lymphocytes are suppressed during pregnancy. Specifically, the number of circulating lymphocytes is decreased during the third trimester. In particular, a lymphocyte referred to as a T helper cell has a decreased proliferative response to antigens (these cells don't reproduce as quickly). There is also a decrease in NK cell activity and a decrease in interleukin-2 release (part of the complement response) (Gennero and Fehder 1996). As a result of these changes, viral, fungal and protozoal infections are often more common in pregnant women, and the symptoms are more severe than they would be in non-pregnant women.

The burgeoning field of psychoneuroimmunology has documented that experiencing stressful events, anxiety and/or depression results in changes in some cell types in the immune system. Studies are often done by studying the cell proliferation response of a particular leukocyte to a known antigen after the subject has experienced a naturally occurring stress. Many studies have shown that this proliferation response has been diminished after stress (Baker, et al. 1985; Linn, Linn and Klimas 1988). Further, many studies have found that stress increases susceptibility to infection. In a classic study Cohen, Tyrrell and Smith (1991) studied 394 healthy subjects in a prospective research design. Their stress responses were measured (negative emotions, perceived stress, negative life events). Subjects were given nasal drops containing either an active virus or a saline solution. The results indicated that the experience of stress was associated with a higher rate of upper respiratory infections (colds) in a classic dose-response manner. (For reviews of this extensive literature see Segerstrom and Miller 2004).

All this work in psychoneuroimmunology, and in the understanding of immulogical suppression during pregnancy, leads to the conclusion that the fetuses of stressed women should be at a higher risk than those of non-stressed women due to immune system compromise. If a pregnant women has an infection, there is a possibility that the neurological development of the child could be compromised by (a) the virus crossing the placental barrier and infecting the fetus, (b) by fever caused by the antigen (e.g., virus, bacteria) or (c) by the medications taken by the mother to combat the infection (Lederman 1995).

Timing of Stressors During Gestation

The animal research, particularly with primates, is among the most supportive of a link between prenatal stress and adverse offspring outcomes. Some of the animal studies were able to isolate specific periods during development in which stress seemed to have the strongest effect. Most often the 'sensitive' period was early in pregnancy. For example, Schneider, Roughton, Koehler and Lubach (1999) demonstrated in rhesus monkeys born to mothers in three groups (early gestational stress, mid-late gestation stress, undisturbed controls) that infants from the early gestation stress condition had a lower birth weight than infants from the mid-gestation stress condition and controls. Further, while both stress groups had lower scores on measures of attention and neuromotor maturity, infants from the early stress group had more severe motor problems than the late stress group.

Most human studies that measure stressor onset or have measured maternal distress repeatedly during pregnancy also find that stressors occurring during the first trimester are most strongly associated with negative outcomes. One of the best studies of timing of stress was by Van den Bergh, et al. (1989) who found that antenatal anxiety between 12 and 22 weeks gestation had the strongest association with hyperactivity, frequent crying, sleeping and feeding difficulties and difficult temperament during the first seven months of life. Van den Bergh and Marcoen (2004) conducted a follow-up of their original sample when the children were eight- and nine-year-old firstborn children. The results again showed that prenatal maternal anxiety was significantly associated with ADHD symptoms, externalizing problems and self-reported anxiety of the children. Also, anxiety assessed at 12 to 22 weeks gestation was the best predictor. Martin, et al. (1999) found that first trimester self-ratings of anxiety/depression, and first trimester mood lability scores were significantly and positively related to maternal rating at age five of inhibition, biological irregularity, negative emotionality, emotionality intensity and the tendency to be unhappy/nonadaptive. In all cases, first trimester maternal distress scores had the strongest associations with outcomes, and the effects were clearest for males. Huttunen and Niskanen (1978) found that adults who had lost a father during prenatal development had a significantly higher incidence of adult psychiatric disorders than age matched peers. In this case the timing of the father's death at three through five months seemed to have the greatest effect.

Early stressors have not always been found to produce the strongest effects. For example, Brouwer, van Baar and Pop (2001) found maternal anxiety was negatively correlated with measures of attention at three weeks and 12 months of age. However, it was maternal anxiety assessed at 32 weeks gestation that had the strongest negative association with infant outcomes.

Methodological Issues

One of the major problems of the maternal stress literature is that mothers are often the reporters of their own prenatal anxiety and the raters of their child's behavior and emotions. This creates the problem that a consistent rating bias could produce the association. For example, a depressed mother during pregnancy may have a higher tendency to be depressed during the postpartum period and, thus, to perceive and rate their child as having a more difficult temperament. This problem has been noted by several researchers in the field (e.g., DiPietro, et al. 2002). Vaughn, et al. (1987) had women in the first trimester of their pregnancy respond to a range of measures concerning her expectations and perceptions about infants, as well as measures of personality and cognitive ability. They found that mothers of infants who were rated as 'difficult' at six-months of age were significantly different from mothers who had rated their infants as 'easy.' Those rating their infants as 'difficult' were more aggressive, suspicious, impulsive, dependent, irritable and anxious before birth. This raises the question of whether the perceptions of the mother of her newly arrived infant are as much a reflection of her personality as they are of the infant's behavior. Of course, it could be that these personality characteristics of the mother affected the neurological development of the infant to produce a more difficult child. The problem is that these effects are confounded; the effect of one cannot be isolated from the effect of the other.

If maternal ratings of the child are viewed as necessary by the researcher, then statistical control for postnatal anxiety/depression is a step toward controlling for this type of bias. It is, of course, preferable to obtain independent ratings of child behavior, a methodology that becomes progressively easier as the child begins to attend day care or preschool.

A closely related interpretation that confounds much current research on maternal anxiety and child behavior involves a genetic link. Mothers who experience an event as stressful during pregnancy may have a heightened predisposition toward adverse (very strong, prolonged) reactions to events that other women might not find stressful. Offspring of these mothers may also have this predisposition due to shared genetic material. Plomin (1990) and Braungart, Plomin, DeFries and Fulker (1992) have consistently found in twin studies that 30 percent to 50 percent of the variation in temperament has a genetic base. Thus, when anxiety or depression of mothers is assessed prepartum, this anxiety would be expected to be related to offspring shyness and anxiety due to genetic similarity. Note that this explanation is weakened if postpartum depression is also assessed and controlled for in the study.

A third mechanism involves the mother's psychological state during the postpartum period and throughout early childhood. Numerous studies have demonstrated the detrimental effects of maternal depression on child development. Bridge, Little, Hayworth, Dewhurst and Priest (1985) found that 80 percent of the women depressed during pregnancy became mildly or severely depressed at some point, up to 12 months postpartum. Thus, associations between prepartum stress responses and child outcomes could result from the effect of postpartum depression.

An often overlooked potential contributing factor in pregnancy depression and its effects on offspring is winter depression or seasonal affective disorder (SAD). In most mammals, when the brain detects shortening of day length, it secretes melatonin for a longer time at night. Melatonin is a hormone that regulates sleep. Wehr, et al. (2001) found that, for most people, melatonin release was steady at nine hours throughout the year However, for persons with SAD, nightly melatonin secretion lasted, on average, 38 minutes longer in the winter than in the summer. This indicates there may be a particular diathesis on the part of some people for prolonged melatonin release and that these people are more prone to seasonal affective disorder.

Summary and Conclusions

There is a rich and growing literature implicating prenatal stress in the production of adverse outcomes among infants, children and adults. These studies indicate that during the prenatal period, maternal stress produces more fetal movement. At the time of delivery, some studies find that maternal stress is associated with preterm delivery and low birth weight. During infancy, prenatal stress is associated with increased negative emotionality (e.g, more crying and more persistent crying). During childhood the data are less clear, but seem to indicate poorer general social and emotional adaptation, as well as increased attention problems. For those studies in which offspring were followed to adulthood, prenatal stress was associated with increased rates of serious mental illness. Across all age groups and in animal studies, first trimester maternal distress seems to produce the strongest effects.

While there is research support for all these generalizations, difficult methodological problems and some inconsistent findings have resulted in a literature that is provocative, but far from conclusive. Similarities in genetic makeup of mother and child, measurement problems, small sample sizes and simply not enough research on many topics (e.g., timing of maternal distress) have weakened the conclusions that can be drawn. Also, there is no agreement on the biological mechanism that links prenatal stress to offspring outcome.

Despite these difficulties it seems prudent to go along with our grandmother's wisdom. That is, happy pregnant women have an increased opportunity to produce contented, happy and well-adapted children.

Section D
Maternal Use of Recreational Drugs

Current estimates indicate that between 10 and 20 percent of pregnant women use cigarettes, alcohol or illegal drugs during pregnancy. Further, these are probably underestimates as most of the data are based on self-reports and most women recognize that there is a social stigma associated with these activities. It is also not known the extent to which women who smoke also drink alcohol or use illegal substances during pregnancy, although the assumption is that poly-substance abuse is common. Thus, despite major public health efforts such as printing warnings on cigarette packaging about the harmful effects to the fetus of smoking during pregnancy, these warnings are ignored. This pattern of behavior makes it important for service providers and researchers to continue to understand the effects on children.

The purpose of this section is to review the literature on the effects of maternal smoking, alcohol use and use of street drugs (e.g., marijuana, cocaine, opiates) during pregnancy. The literature related to long-term effects of prenatal exposure to the compounds in cigarette smoke is large, perhaps the largest of any body of research devoted to one substance. Numerous cognitive and behavioral consequences of prenatal exposure have been identified. Despite this accumulation of evidence, there is considerable controversy about the causative mechanisms. Cigarette smoke contains hundreds of compounds, some of which have been systematically studied. Further, women who smoke during pregnancy share a pattern of sociological and psychological characteristics that seem to contribute to the adverse outcomes for offspring. For example, they tend to be younger than non-smokers, less educated and have higher tolerance for risk. We have included a lengthy discussion of these factors in Chapter 9 to illustrate the complexity of the factors that may affect offspring behavior and learning. The reader should keep in mind that the sociological and psychological characteristics of women who use alcohol during pregnancy or who are poly-drug users are somewhat different from those women who do not use these drugs, so similar caution in interpreting research outcomes should be applied.

Alcohol use and abuse during pregnancy has also been extensively studied, but the literature on effects of moderate to mild use is far smaller than that for extensive use. The mechanisms are somewhat better understood for alcohol use than for cigarette smoking, but confounding sociological and psychological characteristics of the mother still limit our understanding of specific effects. By comparison, the literature on illegal drug use effects on child behavior is small. The illegal nature of the activity makes research difficult since self-reporting of use is still the most common research method for subject recruitment. Further, the sociological and psychological factors associated with illegal drug use during pregnancy make it difficult to recruit and retain these women and their children in long-term research efforts.

Chapter 9
Maternal Smoking During Pregnancy

There is a wealth of literature describing the adverse health effects of smoking. Over the last three decades public health and research has turned its attention to the impact of gestational smoke exposure on offspring outcomes. This literature base continues to expand, with epidemiological and case-control studies identifying the complex interaction of factors that produce both proximal and distal effects following gestational smoke exposure. It is now evident that cigarette smoking represents one of the more controllable environmental risk factors to the overall health of the fetus.

Prior to the late 1950s there was little concern about gestational smoke exposure. With few exceptions, the medical consensus was that the womb protected the developing fetus from environmental insult. However, the thalidomide tragedy that occurred during the late 1950s represented a cognitive shift in the conceptualization of the importance of the prenatal period (Lenz 1962). Following that event, scientists began rigorous investigation of the environmental factors that could adversely effect gestational development. Tobacco and its by-products are some of the most frequently studied teratogens. Gestational cigarette exposure studies have investigated the effect of exposure across multiple stages of development including infancy, childhood, adolescence and adulthood. Overall, these investigations provide evidence that gestational cigarette exposure has an adverse impact on development that persists throughout the early lifespan.

Simpson (1957) sparked interest in gestational smoking research following his report of the increased prevalence of prematurity and low birth weight in infants born to mothers who smoked during pregnancy. Since then, epidemiological studies have consistently demonstrated that gestational smoke exposure is associated with a 150 to 250 gram reduction in birthweight (Stein and Kline 1983), and a strong dose-response relationship. Prenatal smoking research has expanded beyond investigating the association with low birth weight to include psychological and behavioral outcomes. In recent years research has turned its gaze toward the relationship with antisocial behavior, conduct disorder and criminality.

R.P. Martin and S.C. Dombrowski, *Prenatal Exposures: Psychological and Educational Consequences for Children.*
© Springer 2008

Smoking During Pregnancy

According to statistics from the CDC (2004) 11.4 percent of all women giving birth in the United States reported that they smoked during pregnancy. This represents a decrease of 38 percent from 1990, when 18.4 percent reported gestational smoking. Smoking during pregnancy is strongly related to the age of the expectant mother (Mindell 1995), with younger mothers smoking more than older mothers. The smoking rate also varies by ethnicity and socioeconomic status. In general, prevalence of smoking decreases as the woman's education level increases. Outside of pregnancy, Asian-Americans and Hispanics had the lowest prevalence at 11.7 percent and 16.4 percent, respectively. American Indians/Alaska Natives had the highest prevalence at nearly 40 percent. White and African-American smoking rates were at 22.7 and 21.5 percent, respectively. Outside of pregnancy, smoking prevalence was lowest among individuals with a graduate degree (7.4 percent) and highest among those with a GED (44.4 percent). Current smoking prevalence was higher among adults living below the poverty level (33.0 percent) than among those at or above the poverty level (24.2 percent).

Women who smoked prior to pregnancy and were able to stop during pregnancy often relapsed after the birth of the child. This leads to the child being exposed to a good deal of secondhand smoke. Data from several studies indicate that anywhere from 50 percent (e.g., Polanski, Hanke and Sobala 2005) to 70 percent (e.g., Fingerhut, Kleinman and Kendrick 1990) of women who smoked prior to pregnancy relapsed within one year of delivery. This kind of data leads to the estimate that 25 percent to 30 percent of all children experience some exposure to cigarette smoke from mothers during childhood. An additional group of children (perhaps 25 percent) are born into a family in which they are exposed to the smoke of their father. Thus, when considering the effects of smoking during pregnancy, one must also consider the continuous rather than transitory impact of this deleterious behavior via secondhand smoke exposure.

Outcomes

Experimental Animal Studies

Experimental research on animals provides for a more controlled determination of the impact of specific chemicals contained in cigarettes than is possible through research with humans. However, the generalizability of the results of animal models to humans has limitations. Animal and human nervous systems develop according to different timetables. Thus, when discussing the results from animal models, it is important to accurately extrapolate the precise magnitude, timing and duration of an induced teratogenic insult. Furthermore, certain substances may have a differential species-dependent impact.

Nicotine has been the focus of most smoking related research on animals. Much of this research has used animals that were administered nicotine via drinking water or through a surgically implanted osmotic pump. Findings from experimental animal studies (rats, mice, guinea pigs) demonstrated deficits in the areas of learning, behavior and cognition (Ernst, Moolchan and Robinson 2001). These results are thought to be related to the adverse impact of gestational exposure to nicotine on the development and maturation of the central nervous system.

Human Obstetrical and Fetal Outcomes

Women who smoke during pregnancy increase their risk for a number of adverse perinatal outcomes, including spontaneous abortion, placenta previa and obstetric complications (Adams 2003; Dombrowski, Martin and Huttunen 2005; Magee, Hattis and Kivel 2004; Ojima, et al. 2004). The most frequently described outcome is low birth weight and premature birth. Women who smoke during pregnancy have babies who are born 150 to 250 grams lighter than non-exposed babies (Floyd, Rimer, Giovino, Mullen and Sullivan 1993; Hardy and Mellitis 1972; Ojima, et al. 2004). Further, smoking doubles the risk of having an infant born in the low birth weight category (e.g., less than 2,500 grams; United States Department of Health and Human Services 1980).

The smoking threshold necessary to result in intrauterine growth deficiency has yet to be clearly determined (Jones 1989). However, regular smoking of five or more cigarettes per day throughout pregnancy has been consistently linked to decreased birth weight. Studies continue to demonstrate a clear and convincing dose-response relationship, with the most severe effects on birth weight associated with the heaviest maternal smokers (Jones 1989). The relative risk estimates for intrauterine growth restriction among women who smoke ranges from 2.4 to 4.0 (Kramer 1987).

Growth retardation has also been found to persist through at least age 11. For instance, Butler and Goldstein (1973) found in a large British sample that the seven-year-old children of smokers were, on average, one centimeter shorter than the children of non-smokers. At age 11, the difference was 1.6 centimeters. Gestational smoking also increases the risk of reduced head circumference at birth. Kallen (2000), studying the effects of gestational smoking in 1.36 million infants born in Sweden between 1983 and 1996, found a relative risk of 1.65 of head circumference less than 32 centimeters for women who smoked one to 10 cigarettes per day during pregnancy. If they smoked more than 10 cigarettes per day the relative risk was 1.86 for their offspring to have a head circumference less than 32 centimeters.

Effects During Infancy

Prenatal exposure to cigarette smoke has been linked to a variety of effects assessed during the first year of life. These include increased risk of colic (Shenassa and Brown 2004), delayed gross and fine motor coordination (Fried, Watkinson, Dillon and Dulberg 1987), increased activity level (Batstra, Hadders-Algar and Neeleman 2003), decreased scores on a measure of cognitive ability (Gusella and Fried 1984; Saxton 1978) and Sudden Infant Death Syndrome (SIDS) (Hunt and Hauck 2006; Shah, Sullivan and Carter 2006). Two studies have shown cognitive and auditory processing deficits in infancy after prenatal exposure to nicotine. A decrease in motor scores and verbal comprehension was found in 13-month-old offspring (Gusella and Fried 1984), and reduced auditory acuity has also been reported in infants (Saxton 1978)

Some effects relate to the motor skills of the infant. For example, Fried, et al. (1987) studied infants nine to 30 days of age. Offspring of mothers who smoked during pregnancy had deficits in elbow and knee strength, and more motor tremors than offspring of mothers who did not smoke. Fried and Makin (1987) also found greater hypertonicity and increased tremors and startle response among neonates who were gestationally exposed to tobacco. Similarly, Law, et al. (2003) found that gestationally exposed newborns demonstrated greater signs of excitability, hypertonicity and stress on a standard neurobehavioral assessment. These researchers also reported a dose-response relationship. Picone, Allen, Olsen and Ferris (1982) demonstrated poorer habituation, orientation and autonomic regulation among infants whose mothers smoked while they were pregnant.

Some research has documented differences in emotional responsiveness in infants whose mothers smoked. Brook, Brook and Whiteman (2000), as well as Nugent, Lester, Greene, Wieczorek-Deering and O'Mahony (1996) have found that acoustic analysis of the crying of infants three days postpartum were of higher pitch, and of more variable pitch, than infants not exposed. These effects were perceived as an indication of more distress by observers.

Several researchers, however, have found that fetal exposure to maternal smoking was associated with less responsiveness to stress. For example, Ramsay, Bendersky and Lewis (1996) found that two-month-old infants whose mothers had consumed alcohol and cigarettes were hyporesponsive to stress (measured by salivary cortisol). Consistent with this finding, Martin, Dombrowski, Mullis and Huttunen (2006) found evidence for a relationship between maternal prenatal smoking and the temperamental characteristics of distress-to-novelty and biological irregularity at age six months. These researchers found evidence that mothers who smoked during pregnancy rated their infants as less distressed by novelty and less biologically irregular.

Research has also linked gestational smoking with increased risk of colic in infancy. Sondergaard, Henriksen, Obel and Wisborg (2001) described a Danish sample of 1,820 mothers and their infants born between 1991 and 1992. Compared with women who did not smoke during pregnancy, women who smoked more than 15 cigarettes per day or women who smoked continuously had a two-fold risk of having an infant with colic, even when controlling for the sociodemographic factors, low birth weight and advanced maternal age (>35 years old).

In summary, a variety of effects of prenatal smoking have been documented during infancy. These include lower levels of cognitive performance and auditory performance, as well as a higher incidence of colic and SIDS. The evidence regarding muscle tone (hypo- and hypertonic) and responses to stress has been mixed. It is difficult at present to understand why maternal smoking would produce a low reaction to stress in some infants, and high reactivity to stress in others. Some of the explanation may be attributable to differences in the way infant responsivenss is measured. In some cases it is measured using a biological marker and in some cases through maternal report. The relationship of these two different types of measurement is unknown.

Effects Assessed During Childhood

Health Effects There is substantial evidence that maternal smoking during pregnancy has negative affects on the subsequent health of the child. Not surprisingly, the most widely documented association is for respiratory tract illness. Aligne and Stoddard (1997), Chilmoncyzk, et al. (1993) and Martinez, Cline and Burrows (1992) have documented that gestational exposure to cigarette smoke contributes to the later development of respiratory problems. Such exposure has been related to decreased size of lungs and production of less elastin in children (Hanrahan, et al. 1992). Some researchers believe that these children may have congenital damage to the developing respiratory system in the bronchial tree of the immune system that predisposes them to develop respiratory problems (Cunningham, Dockery and Speizer 1994). Additional effects may be the result of the connection between smoking and low birth weight, which is associated with poor prenatal lung development.

Cognitive Ability, Learning, Language and Auditory Processing Several researchers have used measures of cognitive ability as an outcome. Bauman, Flewelling and LaPrelle (1991) surveyed the extant literature and report a clear dose-response relationship– higher levels of smoking are related to lower cognitive scores. For example, Nichols (1977) found reduced cognitive abilities as measured by eight standardized tests, and Olds, Henderson and Tatalbaum (1994) found mothers who smoked more than 10 cigarettes per day were found to have children with lower Stanford-Binet scores. Fried, et al. (1992a, 1992b) reported lower overall cognitive functioning and reduced receptive language functioning at six years of age, following gestational exposure. Cornelius, Ryan, Day, Goldschmidt and Willford (2001) found evidence for deficits in verbal learning, design memory, problem solving and reduced response in hand-eye coordination.

One of the strongest studies was reported by Sexton, Fox and Hebel (1990) who studied three-year-old children born to mothers who either smoked throughout pregnancy or who quit early in pregnancy. Children of mothers who had stopped smoking received a mean General Cognitive Index (GCI) of 107.5 on the McCarthy Scales, while children of persistent smokers received a mean GCI of 102.3. This five-point difference persisted even when children who weighed less than 2,500 grams at birth were removed from the analysis.

Gestational smoke exposure also has been found to predict academic achievement by a number of researchers. For example, Batstra, et al. (2003) found evidence for a dose-response relationship with reading and spelling achievement utilizing a birth cohort of 1,186 children from the Netherlands. Butler and Goldstein (1973) conducted a longitudinal study of 17,000 children born in Great Britain in 1958. An assessment battery was administered when the children were seven and 11 years old. At age seven, children whose mothers had smoked 10 or more cigarettes per day were four months behind in reading attainment. At age 11, the children who had been exposed during the prenatal period were nine months behind in reading and eight months behind in math. In a follow-up analysis in which maternal age, social class (paternal occupation), number of other children living in the home and child gender were statistically controlled, differences remained significant, although both the reading and mathematics score lags were reduced to about four months. In a later study of the same cohort (Fogelman and Manor 1988) it was found that maternal tobacco use during pregnancy was negatively associated with the ultimate level of educational attainment.

Specific aspects of language and reading skills have been found in several studies to be related to prenatal exposure. Naeye and Peters (1984) found reading scores on the Wide Range Achievement Test (particularly in reading comprehension and spelling) were depressed by about 5 percent for children of mothers who smoked during pregnancy, compared to children of non-smoking mothers. Sexton, Fox and Hebel (1990) studied 366 three-year-old children who had been born to mothers who either smoked persistently throughout pregnancy or mothers who quit within their first two months of gestation. Mothers who had smoked throughout pregnancy were more likely to assign lower scores to their children on the Expressive Language and Comprehension/Conceptual Language scales.

As we have seen, several researchers found evidence of auditory processing deficits in infancy for children who were prenatally exposed to cigarette smoke. Similar findings have been reported for offspring in the childhood period (Fried and Watkinson 1988, 1990; Sexton, et al. 1990; McCartney and Fried 1993; McCartney, et al. 1994; Fried, et al. 2003; Lichtensteiger and Schlumpf 1993). McCartney and Fried (1993) recruited six- to 11-year-old children whose mothers had smoked during pregnancy. A negative relationship was obtained between prenatal exposure to cigarette smoke and performance on three measures of auditory processing. None of the children had severe hearing loss, but the authors state that the deficits were severe enough to affect classroom learning. The authors hypothesized that nicotine may damage the outer hair cells of the cochlea. In a related study, McCartney, Fried and Watkinson (1994) assessed the central auditory processing of children gestationally exposed to cigarette smoke using the Screening Test for Auditory Processing Disorders (SCAN). The SCAN assesses the capacity to understand muffled speech, to understand speech in the presence of competing background noise and to understand competing speech signals. The SCAN also is useful in identifying auditory developmental delays and reversed hemispheric dominance for language. When controlling for passive smoke exposure, maternal drug use and demographic variables, the results of this study suggest that maternal smoking during pregnancy was linearly associated with poorer performance on the overall SCAN, and on a measure of competing speech perception.

Behavioral Outcome The relationship with activity level is the most frequently studied behavioral outcome of prenatal maternal smoking in children. For example, Naeye and Peters (1984) studied a group of mothers who had smoked during one pregnancy and did not smoke during another. They found that offspring of pregnancies in which the mothers smoked had children who were reported to have more behavior problems, particularly hyperactivity. Denson, Nanson and McWatters (1975) also reported a connection between high activity level and maternal smoking. Mothers of hyperkinetic children reported a current mean usage of 23.3 cigarettes per day, a level three times higher than the average for the control group. These same mothers reported a mean usage during pregnancy of 14.3 cigarettes per day, a figure that was twice that of the control group.

One of the best designed studies of this association was completed by Kristjanson, Fried and Watkinson (1989) who recruited four- to seven-year-old children to perform the Computerized Continuous Performance Task (CPT). Each child's activity level was electro-mechanically monitored during the task and was observed by researchers blind to the purpose of the study. A significant positive relationship was obtained between prenatal exposure to cigarette smoke and an overall index of activity level during the vigilance task.

Several recent studies have demonstrated that smoking is associated not only with high activity, but with the other two characteristics most often associated with Attention-deficit Disorder/Hyperactivity (impulsivity and distractibility) (Fried, Watkinson and Gray 1992; Milberger, Biederman, Farone, Chen and Jones 1996). These findings are more impressive because outcomes were assessed through numerous measures, including clincial diagnoses, caregiver ratings and laboratory tasks.

A unique study by Thapar et al. (2003) investigated the relationship between maternal smoking during pregnancy and symptoms of ADHD (parent and teacher-rated) using a population-based sample of 1,452 twin pairs. This study used a twin study design capable of controlling for genetic influence on ADHD. The results indicated a significant association with offspring with ADHD symptoms that is in addition to that associated with genetic factors. This study is unique in that it is the first to use a population-based sample and examine the role of genetics.

In the largest population-based prospective follow-up on the relationship between gestational nicotine exposure and hyperactivity in childhood, Kotimaa, et al. (2003) found a positive dose-response relationship between maternal smoking and hyperactivity. Furthermore, the results indicated that maternal smoking, when adjusted for the covariates (sex, socioeconomic status, maternal age and maternal alcohol use) produced nearly a one-third greater relative risk of having a child at age eight with hyperactivity (odds ratio 1.30; 1.08 to 1.58).

Conduct Problems and Aggression Few studies during the childhood period have investigated behavioral outcomes other than hyperactivity and ADHD. However, smoking during pregnancy has been found to be related to conduct problems, oppositionality and aggressiveness in children, as well (Wakschlag et al. 1997). For instance, Fergusson, Horwood and Lynskey (1993), as part of a 12-year longitudinal study, examined the relationship between maternal smoking and the development of behavior problems during middle childhood. Their study of 1,256 children included measures of pregnancy and post-pregnancy smoking, and child behavior at eight, 10 and 12. The authors reported a persistent dose-response relationship, with mothers who smoked the greatest amount having significantly higher behavior problems than those who did not smoke. Smoking during pregnancy was significantly correlated with symptoms of attention-deficit hyperactivity disorder, conduct problems and with a total behavior problem score. None of these outcomes were found when children were exposed only to postnatal maternal smoking.

Three additional studies have found an association with externalizing behavior, including aggression and oppositionality. Orlebeke, Knol and Verhulst (1999) investigated the effects of maternal smoking during pregnancy on behavioral problems in three-year-old children in a sample of 1,377 twin pairs from the Netherlands. Adjusting for the possible confounding effects of birthweight, breastfeeding, socioeconomic status and maternal age, Orlebeke, et al. (1999) found an association with oppositionality, aggression and overactivity on the Achenbach CBCL. Day, Richardson, Goldschmidt and Cornelius (2000) investigated the relationship between prenatal tobacco exposure and behavior problems at age three in 672 children. In particular, there were increased scores on measures of oppositional behavior, immaturity, emotional instability, aggression and activity level on the Toddler Behavior Checklist. Maughan, Taylor, Caspi and Moffitt (2004) investigated the relationship between gestational smoke exposure and conduct problems in 1,116 twin pairs at ages five to seven. These researchers concluded that the strong initial effects were reduced significantly when controlling for personality factors and environmental factors such as socioeconomic status.

All these studies reaffirm that maternal smoking during pregnancy has a range of adverse effects for the developing child. They also clearly affirm that the effects are not transient, relating only to early childhood outcomes. The most well-established outcomes in childhood are for lower cognitive performance, lower achievement, lower language processing skills, increased hyperactivity and a greater risk of conduct problems.

Adolescence and Adulthood

Health Effects Dombrowski, Martin and Huttunen (2005) investigated whether prenatal exposure to cigarette smoke would be associated with increased offspring hospitalization through age 22 for various physical and mental health outcomes diagnosed using the International Classification of Diseases (ICD; World Health Organization). These authors were able to control for any array of confounding factors including parental psychiatric status and maternal somatic health. The results indicated that youth born to mothers who smoked six or more cigarettes per day were more likely to have been hospitalized for neuroses (Odds ratio, OR, 1.97), diseases of the nervous system (e.g., neurological disorders) (OR, 1.47), respiratory infections (OR, 1.28), accidents (OR, 1.44), infections (OR, 1.54), undiagnosed symptoms (OR, 1.65) and total admissions (OR, 1.48). Female offspring prenatally exposed were more likely to experience hospitalization for obstetric complications (OR, 2.94) during the perinatal period. The researchers concluded that the impact of gestational smoking has persistent effects throughout at least the first 22 years of life.

Cognitive Functioning We have seen that maternal smoking during pregnancy is associated with lower cognitive performance in infancy and childhood. The negative effects of maternal smoking would be more convincing if these effects continued into adulthood. Several studies have provided evidence of such long-term effects. Fried, Watkinson and Gray (2003) investigated the relationship between adolescents (13- to 16-years old) prenatally exposed to cigarette smoke and intellectual capacity. Using data from the Ottawa prenatal prospective study, these researchers investigated 145 13- to 16-year olds. The results indicated a mean Short-Form WISC total score of 113.4, 109.8 and 105.2 for non-smokers, light smokers (one to 15 cigarettes) and heavy smokers (16 or more cigarettes). Covariates adjusted for this study included parental education and maternal drug and alcohol use. Fried, et al.'s study is consistent with that of others who reported a persistent long-term impact of gestational smoke exposure on offspring intellectual capacity (Fogelman 1980; Fogelman and Manor 1988).

Mortensen, Michaelsen, Sanders, Reinish and Machoever (2005) report a persistent decrement in intellectual functioning into young adulthood (mean age = 18.7 years). Mortensen, et al. (2005) studied a sample of 3,044 males from the Copenhagen Perinatal Cohort. This study controlled for typical sociodemographic characteristics including socioeconomic status, single mother status, maternal height and age, number of pregnancies, birth weight and gestational age. Maternal cigarette smoking during the third trimester, adjusted for the covariates, displayed a negative association with offspring adult intelligence. The decrement in IQ amounted to 6.2 points when analyzing the relationship between the non-smoking and heaviest smoking category. Another study by Breslau, Paneth, Lucia and Paneth-Pollack (2005) did not find evidence for a relationship between gestational smoking and offspring intelligence at ages six, 11 and 17 using a sample of 798 children from southeastern Michigan. Instead, these authors suggested that smoking contributes to an increased risk of low birth weight in children, and that it is the reduced birth weight and other factors, rather than gestational smoking, that accounts for decreased IQ scores. These authors further suggested that smoking during pregnancy is a mediating factor that has no direct impact on children's cognitive capacity.

Behavioral Effects Within the last decade the research on behavioral outcomes in adolescence has impressively increased. The findings during adolescence are generally consistent with the findings during childhood. In other words, adolescents whose mothers smoked during pregnancy were found to have greater externalizing behavior problems including Attention-Deficit/Hyperactivity Disorder (ADHD) and conduct problems (Ernst, et al. 2001; Maughan, et al. 2001; Schmitz, et al. 2006; Silberg, et al. 2003). Furthermore, there appears to be a consistent dose-response relationship whereby gestational smoke exposure during pregnancy is associated with higher rates of externalizing behavior (Fergusson, Woodward and Horwood 1998). Within the last decade there also has been a considerable body of research on the relationship between gestational smoking and later antisocial behavior and criminality in adolescence and early adulthood (e.g., Brennan, Grekin and Mednick 1999; Brennan, Grekin, Mortensen and Mednick 2002; Silberg, et al. 2003; Wakschlag and Hans 2002; Kemppainen, Jokelainen, Isohanni, Jarvelin and Rasanen 2002). These results have all been found in studies that statistically controlled for a range of variables.

For instance, Brennan, et al. (2002) utilized a large birth cohort of 4,169 males and 3,943 females born in Copehhagen. These researchers found that gestational smoke exposure is related to antisocial behavior outcomes in males and substance abuse in females. Results also indicated higher rates of criminal arrest for both males and females, although hospitalization for substance abuse mediated the relationship between prenatal smoking and criminal arrest for female, but not male, offspring. Brennan's study also revealed a dose-response relationship between maternal prenatal smoking and both criminal arrest and psychiatric hospitalization for substance abuse in male and female offspring.

Fergusson, Woodward and Horwood (1998) investigated the relationship between maternal smoking during pregnancy and the risk of psychiatric symptoms in late adolescence (ages 16 to 18). Participants included a birth cohort of 1,265 children born in New Zealand. Potential confounding variables, including social, family and parental, were controlled for in the analysis. After adjustment for these confounding variables, smoking during pregnancy was associated with an increased risk of conduct disorder symptoms in late adolescence ($p < .001$). The effect was more pronounced for male than female adolescents. Maternal smoking during pregnancy was not significantly related to symptoms of alcohol abuse, nicotine dependence, illicit drug use, major depression or generalized anxiety. There was evidence of a dose-response relationship in which a greater number of cigarettes smoked was associated with higher rates of conduct disorder.

Similar results have been obtained by several other research teams. Wakschlag, et al. (1997) noted an association between maternal smoking during pregnancy and conduct disorder in adolescent boys. Weissman, Warner, Wickramarantne and Kandel (1999) reported more than a 400 percent increased risk of early onset conduct disorder before puberty in boys, and more than a 500 percent risk of increased adolescent onset drug dependence in girls when their mothers smoked more than 10 cigarettes daily during pregnancy. Montreaux, et al. (2006) provided evidence that prenatal exposure to cigarette smoke was associated with increased overt symptoms of conduct disorder in low SES participants, but not in high SES participants.

Regarding the association with criminality and juvenile delinquency, Pratt, McGloin and Fearn (2006) conducted a meta-analysis of the relationship between gestational smoke exposure and later criminal and deviant behavior. These researchers cited more than 17 references on this topic. Pratt, et al. (2006) stated that their investigation showed that prenatal smoke exposure is a moderately important risk factor for criminal and deviant behavior in offspring (Effect Size = .117; $p < .01$). They concluded that gestational smoke exposure is a substantively important predictor of crime/deviance, with an effect size roughly similar to that between socioeconomic status and delinquency. Moreover, there appears to be a consistent dose-response relationship within this literature base.

In general, the data on adolescent and adult sequelae of maternal smoking during pregnancy is consistent with that of infancy and childhood. There are clear adverse cognitive and behavioral effects. The effects assessed in adolescence and beyond are somewhat different than those assessed at earlier ages, simply because of the life tasks and events that are appropriate for each age.

Secondhand Smoke Exposure Occurring During Prenatal and Postnatal Life

Secondhand smoke during prenatal and postnatal life is another type of exposure that can have serious consequences for offspring. Also known as Environmental Tobacco Smoke (ETS), secondhand smoke is a mixture of exhaled smoke and smoldering smoke from a lighted tobacco product. Like inhaled smoke, second-hand smoke contains nicotine, harmful chemicals and substances that cause cancer (Secondhand Smoke *http://www.helpstartshere.org/Default.aspx? PageID=528*). Constant or significant exposure to secondhand smoke is a danger to the health of non-smokers, especially children. Makin, Fried and Watkinson (1991) assert that one-third to one-half of all pregnant women are passively exposed to smoke during pregnancy. DiFranza and Lew (1995) assessed that 284 to 360 childhood deaths per year are due to lower respiratory illness and fires initiated by smoking. Further results of their literature review indicate that between 354,000 and 2 million episodes of otitis media, 529,000 doctor visits for asthma related issues, 1.3 to 2 million visits for coughs, 260,000 to 436,000 episodes of bronchitis and 115,000 to 190,000 episodes of pneumonia are related to tobacco exposure in children.

Makin, et al. (1991) found that the effects of passive exposure during pregnancy was less than direct exposure (mother smoked during pregnancy). However, mothers who were exposed to passive smoke during pregnancy were more than twice as likely to rate their children as having behavior problems in school. Further, these children had lower scores on measures of cognitive ability, motor skills and two measures of language functioning than controls. McCartney, Fried and Watkinson (1994) found that children whose mothers had only been exposed to passive cigarette smoke during pregnancy still performed more poorly on auditory discriminations tasks.

Summary and Conclusions

Animal studies have shown that high doses of nicotine cause slowed brain maturation and hyperactivity in rat pups. In human studies maternal smoking has been linked to increased pulmonary difficulties and increased hospitalizations at all stages of life. Maternal smoking during pregnancy has consistently been shown to be related to low birth weight, decreased cognitive ability, lower achievement and to higher activity levels among children. Other outcomes that have been reported include reduced stature at all developmental periods, motor coordination difficulties, increased impulsivity, attention problems and increased risk of conduct disorder, juvenile delinquency and criminality among adolescents and adults. These effects persist despite control for a host of sociodemographic, environmental and personality factors. Effects of passive smoke have been implicated in a large number of medical conditions, and some negative developmental outcomes such as reduced cognitive performance.

Hypotheses about Causal Mechanisms

There are several mechanisms by which gestational smoke exposure may contribute to adverse developmental outcomes. They can be broadly classified into biological/ physiological and environmental/ psychosocial. These agents act synergistically, with each exacerbating the effect of the other.

Physiological/Biological Explanations

One of the most prominently discussed causal mechanisms is the teratogenic hypothesis. This perspective emphasizes the physiological effects of cigarette smoke on the health of the developing child during the fetal period, and on the health of the child after birth. Within this perspective there are at least four (4) causal pathways by which a child's health could be compromised by cigarette smoke.

1. Toxic Chemicals in Cigarette Smoke Cause Damage to the Developing Fetus
The first hypothesized mechanism investigates the impact of fetal exposure to the toxic compounds contained in cigarettes, including carbon monoxide, ammonia, nitrogen oxide, lead and nicotine. Most studies have investigated the role of nicotine exposure, although other substances are just as likely to be involved. Nicotine crosses the placental barrier and has at least two effects. First, nicotine is a vasoconstrictor and has been found to alter normal placental function by reducing blood flow to the uterus. In effect this contributes to fetal nutritional deprivation and hypoxia, starving the fetus of oxygen and nutrients. Second, nicotine functions as a neurotoxin that interferes with the developing central nervous system (Levin and Slotkin 1998). Ernst, et al. (2001) contend that fetal nicotine exposure triggers a premature switch in the developing brain from cell replication to differentiation of the target cells.

Carbon monoxide in cigarette smoke reduces the oxygen carrying capacity of hemoglobin. About one to five percent of tobacco smoke is carbon monoxide.

Because hemoglobin has a strong affinity for carbon monoxide, it combines with carbon monoxide to form carboxyhemoglobin. When the hemoglobin combines with carbon monoxide, it can no longer carry oxygen, resulting in a hypoxic state for the developing fetus.

Cigarette smoke contains a number of irritant substances that cause bronchial narrowing and stimulate secretion of excessive mucous. Through the actions of these compounds, the lung and circulatory functioning of the pregnant women may be compromised. These effects, in turn, might have indirect effects on the developing fetus. Landesman-Dwyer and Emanuel (1979) reviewed several studies that showed that within minutes of exposure to maternal smoking, fetal breathing movements decrease and fetal heart rate increases. This later effect lasted an average of 90 minutes. Most authorities believe these problems are due to the effect of nicotine on the vascular system of the mother, particularly the placenta. Smoke also increases the carboxyhemoglobin in the blood of the fetus, which could be implicated in fetal hypoxia (Astrup, Olson, Trolle and Kjeldsen 1972; Longo 1977; Spira, Spira, Goujard and Schwartz 1975). Furthermore, Tolson, Seidler, McCook and Slotkin (1995) hypothesize that there is a combined effect of carbon monoxide and nicotine. The actions of nicotine and carbon monoxide decrease oxygen to the developing fetus. Reduced oxygen may be related to intrauterine growth restriction reported frequently in the gestational smoking-low birth weight literature (Dombrowski et al. 2005). Finally, tobacco smoke increases the level of free radicals and depletes levels of antioxidants and zinc. This scenario weakens the fetus's defense mechanisms against free oxygen radicals (Abel and Hannigan 1996).

An additional mechanism related to toxic effects of cigarette smoke has been posited. Fielding (1985) posits that there is a secondary effect of fetal hypoxia. When hypoxia occurs, the level of physiological stress rises, which may contribute to a permanent altering of the adaptive adrenocortical responsiveness of the child. This is consistent with recent hypotheses by Huizink and colleagues who reported that prenatal smoking may dysregulate the HPA axis, later manifesting in psychopathology (Huizink, Mulder and Buitelaar 2004). Although there is an absence of animal models to substantiate Huizink's hypothesis, Ramsay, et al. (1996) reported that two-month-old infants prenatally exposed had higher HPA axis activity and, thus, increased cortisol levels. In turn, this resulted in a reduced stress response among offspring. Hyporeactivity of cortisol responses is associated with less optimal functioning (Gunnar, Porter, Wolf, Rigatuso and Larson 1995) (See Chapter 8).

2. Women Who Smoke Prior to Pregnancy May Have Poorer Health at Conception
This potential causal mechanism, which is seldom remarked upon in the literature, focuses on the woman's health prior to conception. Women who are exposed to cigarette smoke (either active or passive) prior to pregnancy could have increased incidence of respiratory and circulatory problems that set the stage for a less than optimal pregnancy and delivery. For example, uterine blood flow might be reduced by chronic circulatory problems. Such an effect would be most apparent for women conceiving children later in life (age 35 to 45) after heavy exposure to smoke, with the resulting additive effects of advanced maternal age.

3. Men Who Smoke Prior to Conceiving Children May Have Sperm Abnormalities

A third mechanism, also seldom studied, is a male-mediated effect that could cause damage to sperm production or increase sperm abnormalities (Olshan and Faustman 1993). The exposure could be through active or passive smoke ingestion. There is only modest evidence for this mechanism on child behavior, but the evidence that does exist is provocative. Olshan and Faustman (1993) reviewed six studies of fetal loss associated with tobacco use and most found negative results. However, Savitz, Schwingle and Keels (1991) report findings from a study of 14,685 births during 1959-1966 in which the father's cigarette smoking was associated with cleft lip and palate, hydrocephalus, ventricular septal defect and urethral stenosis. Similarly, Krapels et al. (2006) reported an increased risk for orafacial clefts when fathers of offspring were smokers. They concluded that paternal smoking during fetal development may exert a teratogenic effect through passive tobacco exposure of the mother, or via direct impact on spermatogenesis.

4. Passive Exposure to Smoke During Childhood May Have Negative Developmental Consequences

A fourth mechanism by which parental smoking could cause teratogenic effects is through the child's exposure to secondhand smoke (e.g., or smoking of the father or other family members) from the time of birth through the time the child leaves home. It has been estimated that 43 percent of the children in the United States between the ages of two months and 11 years lived in homes where there was at least one smoker (American Academy of Pediatrics Committee on Environmental Health 1997). Further, there is evidence that children are particularly susceptible to the effects of passive smoking (Jin and Rossignal 1993). For example, children of smoking parents have a higher incidence of acute respiratory infections than children of non-smoking parents (Bakoula, Kafritsa, Kavadias and Lazopoulou 1995; Bonham and Wilson 1981; Colley, Holland and Corkhill 1974; Harlap, and Davies 1974; Tager, Weiss, Rosner and Speizer 1979; Wojtacki and Dziewulsha-Bokiniec 1995), have a higher incidence of sudden infant death syndrome (DiFranza, and Lew 1995), of asthma (Beeber 1996; Weitzman, Gortmaker, Walker and Sobel 1990) otitis media (Hinton, 1989; Owen, et al.1993) and a variety of other ailments (see Charlton 1994, for a review).

There has been a twist on the passive smoking hypothesis. The smoking of adults could affect the child's health by increasing their contact with disease if the smokers themselves have a higher incidence of disease. A study by Lebowitz and Burrow (1976) supports the latter hypothesis. They found that while respiratory symptoms among children were related to the smoking habits of adults in their home, the relationship was eliminated when symptoms in adults were controlled.

Psychosocial and Environmental Explanations

Advocates of the psychosocial hypothesis take the position that cigarette smoking is a marker for a lifestyle profile. This lifestyle has its roots in sociological factors (e.g., lower socioeconomic status), and/or in psychological factors (e.g., greater tolerance for risk; impulsive behavioral style). The lifestyle is associated with a cascade of increasing psychological, social and medical risks to women and their sexual partners, which results in increased risks of developmental problems for their children. The direct teratogenic effects of cigarette smoking on the smoker, and indirect effects on the child, are acknowledged. These effects are believed to be weaker in the absence of psychological or sociological issues. Particularly in the realm of long-term child effects, advocates of this position take the position that all the affects attributed to maternal and paternal smoking behavior could be the result of a cluster of psychosocial factors (Eysenck 1991; Rantakallio, Laara, Isohanni and Moilanen 1992).

Eysenck (1991) takes a strong position with regard to this relationship. He believes that much of the smoking research is misleading. Eysenck hypothesizes that smoking is one behavior of a cluster of behaviors that is associated with the personality of the smoker. He argues that smoking is not a necessary or sufficient cause of many health problems. For example, only one of 10 smokers will die of lung cancer. Thus, he posits that there must be many other factors that contribute to this health risk. He contends that smoking is combined with psychological factors such as low IQ, antisocial behavior, use of alcohol and other drugs, all of which have complex interactive effects and contribute to long-term outcomes.

From another perspective, mothers who continue to smoke during pregnancy may place personal desires ahead of concern for the detrimental consequences to their children. In essence, mothers who engage in smoking during pregnancy, despite widespread warnings to the contrary, tend to be less concerned and attentive parents. In the criminality literature, there is the position that maternal smoking during pregnancy is a proxy for later poor parental efficacy (Pratt, McGloin and Fearn 2006).

The Motivation to Smoke

Why do people smoke? Perhaps an exploration of the motivation and life conditions surrounding the habit of smoking can shed light on the psychosocial hypothesis. Of course, one simple answer is that nicotine is generally addictive. However, many people do not ever experiment with tobacco use. Of those that do, many do not continue use after initial experimentation. The problem for researchers becomes how to explain the differential initiation and discontinuation of tobacco use. Thus, what differences in biology and experience account for why some women smoke and some do not?

Age We have already seen that the prevalence of smoking is related to the age of women (O'Campo, Faden, Brown and Gielen 1992). By 1990 29 percent of 18- to 24-year-olds and 18 percent of 35- to 44-year-old women reported they smoked in a national survey (Floyd, et al. 1993). Age is also related to whether women chose to smoke during pregnancy. Mindell (1995) reports data collected in England in

1986 in which 31 percent of pregnant women smoked throughout pregnancy. He found that smoking during pregnancy was strongly related to the age of the women: 44 percent of the 15- to 19-year-olds smoked during prengnacy, compared to 30 percent of the women in the peak childbearing years (20 to 29 years), and only 7 percent of the oldest group (40 plus years).

Culture Among ethnic groups, Asian-Americans and Hispanics had the lowest prevalence at 11.7 percent and 16.4 percent, respectively. American Indians/Alaska Natives had the highest prevalence at nearly 40 percent. White and African-American smoking rates were at 22.7 and 21.5 percent, respectively (Centers for Disease Control 2003). Further, the smoking rates of women in Muslim cultures are very low, while in South America smoking rates among women are high (Floyd, et al. 1993).

Socioeconomic Status According to CDC (2003) data, smoking prevalence was lowest among individuals with a graduate degree (7.4 percent) and highest among those with a GED (44.4 percent). Floyd, et al. (1993) found that women with less than 12 years of education smoke at more than three times the rate of women with 16 years or more of education. Fingerhut, Kleinman and Kendrick (1990) analyzed health questionnaire data from a national sample of 1,918 white women in the United States. They found that women with less education were less likely to discontinue smoking during pregnancy than college-educated women. Similar findings have been reported by Graham (1995), Isohanni, Oja, Moilanen, Kairanen and Rantakallio (1995), and O'Campo, et al. (1992).

Rantakallio (1983) found that Finnish mothers who smoked had less desirable living conditions than their non-smoking peers, and were less likely to be living with their families. Isohanni, et al. (1995) also showed that women who smoke while pregnant tend to occupy the lower socioeconomic classes, and are more likely to be unmarried. Mindell (1995) found that smoking among pregnant women in England was related to employment status (50 percent of unemployed, 18 percent of employed).

Risk Tolerance Eysenck (1991) summarizes several studies in which risk-taking behavior was assessed and an association was found with cigarette smoking. The findings reporting an association between age and prevalence of smoking are also consistent with a risk tolerance hypothesis. That is, younger women are known to be more risk tolerant, and it is younger women who smoke most heavily. Other evidence can be interpreted from this point of view. For example, Mindell (1995) found that, among pregnant women, smoking was related to the timing of the first prenatal visit (21 percent who came in seven to12 weeks of gestation, 47 percent who came to the clinic in the 37th to 42nd week of pregnancy), perhaps indicating an indifference toward risk.

Attitudes Toward Pregnancy and Pregnancy Experience Parity and intention to breast-feed have also been associated with cessation of smoking during pregnancy (O'Campo, et al. 1992). Primiparous women quit at a higher rate than multiparous women, and women who plan to breast-feed quit at a higher rate than those who do not.

Personality Within the United States and similar western cultures, there is evidence that smoking among women is associated with personality. For example, extroversion, rebelliousness, risk taking and antisocial tendencies have been shown to be related to cigarette smoking (Cherry and Kiernan 1976; Eysenck 1991; Hirschman, Leventhal and Glynn 1984). Eysenck (1991) reports the results of a large study of smoking, stress and personality. It was found that if a person smoked and had a cancer-prone personality (low levels of emotional expression, failure to cope successfully with stress), 46 percent died of cancer. Of the 735 smokers who did not have this type of personality, only six died of cancer.

Dunn, McBurney, Ingram and Hunter (1977) cite literature that is supportive of the social manifestations of the personality traits described above. Smokers were found to be less stable and socially responsible than their non-smoking peers. They marry more frequently, change jobs more often, are more likely to use caffeine and hard liquor, and are less likely to use contraceptives to plan the size of their families. Smokers also tend to be sexually active at a younger age than those who do not use tobacco.

Stress Some of the data on factors associated with smoking among women point to a general stress effect. For example, Graham (1995) reported that, among English working class women, those who had more extensive and intensive responsibilities of caring for others (e.g., lived with an adult or child with a chronic illness), had higher rates of smoking. Further, as living standards declined, smoking prevalence increased. A number of sociological factors have been associated with smoking, and many of these raise the stress level of the women. It is reported that 36 percent of unmarried women and 18 percent of married women smoked (Committee on Nutritional Status and Weight Gain during Pregnancy 1990).

Role Models One of the most stable findings in the smoking literature is that smoking is initiated more frequently, and takes place more frequently, in the presence of others who smoke (parents, peers, cultural role models). Williams and Covington (1997) reported that having family members and friends that smoked was a strong predictor of smoking among adolescents. Some evidence suggests that females are more affected by the presence of others who smoke (Silverstein, Feld and Kozlowski 1980), but this is a finding that has been challenged vigorously (see Grunberg, Winders and Wewers 1991, for a review).

It has been argued that advertising has contributed in important ways to the tobacco use of women (Ernster 1983). Females are presented in advertisements as sexually attractive, young, competent and healthy (e.g., the Virginia Slims ads). It is difficult to demonstrate a direct link between advertising and smoking behavior. However, the continued use of sophisticated advertising by tobacco companies speaks to the fact that they believe it increases either the baseline of use or their market share in competition with other companies.

Perceived Advantages of Smoking Smokers most often report three benefits of smoking. One is reduction in body weight. The relationship of smoking to body weight is well-documented (Grunberg 1990); smoking, on average, lowers body weight by seven pounds. Given the emphasis placed on a slender body, particularly for women in many cultures, it is not surprising that this perceived benefit is often cited.

The second benefit is stress reduction. Nicotine, one of the many compounds in cigarette smoke, seems to have a calming effect on some smokers, although the scientific evidence on this point is not clear (Grunberg, et al. 1991). The third benefit is somewhat contradictory to the second. That is, nicotine serves as a stimulant to most people, with the side effect of improving attention.

Use of Other Drugs Eysenck (1991) posits that cigarette smokers use tobacco because they derive benefit from this use, and the physiological "benefits" are related to personality. Thus, it seems likely that they would use other substances in a self-medicating fashion. Indeed, in the United States smoking is associated with use of other substances that are known to have deleterious effects on health (Jacobson, Fein, Jacobson, Schwartz and Dowler 1984; Kuzma and Kissinger 1982). This association has often not been found in European studies. For example, Nugent, Lester, Greene, Wieczorek-Deering and O'Mahony (1996) found no relation between cigarette smoking and alcohol use in a sample of pregnant women in Dublin.

The effects on maternal health of multiple drug use may not be additive, but multiplicative. Hill (1995) has shown from studies of French smokers that the association of cigarette smoking on cancers of the mouth, pharynx, larynx and esophagus are five times greater than population averages for heavy smokers, 18 times higher for heavy alcohol users and 44 times higher for heavy users of both. Poly-drug use confounds individual effects since it is difficult to tease apart whether tobacco smoke or some other substance contributes to the adverse outcome.

In summary, there a large number of sociocultural and personality factors that are associated with smoking, maternal age, ethnicity and socioeconomic status are strong predictors of this behavior, as are maternal personality factors, presence of role models, maternal stress and the perceived advantages of smoking. All of these factors undoubtedly contribute to the decision to smoke during pregnancy, and continue to affect the interactions of the child and parent throughout postnatal development. Further, some of these variables have been shown to be heritable (e.g., risk tolerance), thus offspring may share these dispositions with parents. While the case for sociocultural and personality factors is strong, it does not indicate that there is no direct biological teratogenic effect of toxins in cigarette smoke on the development of the fetus. Thus, it is our view that these two sets of factors, the biological and the psychosocial, are complementary and work side by side to produce the majority of effects observed.

Summary and Conclusion

The gestational smoking research is fairly well-trodden, with outcomes reported from birth through adulthood. The preponderance of gestational smoking research indicates that smoking during pregnancy contributes to adverse cognitive, behavioral and psychological outcomes. There is evidence for a dose-response relationship. Sociodemographic, personality and environmental factors attenuate, but do eliminate, the adverse impact. Experimental animal research points to a physiological explanation for the adverse outcomes. Further, human studies suggest a gradient relationship, such that the higher the number of cigarettes, the more adverse the impact. Future studies should be targeted at more precisely defining the magnitude of cigarette exposure necessary to produce an outcome. Furthermore, research attention should focus more fully on exposure to secondhand smoke. There is a smaller research base addressing this topic, but it deserves additional research attention due to its possible contributing role in effects on the behavioral, cognitive and psychological functioning of offspring.

Chapter 10
Gestational Exposure to Alcohol

For centuries it has been commonly understood that certain substances, when consumed during pregnancy, are harmless to the pregnant mother, but toxic to the developing fetus. Alcohol is one example. As a result, admonitions against its use are commonplace in the historical, philosophical and religious literature. In the Old Testament Judges 13:7 warns: "Behold, thou shalt conceive and bear a son; and now drink no wine or strong drink." Carthage and Sparta prohibited newlyweds from consuming alcohol, perhaps to protect against the possibility of alcohol-related birth defects. Aristotle recognized that drunken women conceive children with developmental problems, saying that "foolish, drunken, or hare-brain women, for the most part, bring forth children like unto themselves" (as cited in Mattson and Riley 1998).

During the first half of the 18ᵗʰ Century in Britain the working class consumed excessive quantities of gin. Some physicians during that period warned that alcohol consumption during pregnancy was the cause of weak, feeble-minded and distempered children. However, this warning was generally dismissed until the second half of the 20ᵗʰ Century, following the thalidomide tragedy of the late 1950s. Up until that point the medical consensus was that the placenta protected the developing fetus from noxious or toxic substances such as alcohol.

It is now known that when consumed during pregnancy, alcohol can have deleterious physical and psychological effects on the developing fetus. Recent data indicate that anywhere from 10 percent to 16 percent of children have been gestationally exposed to alcohol (Centers for Disease Control and Prevention 1991 and 1995). Approximately 30 percent of children prenatally exposed to heavy alcohol exposure will manifest Fetal Alcohol Syndrome (FAS) (Streissguth 1991, Sampson and Barr, 1989).

While the data that will be reviewed in this chapter provides a convincing case for the adverse affects of alcohol consumption during pregnancy, the research is constrained by several factors. First, maternal report of alcohol use is not completely accurate, given the tendency to underreport or inaccurately recall the level of alcohol consumption (Ernhart, Morrow-Tlulack, Sokol and Martier 1988). Also, women who consume alcohol during pregnancy may use other drugs such as tobacco and marijuana, making it difficult to tease apart the impact of alcohol use from the impact of other drug use. At present, there is not a reliable biological

R.P. Martin and S.C. Dombrowski, *Prenatal Exposures: Psychological and Educational Consequences for Children.*
© Springer 2008

marker of prenatal alcohol exposure (Sokol, Delaney-Black and Nordstrom 2003). The measurement of alcohol use during pregnancy is further constrained by how drinking is defined (e.g., light, moderate and heavy). These levels of alcohol use have been defined differently by different investigators. Generally, researchers define light drinking as 1.2 ounces per day, moderate as 2.2 ounces and heavy as 3.5 ounces or more (Abel, Kruger and Friedl 1998), but these categories are not universally used. Another important issue with regard to the measurement of prenatal alcohol exposure is the lack of a precise threshold of teratogenesis. Hankin and Sokol (1995) posit that the risk threshold is consistent with daily use of one or more drinks per day, or a five drink or more one time binge episode. Sood, et al. (2001) report that children have experienced adverse outcomes following 0.5 drinks per day. As a result of the lack of research and clinical consensus regarding the ill effects of prenatal alcohol exposure, both the American Academy of Pediatrics and the American College of Obstetrics and Gynecologists recommend completely abstaining from any alcohol use during pregnancy.

There is an extensive body of research that investigates heavy alcohol use under the rubric of fetal alcohol syndrome (FAS). This condition is generally associated with heavy maternal alcohol consumption during pregnancy, although some offspring of heavy users appear unaffected. Since the effects of prenatal alcohol exposure exist on a continuum, with FAS lying at one end, we provide a brief review of the literature on FAS, recognizing that numerous books and articles on this topic are readily available elsewhere (e.g., Soby 1994; Spohr and Steinhausen 1996). We place primary emphasis upon the literature that has examined the impact of light to moderate alcohol use. The field has now recognized that alcohol produces a continuum of effects and has adopted the term Fetal Alcohol Spectrum Disorder (FASD). FASD covers all exposures to alcohol during pregnancy. FASD has recently supplanted other commonly used terms, including fetal alcohol effects, alcohol-related birth defects and prenatal alcohol effects, as the term of choice to describe the range of physical, mental and behavioral outcomes that lie on a continuum from florid FAS to subtle psychological and behavioral outcomes.

Fetal Alcohol Syndrome

Lemoine, Harousseau, Borteyru and Menuet (1968) of France were the first researchers to report the characteristics of a large sample (n = 127) of children born to alcoholic parents. Gestational alcohol research went unnoticed in the United States until Jones and Smith (1973) reported on a cluster of congenital birth defects linked to maternal alcohol consumption. Since then, this topic has been extensively studied. Although FAS represents a range of neurological and physical symptoms, it is generally diagnosed when the following three characteristics are identified in the child: facial anomalies, growth deficiency and mental retardation (Jones and Smith 1973; Streissguth, Bookstein, Sampson and Barr 1989). However, recognition of prenatal alcohol exposure is often difficult until after age four, with the exception of the most profoundly impacted who display obvious physical characteristics. Diagnosis based on dysmorphic characteristics often involves considerable judgment, in part because certain physical features characteristic of FAS, such as epicanthal folds, are common in some ethnic groups who were never gestationally exposed (Stoler and Holmes 1999).

Adverse outcomes observed among samples of FAS children include premature birth, failure-to-thrive, reduced stature, small head circumference, flattened midface, small wide-set eyes and drooping eyelids. There also is a broad range of neurological difficulties which include mental retardation, speech and language disorders, learning disabilities, decreased attention span, visual-motor integration difficulties, head and body rocking, strabismus and hearing impairment. Specific educational and behavioral effects include IQ scores in the mildly retarded range (e.g., mean IQ=68; Streissguth, Randels and Smith 1991). FAS is thought to be the primary contributor to mental retardation in the United States, with approximately 25 percent of IQ scores less than 70 (Abel 1984; Abel and Sokol 1987; Streissguth, Barr, Kogan and Bookstein 1997). Generally, IQs among children with FAS range from 65 to 72, with children with more dysmorphic features evidencing lower IQs (Mattson and Riley 1998).

A hallmark of FAS is impaired judgment and difficulty with abstract reasoning. Also, impaired memory exacerbates difficulties with academic and social functioning. Finally, FAS is characterized by attentional difficulties and conduct problems in adolescence.

The preponderance of research evidence suggests that children with full FAS are born to mothers who are chronic, heavy alcohol abusers during pregnancy (Streissguth, Martin, Martin and Barr 1981). Among chronic alcohol drinkers during pregnancy, the estimated risk of having a child with FAS is one in three (Streissguth 1986). There are a number of factors that moderate which child ultimately receives a diagnosis of FAS, but it is difficult to precisely predict who will manifest the syndrome.

Effects of Mild to Moderate Alcohol Use During Pregnancy

As indicated earlier, there is no consensus regarding what constitutes light, moderate or heavy alcohol consumption. The cut-point separating moderate from heavy use serves as an example. Some reports suggest as little as two to three drinks per day (e.g., Marbury, et al. 1983), or 4.6 ounces per day (Rosett, et al. 1983) constitutes heavy use. Others indicate that the threshold of heavy use is eight to 11 drinks per day (e.g., Diav-Citrin and Ornoy 2000; Davis, Partridge and Storrs 1982). Despite these inconsistencies, there is a growing body of research related to the effects of mild to moderate alcohol consumption during pregnancy.

Most researchers now believe that there is a dose-response relationship between maternal use of alcohol during pregnancy and the adverse outcomes that occur for offspring. Thus, outcomes are thought of as being on a spectrum from very severe (exemplified by FAS) to relatively minor. Placing a child's symptoms on this spectrum is an inexact science at present for several reasons. First, the diagnosis is often done retrospectively, since two of the three other characteristics (e.g., growth restriction and facial dysmorphology) of FAS are subjectively determined. Further, the diagnosis is often contingent upon findings of neurobehavioral deficits, which typically do not manifest until later in development. Further complicating the diagnosis is that individuals with less than heavy alcohol use during pregnancy can manifest a spectrum of fetal alcohol effects, evidencing some combination of outcomes typically associated with FAS, or some effects that are usually associated with mild use. For all these reasons placement of a given child on the spectrum is problematic.

Cognitive Ability and Neuropsychological Outcomes

The work of Ann Streissguth over the past three decades has contributed considerably to the understanding of the more subtle psychological and behavioral outcomes that can emerge following gestational alcohol exposure. Her studies and numerous others show that adverse effects persist from the neonatal period through early adulthood.

Intellectual functioning is the most frequently studied outcome in the fetal alcohol spectrum research. The consensus finding is that there is a dose-response relationship with heavier gestational exposure related to greater intellectual deficits, even within the mild/moderate range. Also, intellectual decrements are observed across most stages of development investigated. Academic achievement is also affected, although the research in this area is fairly sparse.

Testa, Quigley and Eiden (2003) conducted a meta-analysis of literature on infants (defined as two years old or less) who were assessed prospectively using the Bayley Mental Development Index (MDI). This review suggested that at six months and 18 to 24 months of age, there was no discernable difference between prenatally exposed infants and controls on the Mental Development Index (MDI). However, at one year a dose-response relationship became evident. When adjusting for covariates (e.g., other drug use; SES; education; smoking), Testa, et al. (2003) found evidence that the highest exposure level was associated with MDI deficits. There was an 8.32 point average decrease in MDI scores among children following maternal consumption of two or more drinks per day during pregnancy (at the margin of moderate to heavy drinking). The effect of alcohol exposure less than two drinks per day was not significant. Streissguth, et al. (1989) found evidence that alcohol use during early pregnancy was significantly related to offspring IQ scores at age four. In particular, the use of more 1.5 oz. (44 ml), or approximately three drinks of alcohol, per day during pregnancy was associated with nearly a five point decrement (p = .008) in IQ, even after controlling for maternal and paternal education, race, prenatal nutrition, aspirin and antibiotics use, child gender, birth order, mother-child interaction and preschool attendance.

When investigating the relationship between cognitive ability and moderate prenatal alcohol exposure at age seven Streissguth, Barr and Sampson (1990) found that moderate alcohol use during pregnancy was significantly related to child IQ, achievement test scores and classroom behavior. Consumption of 1 oz. (two drinks per day) or more was related to an approximate seven point decrement in IQ in exposed children, even after controlling for more than a dozen covariates including breastfeeding, SES and race. Carmichael-Olsen, et al. (1997) also demonstrated that drinking slightly less than two drinks per day can contribute to learning problems at age 14.

In adolescence Howell, Lynch, Platzman Smith and Coles (2006) reported that moderate prenatal alcohol exposure had a significant negative effect on cognitive ability and academic achievement. Their results demonstrated that moderate drinking was related to an approximate eight point decrement in full-scale IQ, as measured by the WISC-III, and an approximate seven point decrease in academic achievement, as measured by the WIAT Screener. These differences were found in the group that manifested alcohol-related dysmorphic features, while the alcohol exposed non-dysmorphic group was not significantly different from the other groups analyzed.

The research of Streissguth and colleagues (1990) also addressed the effects of binge drinking. A binge drinking episode of five or more drinks on at least one occasion resulted in a three standard score decrement on the WRAT, a standardized test of achievement. Goldschmidt, Richardson, Cornelius and Day (2004) found that children gestationally exposed to alcohol had lower overall academic achievement scores, and that binge drinking during the second trimester predicted deficits in reading. The finding that reading skills were particularly sensitive to the effects of maternal alcohol consumption is consistent with findings of Streissguth, Barr, Bookstein, Sampson and Olsen (1999) and Olsen et al. (1997) who reported in both studies that they found deficits in phonological processing.

Not all research has found adverse cognitive and achievement effects, particularly if the dosage was small. For example, Fried and colleagues (e.g., Fried and Watkinson 1990; Fried, O'Connell and Watkinson 1992) found that gestational exposure to low levels of alcohol was not related to cognitive outcomes in three- to six-year-old children. Other researchers have found that sociocultural variables moderated the relationship between prenatal alcohol exposure and cognitive performance. Willford, Richardson, Leach and Day (2004) found a relationship at age 10 in African-American, but not Cacausian participants, who were assessed via the Stanford-Binet, Fourth Edition.

Neuropsychological Sequelae

Studies investigating the relationship between prenatal alcohol exposure and neuropsychological sequelae have found a relationship with executive function, learning and memory, attention, language and fine and gross motor skills. Most of this literature is based upon heavy prenatal alcohol exposure. There is considerably less research on mild to moderate exposure.

Deficits in the executive functioning domains are commonly reported following heavy gestational exposure to alcohol. Several studies have reported an association with higher order cognitive function including planning, problem solving, cognitive flexibility and reasoning (Mattson, Goodman, Caine, Delis and Riley 1999; Mattson and Riley 1998; Rasmussen 2005). For instance, Mattson, et al. (1999) examined executive functioning in children with FAS following heavy prenatal exposure to alcohol and found reduced levels of functioning across the executive domains of cognitive flexibility, response inhibition, planning and concept formation/reasoning.

There is little available research regarding executive function and light to moderate alcohol exposure. One study of light to moderate alcohol exposure did not find an association. Richardson, Ryan, Willford, Day and Goldschmidt (2002) followed 593 children gestationally exposed to light to moderate levels of alcohol. The children were assessed at age 10 using a neuropsychological battery, which focused on problem solving, learning and memory, mental flexibility, psychomotor speed, attention and impulsivity. Richardson, et al. found no evidence for executive functioning deficits. These authors explained their findings on the grounds that the dose level was light to moderate. Further, they suggested that deficits in executive functioning may not have manifested at age 10 since many aspects of executive function do not appear until around age 12.

Learning and Memory

Deficits in learning and memory are frequently reported in the gestational alcohol exposure literature (e.g., Carmichael-Olsen, Feldman, Streissguth and Gonzalez 1992; Gray and Streissguth 1990; Mattson, Riley, Delis, Stern and Jones 1996). Generally, prenatal alcohol exposure has been associated with deficits in verbal/auditory memory, recall and recognition of verbal information, memory for stories or designs, and spatial memory (Carmichael-Olsen, et al. 1992; Mattson and Riley 1999). There is a dose-response relationship whereby heavier alcohol exposure is associated with greater impairment (Richardson, et al. 2002). However, even light to moderate consumption during pregnancy has been implicated. For example, in a study of prenatal exposure among 14-year-old adolescents, Willford, Richardson, Leech and Day (2004) found that light to moderate exposure to alcohol during the first trimester predicted deficits in verbal learning, short-term memory and long-term memory as measured by the Children's Memory Scale.

Fine and Gross Motor Skills

Delays in fine and gross motor skills are also apparent in children prenatally exposed to alcohol. Some of the earliest studies of prenatal alcohol exposure found increased risks of weak grasp, tremors and poor fine motor coordination (Jones, Smith,

Ulleland and Streissguth 1973). Later studies reported motor delays in infants, and fine and gross motor delays in children (Autti-Ramo and Granstrom 1991; Kyllerman, Aronson, Sabel, Karlberg, Sandin and Olegard 1985). In a recent study Kalberg, et al. (2006) indicated furthermore that there is a continuum of adverse outcomes in some areas of motor development, depending upon the degree of alcohol exposure. In addition, children's vestibular systems appear to be impacted as this study demonstrated impairments in balance and gross motor coordination.

Behavioral Outcomes

The FAS literature is replete with reports of greater behavioral, social and psychological problems among offspring exposed to heavy alcohol during pregnancy. Maladaptive behaviors such as poor judgment, difficulty perceiving social cues, decreased attention span, increased activity level and greater risk for psychiatric problems have been reported repeatedly in the literature (e.g., Kelly, Day and Streissguth 2000). These effects have been found to persist into adulthood, with adverse outcomes that include contact with the law, inappropriate sexual behavior, higher risk for suicide and improper parenting (Kelly, et al. 2000).

Psychiatric diagnoses, including those of both an internalizing and externalizing nature, attention-deficit/hyperactive disorder, depression, oppositional defiant disorder, conduct disorder, anxiety disorder, obsessive compulsive disorder and bipolar disorder (Green 2007; O'Conner, et al. 2002) have been found at higher rates for prenatally exposed persons than in control groups.

Attention and Activity Related Deficits

Attention deficits and hyperactive behavior are considered to be a hallmark of prenatal alcohol exposure and may be as sensitive an indicator of prenatal alcohol exposure as physical features (Landesman-Dwyer and Ragozin 1981). Gestational exposure produces deficits in activity and attentional regulation, and these deficits persist through adolescence and into adulthood. The effects of prenatal exposure to alcohol also appears to be dose-dependent, with more moderate to light exposure resulting in slightly lower reports of attention deficits and hyperactive behavior than those found in heavy exposure.

For instance, Streissguth, Sampson and Barr (1989) reported elevated levels of maternal reported hyperactivity at age four in offspring prenatally exposed. Similarly, Landesman-Dwyer and Ragozin (1981) found that daily drinking of an average of 0.45 fluid ounces of alcohol throughout pregnancy increased the likelihood of higher maternal reported ratings of hyperactivity or inattention, compared with a non-drinking or an occasional drinking control group. Leech, Richardson, Goldschmidt and Day (1999) reported increased deficits in attention following prenatal exposure to light to moderate alcohol use. Burden, Jacobson, Sokol and Jacobson (2005) found deficits in working memory among a total of 337 black children who were aged 7.5 years and exposed to prenatal alcohol at moderate to heavy levels.

Although the preponderance of studies found an association with deficits in attention, several studies did not yield such findings. Hill, Lowers, Locke-Wellman and Shen (2000) conducted a longitudinal prospective study of 150 children and adolescents investigating factors that might contribute to childhood psychopathology. They found that familial loading for alcohol dependence, rather than prenatal alcohol exposure, explained the association with adolescent psychiatric disorders. Boyd, Ernhart, Greene, Sokol and Martier (1991) investigated sustained attention in 245 four-year-old preschool children from lower SES backgrounds that were exposed gestationally to alcohol. These researchers did not find evidence for deficits in sustained attention following gestational exposure. Further, Coles, et al. (1991) reported no differences in adaptive behavior among alcohol exposure groups (none, low, moderate).

Aggression and Conduct Problems

There is a relationship between prenatal alcohol exposure and greater externalizing behaviors including aggression and conduct problems (Mattson and Riley 2000; Nanson and Hiscock 1990). Paley, O'Connor, Kogan and Findlay (2005) found that prenatal alcohol exposure was related to higher levels of externalizing behavior in four- to six-year-old children. This relationship persisted even after control of current maternal alcohol use and other sociodemographic factors. This study also reported greater externalizing behaviors with higher levels of alcohol consumption during pregnancy. The authors found, contrary to expectations, that present alcohol consumption had no effect on externalizing behavior. The authors also found that higher levels of externalizing behaviors were associated with higher levels of maternal stress. In a similar study Sood, et al. (2001) investigated a large African-American cohort of 665 families at six years of age. They categorized alcohol exposure into a no exposure, low exposure (>0 but less than 0.3 fluid ounces per day) and moderate/heavy (>0.3 fluid ounces per day) group. The results of this study indicated that low levels of prenatal alcohol exposure produced higher ratings of externalizing and aggressive behaviors on the Achenbach CBCL. Moderate to heavy levels of exposure resulted in elevated total problems and delinquency scores. In fact, children gestationally exposed to alcohol were more than three times likely to have delinquent behavior scores in the clinically significant range than non-exposed children. Sood, et al. concluded that no level of alcohol exposure is safe and identified a dose-response relationship.

This conclusion was supported by the research of Olson, et al. (1997) who reported that even social drinking of slightly under two drinks per day would produce behavioral effects. This study investigated the relationship between gestational exposure and adverse outcomes 14 years later in 464 children. Effects included antisocial behavior, poor self-esteem, impulsivity, disorganization and substance abuse.

Other researchers, however, have concluded that prenatal alcohol exposure is unrelated to later delinquent behavior. Lynch, Coles, Corley and Falek (2003) analyzed a sample of low income, largely African-American children (n=250) who were prenatally exposed. These authors did not find in the dysmorphic, non-dysmorphic or non-exposed groups any difference with respect to delinquent behavior.

Social Skills Deficit

Until the arrival of longer term studies that focused on outcomes beyond childhood, it was difficult to discern social skills deficits in children with FAS, since these children tended to be affectionate, extraverted and talkative. Several researcher studies now conclude that children gestationally exposed to alcohol are at-risk for greater social skills deficits, even after controlling for the potential mediating effects of intelligence (e.g., Roebuck, Mattson and Riley 1999; Steinhausen, Williams and Sphor 1993; Streissguth, et al. 1991; Thomas, Kelly, Mattson and Riley 1998). These deficits become pronounced over time as children with FAS have been found to experience a plateau in their social abilities around the time of school entry (Steinhausen, et al. 1993). Also, there is an elevating standard of behavior for older children and adolescents. Certain socially unacceptable behavior that may be considered customary in early childhood may not be well-tolerated at later developmental stages. In a recent study Schonfeld, Mattson and Riley (2005) found that nearly 50 percent of children prenatally exposed to alcohol, but not experiencing FAS, were later diagnosed with conduct disorder. These researchers found that poor moral development was related to these children's delinquency.

Social skills deficits do not seem relegated solely to heavy gestational alcohol exposure and florid FAS, as children without dysmorphic feature also manifest social skills deficits (Roebuck, Mattson and Riley 1999). Specific instances of social skills deficits include difficulty with following rules in simple games, sharing, taking turns, weighing consequences of actions and behaving impulsively. These psychosocial impairments persist throughout the lifespan, resulting in a cascade of adverse behavioral and emotional effects, including increased contact with the law, inappropriate sexual behavior, greater risk for emotional problems, including suicide, and reduced moral maturity (Green 2007; Schonfeld, Matson and Riley 2005).

Alcohol and Drug Use

Recent research reports a relationship between prenatal exposure and later predilection for drug and alcohol use. Much of the research in this area did not distinguish heavy from light or moderate drinking. Yates, Cadoret, Troughton, Stewart and

Giunta (1998) investigated the relationship between fetal alcohol exposure and later substance dependence using a sample of 197 children who were adopted. Adoptees with fetal alcohol exposure had higher symptom counts for alcohol, drug and nicotine dependence. This relationship persisted even when controlling for gender, biological parent alcohol dependence, birth weight, gestational age and other environmental variables. In a longitudinal investigation Baer, Sampson, Barr, Connor and Streissguth (2003) found that prenatal alcohol exposure is significantly associated with alcohol-related problems in offspring at 21 years of age. This relationship remained even after control for sex, family history of alcohol problems, prenatal exposure to nicotine and other drugs and other aspects of the family environment.

Summary

Reported outcomes following gestational alcohol exposure include deficits in intelligence, attention, visual/spatial abilities, school achievement and executive functioning including planning, problem solving and reasoning. There is presently little available research on the relationship between light to moderate alcohol use and associated cognitive and learning outcomes. What is available does suggest that exposure at even low levels has an adverse effect on children's cognitive and academic functioning. There also appears to be a dose-response relationship such that the heaviest alcohol use results in the most deleterious outcomes, with moderate use intermediate between light use and no use.

Increasing research evidence also points to greater attentional, behavioral and social deficits among youth prenatally exposed even to light/moderate levels of alcohol. The research reports a consistent dose-response relationship such that heavier alcohol exposure produces greater social and behavioral problems, with moderate exposure generally producing lesser effects and light exposure even less effects.

Mechanisms of Teratogenesis and Resulting Brain Morphology

Following Jones and Smith's (1973) seminal article on FAS, experimental animal models began to elucidate the mechanisms of the neurodevelopmental impact of maternal alcohol consumption during pregnancy. Alcohol freely crosses the placental and blood brain barrier, directly entering fetal physiology (Julien 1998). Experimental animal studies have found that gestational exposure to alcohol adversely affects the corpus callosum, glutamatergic neurotransmitter function in the hippocampus and development of the neural tube. Exposure during the human equivalent of the second and third trimester in rodent studies produced alterations in brain development, including altered neuronal circuitry, neuronal loss and perturbations to the developing forebrain (Huizink and Mulder 2006).

Human brain imaging studies have revealed differences between individuals gestationally exposed to alcohol and those non-exposed. The findings of these studies, mostly based on heavy alcohol exposed children, suggest that prenatal exposure results in reductions in the basal ganglia, primarily in the caudate nucleus. Since the caudate nucleus has been implicated in higher order thinking and executive functioning, a perturbation to this structure has been linked to decreased cognitive functioning after prenatal exposure. In addition, the corpus collosum appears adversely impacted following gestational exposure. Individuals prenatally exposed experience corpus callosum thinning and displacement, as well as reduced cerebellar size (Sowell, et al. 2001). Disruptions to these structures have been linked to verbal and learning deficits (Sowell, et al. 2001). Another affected brain structure is the hippocampus. Prenatally exposed children were found to have volume asymmetries in the hippocampus, which is thought to be associated with memory deficits (Riikonen, Salonen, Partanen and Verho 1999). Finally, brain mapping techniques have revealed reductions in white matter of the brain, particularly in the parietal lobe. The parietal lobe is involved in visual-spatial processing and the integration of sensory information (Sowell, et al. 2001).

In the end all fetal damage will involve a disruption to the cellular processes of growth, differentiation, proliferation, migration and apoptosis. Abel and Hannigan (1996) indicate that there is not a specific pathway of adverse impact, but rather prenatal alcohol exposure is acting through a relatively general mechanism that potentially has a wide-ranging impact.

Abel and Hannigan (1996) hypothesize that the deleterious impact of prenatal exposure to alcohol is the result of two probable mechanisms: hypoxia and free radicals. Citing the importance of cellular oxygenation for physiological processes, Abel and Hannigan (1996) suggest that any factor which reduces cellular oxygenation can adversely affect a living organism, particularly those in gestation. Decreased fetal oxygenation can arise as a result of many factors, including maternal alcohol consumption.

A second mechanism of teratogenesis involves a free radical theory. Abel, et al. suggest that alcohol's teratogenic effects may also occur as a result of damage to cells through the generation of free oxygen radicals. Free radicals are highly reactive within the cells and contribute to the peroxidation of cell membranes (Riley and Behrman 1991). To protect the body against the deleterious impact of free radicals, the body utilizes antioxidants and enzymes. Through particular enzymatic action, the element Zinc is depleted in the body. Zinc deficiency is accelerated when consuming alcohol and has been associated with FAS (Assadi and Ziai 1986).

Summary and Conclusion

The preponderance of research evidence indicates that gestational alcohol consumption is harmful to the developing fetus. The evidence is clear and convincing regarding heavy alcohol consumption. Some research suggests "caution" about taking too conservative a stance toward alcohol use during pregnancy. In other words, this perspective suggests that additional research on light and occasional gestational use should be undertaken prior to concluding that absolutely no alcohol should be consumed during pregnancy. Despite this minority perspective, the preponderance of research suggests that women who are pregnant should avoid even low levels (e.g., one to two drinks per day) of alcohol during pregnancy, and even the occasional social drink. Despite measurement difficulties of alcohol exposure levels, and the often multiplicative effects of other factors associated with women who drink during pregnancy, the evidence for adverse educational and behavioral outcomes following gestational exposure is accumulating.

Alcohol use during pregnancy is undoubtedly influenced by individual differences in personality (e.g., risk tolerance) and a variety of sociocultural factors, just as is cigarette smoking during pregnancy (see Chapter 9). Future research should be focused on teasing apart the impact of alcohol exposure from the impact of other environmental and chemical factors, including sociodemographics, poly-drug use and individual differences in such variables as maternal risk tolerance. Additional attention should also focus on alcohol consumption in the light to moderate levels.

Chapter 11
Maternal Use of Illicit Drugs

In this chapter we focus on the impact of used drugs, such as marijuana, cocaine, opiates and amphetamines, on later developmental outcomes. The earliest studies of the effects of recreational substance used in pregnancy occurred for alcohol, and these studies began to appear in the 1970s. In the 1980s gestational smoke exposure research accelerated and now is one of the most extensive body of research in the prenatal exposures literature. During the first part of the 1990s gestational cocaine research accelerated, and a small body of research exists on a variety of other recreational or street drugs. Finally, there are many studies that report on the topic of "prenatal drug use," often meaning poly-drug use. For the purpose of clarity, we have broken out each of the illicit substances, although the more common scenario is for users to ingest not just a single substance, but multiple substances.

Marijuana

Marijuana is the most widely used illicit drug among women of reproductive age. Reports of marijuana use during pregnancy range from 10 percent to 14 percent (Fried 1982). Despite the potentially high rate of use, there is little research dealing with gestational exposure to marijuana and the associated short- and long-term effects. One can only speculate that perhaps the lack of physical teratogenesis following gestational marijuana exposure has contributed to this lack of research.

Marijuana crosses the placental barrier and appears in mother's milk (Dalterio and Bartke 1979; Vardaris, Weisz, Fazel and Rawitch 1976). Thus, it has the potential to adversely impact development. However, there are only two longitudinal birth cohort studies that have investigated the impact of gestational marijuana exposure. This includes Fried's Ottawa Prenatal Prospective Study (OPPS) birth cohort study (Fried and Watkinson 1988, 2000, 2001; Fried, Watkinson and Gray 2003) and the Maternal Health Practices and Child Development Study (MHPCD) based in Pittsburgh (Goldschmidt, Day and Richardson 2000; Richardson 1998; Richardson and Day 1998).

R.P. Martin and S.C. Dombrowski, *Prenatal Exposures: Psychological and Educational Consequences for Children.*
© Springer 2008

The OPPS examined the consequences of prenatal marijuana and smoke exposure in a sample of 180 White, middle-class offspring followed through ages 18 to 22 years of age. This study began in 1978 and continues to the present. The OPPS collected data on prenatal exposure to marijuana, cigarettes and alcohol. The MHPCD involves a high risk, low socioeconomic status birth cohort through age 10, which was initiated in 1982. The MHPCD collected data on the consequences of prenatal use of marijuana, alcohol and cocaine. Over half of the participants are African-American. The field's perspective has been influenced to a large degree based on these two studies.

Growth Indicators

There is some conflicting evidence regarding the impact of gestational cannabis exposure on growth parameters. Several studies have reported that prenatal exposure to cannabis is related to smaller stature and reduced weight at birth. For instance, Hingson, et al. (1982) found that infants of mothers who smoked marijuana during pregnancy weighed significantly less than infants who were unexposed. Similarly Qazi, Mariano, Milman, Beller and Crombleholme (1985), in a small sample of five infants, indicated that reduced birth weights and head circumference were linked to intrauterine exposure to marijuana.

However, there have also been studies reporting no effect on growth parameters. Linn, et al. (1983) did not find any difference between marijuana-exposed groups and controls when socioeconomic characteristics were controlled for in their analysis. Fried (1980) identified 291 women, the majority of whom reported irregular or moderate use of marijuana during pregnancy. He did not find that marijuana use had any measurable effect on infant size. Finally, findings from the most rigorous and extensive studies in the literature (the OPPS and MHPCD) have not reported reductions in any growth parameter (e.g., Fried, Watkinson and Gray 1999), with one exception. Head circumference was lower for marijuana-exposed infants in the OPPS cohort from birth to six years of life (Fried, James and Watkinson 2001).

Studies that have examined growth parameters beyond the neonatal period also have not found a significant association. This includes research on youngsters ranging from eight months to six-years-old (Day, et al. 1992; Fried, Watkinson and Gray 1999). Of all the growth parameters investigated, head circumference was smaller in the OPPS cohort. This trend occurred until age six, but was no longer significant during mid-adolescence (Fried, James and Watkinson 2001). Fried, James and Watkinson (2001) did not find any impact of prenatal marijuana exposure on puberty onset or characteristics. Thus, the preponderance of the evidence would suggest that prenatal cannabis exposure has a very limited impact, if any, on growth parameters, including birth weight, birth length and puberty milestones. Head circumference appears to be initially reduced, but this effect is non-significant after age six.

Behavioral Outcomes

Prenatal exposure to marijuana seems to affect the neurobehavioral responses of the infant during the neonatal period. In the first week of life prenatal marijuana exposure has been associated with increased tremors, exaggerated and prolonged startle response, altered sleep patterns and reduced habituation to visual stimuli (Fried and Makin 1987; Richardson, Day and Taylor 1989). Consistent with this finding, Lester, et al. (2002) reported greater signs of stress in one-month-old infants following low to moderate gestational marijuana exposure. Fried (1980, 1982) found a decrease in responsiveness to light shined at the eyes in neonates assessed at 60 to 80 hours postpartum on the Brazelton Neonatal Scales. Lester and Dreher (1989) also found that infants born to cannabis smokers emitted a higher pitched cry than non-smokers.

Surprisingly, five other studies have reported no evidence for a relationship in infancy between habituation to visual stimuli and gestational cannabis exposure (Hayes, Dreher and Nugent 1988; Dreher, Nugent and Hudgins 1994; Dreher 1997; Tennes, et al. 1985; Richardson, Day and Taylor 1989). Whether this is a measurement issue or one of level of prenatal marijuana exposure is unclear.

At later developmental stages attention related deficits have been regularly found. Evidence for this association is provided via parent and teacher behavior ratings, as well as performance on continuous performance tests. In the OPPS Fried, O'Connell and Watkinson (1992) found that prenatal marijuana exposure was predictive of increased inattentiveness at age six. Fried and Watkinson (2001) also found that smoking greater than five marijuana cigarettes per week adversely impacted attentional capacity in youth 13- to 16–years-old. Additionally, these researchers evidence for a dose-response relationship between the extent of the prenatal exposure to marijuana and sustained attention, as measured by a Continuous Performance Task.

The researchers in OPPS asked mothers to rate their six-year-old children on the Connors (1989) Behavior Symptoms Checklist. Children exposed to marijuana were rated as more impulsive and hyperactive by mothers than controls. Leech, Richardson, Goldschmidt and Day (1999) also found that MHPCD children six years of age displayed greater impulsivity on a continuous performance task. By age 10, using the same sample, Goldschmidt, et al. (2000) found elevated parent and teacher ratings of hyperactivity, inattentiveness, impulsivity and delinquency in the MHPCD sample. The few studies investigating conduct problems in offspring are inconsistent. Six-year-old children in the MHPCD birth cohort were rated by teachers as more delinquent (Leech, et al. 1999). However, when controlling for extraneous variables, O'Connell and Fried (1991) did not find evidence for a higher rate of conduct disorder in nine- to 12-year-old children from the OPPS cohort.

Cognitive Outcomes

The evidence so far suggests that there is no relationship between gestational exposure to marijuana and global IQ scores. In the OPPS no association was found between marijuana exposure and infant mental and motor development at one year of age (Fried and Watkinson 1988). For the MHPCD cohort, gestational cannabis exposure was associated with a decrement in mental scores on the Bayley at nine months of age, but not at 18 months (Richardson and Day, 1998).

Fried (2002) cites an accumulated body of research observations regarding more specific cognitive deficits, however, including visuospatial reasoning capacity, short-term memory, sustained attention and attentional deficits. These deficits were consistent across several different ages studied in the OPPS (ages four; five to six; ages nine to 12), and the MHPCD (ages three and 10). For instance, at age four, children in the OPPS born to women who had smoked five or more marijuana cigarettes per week scored lower on the verbal and memory outcome measures from the McCarthy Scales of Children's Abilities (McCarthy 1972). Similarly, the MHPCD found that three-year-old children prenatally exposed had impairment on the short-term memory, verbal and abstract/visual reasoning subscales of the Stanford-Binet Intelligence Scales (Thorndike, et al. 1986). Fried, et al. (1999) reported that children aged nine- to 12-years old performed more poorly on the WISC-III subtest of Block Design and Picture Completion, which are purported to measure visual-spatial reasoning. The findings using the WISC-III are consistent with those of the MHPCD cohort when participants were assessed at 10-year-olds. Gestationally exposed youth displayed greater difficulties with abstract and visual reasoning, and increased deficits in attention and impulsivity following prenatal exposure to marijuana (Richardson, et al. 2002). In a more involved analysis of visuoperceptual functioning, Fried and Watkinson (2000) found that OPPS youth (ages nine to 12) experienced greater deficits in visual-motor integration, nonverbal concept formation and capacity to inhibit a prepotent response. However, at age 13 to 16 years, Fried, et al. (2003) found that prenatal marijuana exposure was not associated with several aspects of attention (e.g., flexibility, encoding, focusing).

Although prenatal exposure to marijuana does not appear to impact global intellectual functioning, Fried and Smith (2001) make the case that the performance areas most affected by gestational exposure can be best thought of as deficits in executive functioning. Executive functioning is a construct associated with the capacity to engage in behaviors such as problem solving, sustained attention, inhibition of prepotent responses and capacity to monitor, evaluate and adjust responses.

Mechanisms

Cannaboids cross the placental barrier and have the potential to affect the expression of genes important for neural development. This impact is thought to contribute to behavioral and neurotransmitter disturbances. Researchers hypothesize that because of the presence of cannaboid receptors in the placenta and in the CNS of the fetus, its presence in the fetal environment via gestational exposure might provide a mechanism by which derivatives of marijuana smoke adversely impact development. Glass, Dragunow and Faull (1997) reported that some parts of the forebrain are among the major receptor sites for cannaboids. The forebrain is associated with higher cognitive function. Thus, the hypothesis that executive functioning is impacted is consistent with this hypothesis. Further contributing to this hypothesis is an fMRI study conducted by Smith, Fried, Hogan and Cameron (2004). These authors scanned 18- to 22-year-old OPPS offspring and found increased activity in the left orbital frontal gyrus and right dorsolateral area of the prefrontal cortex, suggesting delayed development in these areas of the brain are related to an increased effort to perform an inhibition task.

Animal models also elucidate the possible mechanism of teratogenesis. Such models indicate that gestational cannabis exposure influences expression of a protein important for brain development (e.g, L1). This molecule is critical to the cellular processes of proliferation, migration and synaptogenesis (Rodriguez de Fonseca, Cebeira, Fernandez-Ruiz, Navarro and Ramos 1991). Also, prenatal cannabis exposure altered dopiminergic system neurons in several brain areas (Rodriguez de Fonseca, et al. 1991). Whether analyzed at the biochemical level or at the level of organogenesis, there is currently not enough information to lay out the pathway through which marijuana use during pregnancy influences child development.

Summary

There do not appear to be any morphological deficits associated with prenatal cannabis exposure. Further, up until age three, no consistent evidence for deleterious effects on behavior emerges. The one possible exception to this generalization is the adverse affects on emotional arousal of the neonate. Prenatal exposure to marijuana also does not appear to impact global cognitive functioning. However, after age three, there is increasing evidence that prenatal exposure increases impulsivity and inattentiveness. It also appears to impact aspects of Executive Function. In particular, two domains of executive functioning—problem solving and attention/impulsivity— appears adversely affected. This relationship persists across studies even when controlling for such confounding variables as socioeconomic status, parental drug use and home environment characteristics. There is an accumulating body of evidence for a deficit in attention and impulsivity, as measured not only be a continuous performance test, but also by parent and teacher ratings.

Cocaine

Despite media concerns about the looming epidemic of crack/cocaine exposed babies who will later develop without regard for morality or the consequences of their behavior, there is little evidence this has occurred. The initial ominous predictions of later developmental outcomes were grounded more in hyperbole than in scientific inquiry. The scientific reality is that prenatal cocaine exposure has not consistently been linked to adverse postnatal affects.

The prevalence of cocaine use in the United States during pregnancy has never been convincingly documented. Since use of the drug in general is illegal, and since there is strong social pressure against drug use during pregnancy, self-reports are unreliable. The profile of the women who are most likely to use cocaine during pregnancy, however, is well-known. These women are typically urban and impoverished. About 30 to 50 percent of women who lack prenatal care will have positive evidence of cocaine use at the time of delivery. Thus, those most likely to use cocaine during pregnancy are beset by a host of complicating environmental, personality and sociodemographic factors that, in themselves, might account for any longer term outcomes. This feature, in particular, was overlooked in first generation cocaine studies where an association with a host of adverse outcomes was reported.

Growth Outcomes

The relationship between prenatal cocaine exposure and low birth weight is inconsistent. Several reports have documented a relationship (e.g., Bingol, Fuchs, Diaz, Stone and Gromish 1987), including an older meta-analysis (Lutiger, Graham, Einarson and Koren 1991). Hulse, English, Milne, Holman and Bower (1997) conducted a meta-analysis of five studies which produced a pooled relative risk estimate of low birth weight of 2.15. The mean reduction in birth weight was 112 grams. This meta-analysis included studies that were adjusted for tobacco use, and excluded studies that did not contain an unexposed comparison group or account for poly-drug use. Based on their analysis Hulse, et al. (1997) concluded that cocaine use has an effect over and above that due to socioeconomic, health and other lifestyle factors associated with illicit drug use. They further supported their conclusion by indicating that the results of their meta-analysis were consistent with the experimental animal literature in which gestational cocaine exposure causes a reduction in offspring birthweight (e.g., Church, Overbeck and Andrzejczak 1990).

Coming to a different conclusion, Frank, Augustyn, Knight, Pell and Zuckerman (2001) concluded that several studies that found a relationship between gestational cocaine use and birth weight did not control for dose of prenatal exposure to tobacco and alcohol. In their meta-analysis of studies that controlled for tobacco and alcohol use, no association was found between gestational exposure and birth weight. Subsequent research since 2000 also has not found any decrements in mean weight, height or head circumference through early school age (Kilbride, Castor and Fuger 2006).

Thus, the preponderance of the evidence is consistent with the conclusion that there are few detrimental effects on growth of prenatal cocaine use. It appears that studies that found an association with birth weight or growth had not accounted sufficiently for confounding factors. Still, more research is needed considering the sometimes inconsistent results (e.g., Behnke, et al. 2006) and the experimental animal literature which reports intrauterine growth restriction.

Cognitive Outcomes

The Robert Wood Johnson Foundation has compiled much of the published literature on prenatal cocaine exposure and child outcomes. Lester, LaGasse and Seifer (1998) analyzed this literature. Of the studies investigated, 101 met methodological inclusion criteria (e.g., inclusion of a control or comparison group with statistical analyses). Only eight of these more rigorous scientific studies were conducted on children at school age. Intellectual ability was measured in five of these studies. Lester, LaGasse and Seifer (1998) analyzed these five studies, producing an effect size account (ES = 0.33) of the influence of gestational cocaine exposure. These authors suggested that the IQ difference between prenatally cocaine-exposed and control groups in the studies analyzed amounted to 3.26 IQ points. Lester, et al.'s article was important for the general public in that it countered the dramatic claims of the prior decade. While the scientific community for some time had recognized that cocaine impact was not as profound as first thought, this insight had not yet caught up with public perception. Lester, et al.'s work offset this perception by indicating that the effects are subtle, rather than severe. The Frank, et al. (2001) meta-analysis tempered even further the consensus that gestational exposure was related to severely adverse cognitive and behavioral outcomes. These authors, being even more conservative, concluded that there is little impact of prenatal cocaine exposure on children's standardized tests scores of cognitive ability. Instead, they indicated that findings of cocaine effects are related to contextual factors such as prematurity and prenatal exposure to other substances.

In the preponderance of studies there was no effect on intellectual capacity, no matter what age period was analyzed. In infancy, five of the nine available studies found no effect. In one study that reported an effect, mothers who used cocaine, alcohol and marijuana had lower scores than infant controls, but similar scores to infants who were gestationally exposed to marijuana and alcohol without cocaine (Chasnof, et al. 1998). Through the preschool period and into early school age, several studies reported no cocaine effect (Arendt, et al. 2004; Behnke et al. 2006; Kilbride, et al. 2006). Thus, the literature regarding gestational exposure to cocaine and cognitive ability has not shown an effect on tests of cognitive ability.

Behavioral Outcomes

Like the association with cognitive outcomes, most of the well-controlled cohort studies that provide for covariate or case-control of confounding influences have not found significant evidence for behavioral effects of prenatal cocaine exposure. In infancy the literature reports a transient period of insomnia, irritability and inconsolable crying (Chiriboga 2003). This is thought to be the result of cocaine's effect on the monoaminergic system. Conceptually, this was thought to presage later difficulties with attention, aggression, impulsivity and mood lability. However, the evidence on long-term outcomes research remains inconsistent. Some research reports increased levels of inattention and poor impulse control (e.g., Bandstra, Morrow, Anthony, Accornero and Fried 2001). Other studies have demonstrated negative effects on behavioral functioning during childhood (e.g., Chasnoff, et al. 1998; Richarson 1998). For instance, Delany-Black, et al. (2000) found that boys gestationally exposed to cocaine experienced more externalizing behaviors at age six, as measured by the Child Behavior Checklist. These researchers also found that children prenatally exposed displayed more teacher rated classroom behavior problems. Linares, et al. (2005) reported that cocaine-exposed children self-report more symptoms of Oppositional Defiant Disorder and Attention-Deficit/Hyperactive Disorder than non-exposed children. However, this same study reported no effects when caregivers rated the children on the Child Behavior Checklist (CBCL). The preponderance of research studies, including some that use sophisticated modeling techniques (e.g., Behnke, et al. 2006), suggest that any association with behavioral outcomes– including impulse control, attention deficits, aggressive tendencies and anger control– is more likely influenced by other pre- and postnatal influences on the child, mother and caregiver-child interaction (e.g., Accornero, Morrow, Bandstra, Johnson and Anthony 2002; Arendt, et al. 2004; Behnke, et al. 2006; Messinger, et al. 2004). For instance, it is now well-known that caregiver prenatal drug use is a marker for maternal psychopathology, poor parenting, child abuse/ neglect and increased exposure to violence and crime (Bays 1990).

Mechanisms of Teratogenesis

Cocaine crosses the placental barrier and is postulated to impair brain development through both direct and indirect mechanisms. Cocaine alters the developing neuro-transmitter systems critical to neuronal differentiation and brain structure formation by blocking the reuptake of monoaminergic neurotranmitters. This disruption, in turn, is thought to disrupt the development of neuronal circuitry in the fetus (e.g., Lidow 1995). When monoamniergic neurotransmitter systems are impaired, the neurodevelopmental functioning of children is thought to be deleteriously impacted in the functional areas of reactivity, arousal and attentional regulation. Vasoconstriction of the maternal uterine artery is also a more indirect mechanism by which gestational cocaine exposure can produce adverse outcomes.

Summary

Most of the literature in regard to growth outcomes has not reported an association with prenatal cocaine exposure. Initial reports of adverse impact now appear related to the confounding influence of poly-drug use, environmental characteristics and sociodemographic factors. Most studies found no negative impact of prenatal cocaine exposure on global or specific cognitive outcomes. The preponderance of research evidence suggests that initial discernable effects of prenatal cocaine exposure may be more related to environmental, personality, poly-drug use and sociodemographic factors. Recent studies that follow children through early school age and that better account for confounding influences have not yielded a significant effect.

The literature on gestational cocaine exposure in relation to behavioral outcomes is equally equivocal. Several studies have reported an association with attention-related deficits, oppositionality and overall behavioral problems. Other studies, including more recent ones that have controlled for confounding environmental and poly-drug influences, have not reported an association.

Within the gestational cocaine literature it is interesting to note that the tenor of the discussion of the literature has swung from worries about ominous outcomes to a more balanced perspective regarding potential long term effects. This is important because the mechanisms of teratogenesis for later developmental effects are plausible. First, cocaine crosses the placental barrier and has the potential to harm the developing fetus. Second, the indirect mechanisms of uterine artery vasoconstriction and maternal cardiovascular and neurological effects may potentially disrupt fetal development. Finally, animal experiments with cocaine show that it produces alterations in cortical neuronal development which lead to permanent changes in brain morphology and neurobehavior (Harvey, et al. 2003; Lidow 2003). Thus, despite inconsistent research findings, additional research is clearly warranted before cocaine is summarily dismissed as a harmless substance during pregnancy.

Opiates

Maternal use of opiates such as heroin, morphine and methodone during pregnancy has been studied infrequently, and mostly during the neonatal period. It has been long known that opiates readily and freely cross the placenta barrier (Bureau 1895). Happel reported in 1892 that opium passes through maternal breast milk and is associated with drug dependency in normal infants and ameliorates withdrawal symptoms in congenitally addicted infants. Even prior to this time period, Hippocrates reported that opium is associated with "uterine suffocation" (as cited in DeCristofaro and La Gamma 1995). Since the late 19th Century opiates such as morphine, heroin and paregoric have been used to ameliorate passive narcotic addiction in the fetus and newborn (Zagon 1985).

Outcomes

Opiate-addicted mothers have offspring who experience neonatal abstinence syndrome, with features of acute withdrawal (see Table 11.1). These symptoms begin shortly after birth, with most effects occurring 48 to 72 hours after birth. Withdrawal

Table 11.1 Opiate Withdrawal Features

Central Nervous System
   Jittery movements/tremors
   Hypertonicity
   Irritability
   High-pitched Cry
   Convulsions
Autonomic
   Fever
   Sweating
   Accelerated respiratory rate
   Skin blotches
Gastrointestinal
   Diarrhea
   Vomiting
   Poor feeding

symptoms include tremors, hypertonia, irritability, a high-pitched cry, rapid respiration and gastrointentinal upset (Chiriboga 2003). There is also a four to 10 time greater prevalence of SIDS in opiate-exposed infants (DeCristofaro and LaGamma 1995).

Over two dozen studies have investigated the relationship between opiate use and low birth weight. A group from Australia (e.g., Hulse, Milne, English and Holman 1997) conducted a meta-analysis on this literature. This review also produced data on heroin use, methadone use and any opiate use. Prenatal heroin use is associated with mean birth weight reduction of 489 g (95 percent CI 284-693), reflecting a 461 percent relative increased risk of low birth weight. Methadone use is associated with a 279 g (95 percent CI 229-328) reduction in birth weight, reflecting an 136 percent increased relative risk of low birth weight. Combined heroin and methadone use produced a pooled mean reduction in birth weight of 557 grams, reflecting a pooled relative risk of 3.28. Any opiate use produced a mean reduction in birth weight of 395 grams, resulting in a relative risk estimate for low birth weight of 3.81.

Studies on outcomes beyond the neonatal period are considerably less common. Those that are available show a lack of consistency in specific psychological or behavioral outcomes, and demonstrate that environmental factors play a significant role in many of the reported delays. Early reported outcomes initially associated gestational opiate exposure with poor attention span, greater risk for mental retardation, learning disabilities and impaired speech and language development (Messinger, et al. 2004). However, such delays appear to remit over time and after control for confounding variables. This suggests that sociodemographic and postnatal environmental factors account for the delays.

In the largest sample observed longitudinally to date, Messinger, et al. (2004) investigated the relationship between gestational opiate exposure and cognitive, motor and behavioral outcomes through age three years. These researchers concluded that gestational opiate exposure was not associated with deficits after controlling for birth weight and environmental factors. In addition, Lifshitz and Wilson (1991) reported no difference on the McCarthy Scales of Children's Abilities when assessed on a cohort of three- to six-year-olds.

Mechanisms of Teratogenesis

Opiates are thought to inhibit cellular proliferation and differentiation (Zagon McLaughlin, Weaver and Zagon 1982). Gestational opiate exposure is also postulated to adversely affect astroglial cells which are important for providing the foundation for neuronal migration, and the cytokines and peptides responsible for brain growth (DeCristofaro and LaGamma 1995). A more complex conceptualization of the role of opioids on opioid-induced changes on cellular development is available elsewhere (e.g., Hamill and LaGamma 1992).

Summary

Maternal opiate use during pregnancy doubles the risk of having a low birth weight baby, with mean reductions in birth weight ranging from 279 grams to 550 grams. Adverse effects beyond the neonatal period appear to remit. Despite initial speculation that prenatal opiate exposure was related to later effects on learning and behavior, no well-controlled or longer term study has produced this association. Still, the potential impact of gestational opiate exposure is plausible considering experimental animal models which reveal its biochemical action on the developing nervous system. Additional studies are clearly warranted before concluding that there are no longer term effects of prenatal opiate use on offspring.

Amphetamine/Methamphetamine

Methamphetamine

A derivative of the stimulant amphetamine – methamphetamine (MA) – was first synthesized from ephedrine by the Japanese pharmacologist Nagayoshi Nagai in 1893. MA emerged as a problem in the United States during the late 1990s, and has recently reached epidemic proportions. Despite the present epidemic, whereby even pseudophedrine purchase is carefully monitored by pharmacies, knowledge about the effects of prenatal MA is limited. A 1993 study by the National Institute on Drug Abuse determined that less than 1 percent of pregnant women used MA during their pregnancy. A later large scale investigation of MA use during pregnancy reported a 5.2 percent rate in areas where MA has been reported as a problem (Arria, et al. 2006). The few studies reporting on the impact of MA are hampered by the same methodological problems faced by first generation gestational cocaine studies, including small sample size and a failure to control for poly-drug use and other environmental problems.

With these limitations in mind MA has been associated with an increased incidence of premature birth and placenta abruption (Ericksson, Larsson, Windbladh and Zetterstrom 1978). A recent study indicated that MA (along with nicotine) use is associated with a higher number of small-for-gestational-age infants born at term (Smith, et al. 2003). The authors concluded that other factors including tobacco, marijuana and alcohol exposure likely contributed to their findings.

Amphetamine

The available research regarding prenatal exposure to amphetamine is equally sparse and inconsistent. One group of researchers has followed a small Swedish cohort of 65 children gestational exposed to amphetamine. The children were assessed at various stages of development including ages four, eight, 10 and 14 to 15 years of age. This group indicated that, at age four, maternal alcohol and drug abuse during pregnancy, paternal criminal convictions, maternal stress and maternal parity were correlated with children's adjustment (Billing, Eriksson, Steneroth and Zetterstrom 1988). No specific association with amphetamine use was found at this age. At age eight aggressive behavior, peer-related problems and overall behavioral adjustment was associated with prenatal amphetamine use, with greater levels of behavioral difficulty associated with the magnitude and duration of this drug's use (Billing, Eriksson, Jonsson, Steneroth and Zetterstrom 1994; Eriksson, Billing, Steneroth and Zetterstrom 1989). Eriksson, et al. (1989) reported that IQ performance was within normal limits, while school performance at age 10 was below normal levels. Eriksson and Zetterstrom (1994) reported that 12 percent of this cohort were retained, compared to a normal of 5 percent in Sweden. They concluded that amphetamine abuse during pregnancy influenced the development of exposed children up until at least age 10. School-related difficulties persisted through age 14 in this same Swedish cohort (e.g., Cernerud, Eriksson, Jonsson, Steneroth and Zetterstrom 1996). When cohort children were in eighth grade 15 percent were performing one grade lower than expected levels, compared to a norm of 5 percent.

A significant limitation of this group of studies is its small sample size and the possible confounding of the results with other sociodemographic factors. The overall conclusion from prenatal amphetamine use is that the literature is too sparse to draw anything but tentative conclusions about whether it is detrimental to offspring (Middaugh 1989).

Mechanism of Teratogenesis

The mechanism of teratogenesis has not been well elucidated for amphetamine/ methamphetamine. Amphetamine can have long-term effects of monoaminergic systems in the brains of adults, including neural degeneration (Middaugh 1989). Middaugh (1989) contends that, since amphetamines can cross the placenta, it is plausible that exposure can have simlar consequences for the developing fetus. The rationale for a potential adverse impact during prenatal development is linked to the potential impact of amphetamine/methamphetamine on the monoaminergic and pituitary-adrenal systems, which are undergoing rapid development during late gestation and early in the neonatal period.

Summary and Conclusion

The literature regarding gestational amphetamine and MA use is far too scant to make any conclusions about its ill-effect on later developmental outcomes. The research available to date is confounded by poly-drug effects, sociodemographic characteristics and other environmental characteristics that may account for much of the reported outcomes. Additional research regarding gestational amphetamine and MA use is warranted, particularly given the recent rapid increase in MA abuse.

Section E
Pollutants and the Development
of the Human Fetus: An Introduction

All human beings are being exposed to a wide range of man-made chemicals to which their parents and grandparents were not exposed. Estimates by the United States Environmental Protection Agency (EPA) are that 10 new chemicals are currently being introduced each day, adding to the 87,000 such chemicals that are currently in use. The plastics industry, for example, has an annual production in the United States of 85 billion pounds, or approximately 340 pounds for each person per year (Colburn 2004). Plastics are used in a wide range of products from toys, cosmetics, cleaning compounds and clothing, to construction materials for buildings and automobiles. Thus, almost every human being comes in contact with these products on a daily basis.

In the agricultural realm there are currently more than 900 active ingredients registered as pesticides by the United States EPA. These pesticides have been combined with other materials into more than 21,000 pesticide products (Colburn 2004). In 1995 Short and Colburn (1999) estimated that the United States produced 1.3 billion pounds of pesticide active ingredients, of which herbicides (weed killers) are the most widely used. It is estimated that herbicides cover 14 percent of the land surface within the United States. This does not count lawns, gardens, golf courses, parks and uses by governmental agencies (such as on rights-of-way).

Colburn (2004) has outlined the history of exposure to synthetic chemicals in the United States. In the 1920s and '30s DDT (dichlorodiphenyltrichloroethane) and PCBs (polychlorinated biphenyls) were first produced, creating a discrete prenatal exposure for the first time. As a result of industrial expansion before and after World War II, production of these chemicals and others were greatly expanded. In the period from the 1950s to the 1970s the first generation was born that was widely exposed prenatally. From the 1980s to the present the generation exposed prenatally gave birth to the second generation that themselves were at high risk of prenatal exposure. Thus, in the past 30 to 40 years there have been two generations of prenatal exposures, in the context of rapidly (almost exponentially) increasing production of synthetic chemicals.

In addition to man-made chemical products, toxic pollutants are emitted by industrial plants, mining operations, petroleum processes and many other industrial concerns. For example, the EPA estimated that in 2003 the five largest releasers of toxic chemicals by industrial type (metal mining industry, chemical and allied products industry, primary metal industries, the paper industry and chemical wholesalers) released approximately 2.5 billion pounds of toxic chemicals into the air or water as part of production or storage of materials. The majority of these releases were on site, exposing primarily workers in that industry. However, across all industries in 2003, 518 million pounds of toxic pollutants were released into the air, water or soil of the United States (United States Census Bureau 2006).

In addition to increasing synthetic chemical production, and toxic by-products of industrialization, the increase in the number of human beings on the planet, and the tendency for human beings to live in larger and larger cities, creates more opportunities for exposure to toxins. In 1975 there were only four megacities (e.g., cities with more than 10 million inhabitants): Tokyo, New York, Shanghai and Mexico City. By the year 2015 there will be 22. Five of these cities will have more than 20 million inhabitants, all but Toyko being in the developing world (e.g., Mumbai, India; Delhi, India; Mexico City, Mexico; Sao Paulo, Brazil). In the United States only New York and Los Angeles are expected to have more than 10 million inhabitants by 2015 (Marshall 2005).

The control of toxic wastes in such cities is a problem of staggering proportions. The Indonesian capital of Jakarta, for example, has a population of 12 million (21 million if you count the surrounding suburban towns). Air pollution contributes to thousands of deaths and millions of asthma attacks per year. In Jakarta 12.6 percent of deaths are due to respiratory inflammation. This is twice the rate of the rest of the country (Marshall 2005). Most of these deaths are due to airborne particulate matter caused by a lack of emissions controls on cars. Automobile, truck and motorcycle emissions account for 70 percent of the nitrogen oxides and particulate matter emitted into Jakarta's air (Marshall 2005). Swamps and rivers in the city serve as sewers and trash disposal sites. In Jarkata less than 3 percent of the city's sewage reaches a sewage treatment plant. Yet 1.3 million cubic meters of sewage are created each day in the greater Jakarta area.

Further, pollutants in one region of the world affect persons in other regions of the world. This is known to be the case with air pollution, as it is easy to understand the worldwide distribution of air and suspended particles such as dust. However, there are other examples that have not become apparent until the past few decades. For example, people around the world are being exposed to more and more man-made chemicals that are designed to control pests (insecticides, fungicides). This is a major issue in food contamination. A report by the BBC in 2002 (June 19, 2002) indicates that a committee of the government of the United Kingdom that oversees pesticide levels in food found that of 15 types of fruit and vegetables tested, 11 had pesticide residues in excess of the maximum recommended levels. The fruits included strawberries and grapes, and the vegetables included potatoes. Residues of pesticides were found in 25 of 27 samples of lemons examined, 71 of the 73 fresh salmon samples and 115 of the 179 strawberries tested. Pesticides that are not approved by the British government were found on strawberries, mushrooms and lettuce. In many cases, these foods were grown outside the United Kingdom.

Given the worldwide marketing of food and produce, contaminants in one region can easily affect consumers in other regions. Woolf (2005) found, for example, that some imported spices from India and the Republic of Georgia contained levels of lead that were hundreds of times greater than the limits set by United States food standards.

Another example of the effects of worldwide circulation of pollutants has recently been documented by Cone (2005) in her book on contamination of the Arctic region. The Arctic is generally thought to be a pristine environment, free of factory and most agricultural contaminants, as well as having low levels of vehicular-based pollutants. However, recent data from the Arctic Monitoring and Assessment Program indicate that pesticides and industrial pollutants are found in high concentrations in whales and seals in the Arctic. The pollution is contained in food sources ingested by these animals as they migrate from south to north. Whales and seals are the traditional food source for the Inuit peoples of the region. Due to high levels of contamination of these food sources, there are negative effects on the human immune system resulting in high rates of infections in the Inuit population. Further, high levels of mercury in the primary food animals have been shown to relate to neurological damage to fetuses and later learning problems (see heavy metal pollution in Chapter 14).

The majority of research on environmental hazards to health is concentrated on outdoor contamination. However, most people spend the majority of their time indoors. Perhaps for this reason, the level of risk due to indoor contamination is generally considered to be less than those generated by outdoor risks. However, new research has questioned this assumption. One group of man-made chemicals that is known to increase health risks are volatile organic compounds (VOCs) that arise from sources such as air fresheners, cleaning agents and cigarette smoke. Adgate, et al. (2004) outfitted 71 non-smoking volunteers in Minneapolis and St. Paul with lapel-mounted air filters from which concentrations of VOCs were tested. Of 15 VOCs that were designated by the Clean Air Act as hazardous, these researchers found that 14 were present in much higher concentrations in indoor samples than outdoor samples had previously suggested. For example, in the Adgate, et al. study the median exposure to benzene was 3.2 micrograms per cubic meter of air among the volunteer subjects, whereas outdoor concentrations were 1.3 micrograms per cubic meter of air. VOCs that were tested included chloroform, a by-product of chlorination of household water, and d-limonene and 1- and b-pinene, both of which are common in deodorizing chemicals. Of the 14 compounds tested in which high concentrations were found, the concentrations were three to 60 times the concentrations obtained in outdoor monitors.

Despite the alarming increase in the number of man-made chemical compounds and the rise of mega-cities with all the problems of air and water contamination that these trends imply, there has been steady progress in controlling and reducing some of the better known types of air and water pollutants in the wealthier countries of the world. For example, carbon monoxide as measured by 387 air monitoring stations in the United States has been reduced from six parts per million in 1990 to 2.8 parts per million in 2003. Particulate matter has been reduced from 30.8 micrograms per square meter of air to 23.5 micrograms per square meter (United States Census Bureau 2006). The data over longer periods is even more impressive. For example, lead contaminants in the air have been reduced from more than 220,000 tons in 1970 to less than 2,000 in 2003 (United States Census Bureau 2006).

Despite the impressive nature of these advances it is clear that progress has been made for only a few chemicals, those for which there has been a long history of toxic effects. The sheer number of toxic substances produced and emitted into the air and water are currently so large and increasing so rapidly, that it is clear that the toxic effects of the vast majority of chemicals in the marketplace are unknown. Further, the effects on pregnant women and their offspring have just begun to be studied, so there is a vast amount of work to be done in order to understand the relative risks of exposures to a wide range of man-made substances.

In order to get a better appreciation for the complexity of the problem faced by the research community in determining fetal toxicity of any given chemical, it is important to have a brief introduction to the variables that contribute to toxic reactions.

An Introduction to Toxicology

Over the past 15 years there has been a dramatic increase in recognition of the susceptibility of children, particularly very early in life, to exposure to environmental toxins (Colburn and Clement 1992; Daston, et al. 2004). As a part of this recognition there have been attempts to understand the many factors that affect the toxicity of a particular agent for children at a given stage of development. One useful framework for understanding risks of exposure to toxins has been developed by the Risk Science Institute of the International Life Sciences Institute. This framework has been summarized by Daston, et al. (2004). Its focus was understanding toxicity in children and adolescents. For the purposes of this book we will address the fetal and perinatal periods of development.

One of the first issues in ascertaining risk to an individual is to determine the amount of a potentially toxic substance that was brought into contact with the physiology of the developing individual. In almost all toxic reactions, a dose-response curve is expected in which a greater toxic reaction is expected as the dose is increased. Determining the dose is a complex process. In the case of air pollution, for example, most researchers simply chart the air quality in a given region on one or more occasions, then correlate that air quality with physiological responses or behavioral changes. But the dose that a pregnant woman and her fetus are exposed to might vary by (a) time spent outdoors, (b) proximity of the home to a point source of air pollutants (e.g., petrochemical plants; a busy street), (c) how deeply the mother breathes the air and the volume of air that is breathed during a given period of time (e.g., mothers who jog early in pregnancy versus those that are sedentary) and (d) the health of the lung and cardiovascular systems of the mother. Thus, even if the mother wears an air quality monitor, which is a major improvement in measuring the dose of air contaminants, this does not represent the exact dose that this mother receives at the physiological level.

Another complication of this type of research involves the issue of whether to measure the amount of the focal compound that the mother received (e.g., a compound in an insecticide), or to measure metabolites of the compound once the biochemical processes of the body have broken this compound down and the active ingredient is metabolized in the body. A third complication is that toxicologists differentiate exposure scenarios; that is, was maternal exposure sporadic (e.g. maternal alcohol ingestion), continuous (e.g., air pollution) or did it occur during a single occurrence (e.g., ingestion of contaminated food). A further issue is how maternal exposure scenarios relate to the exposure scenarios of the fetus. A one-to-one correspondence cannot be assumed. For example, a sporadic or even one-time exposure of the mother may expose the fetus on a more continuous basis. Such an event would occur if a compound whose toxic ingredient is fat soluble and accumulates in the fatty tissues of the mother and then leaches out into the blood stream exposing the fetus.

After issues of dose are considered, a researcher must address the route of uptake of the agent. For children and adults, there are three primary mechanisms of uptake: gastrointestinal absorption, dermal penetration or respiratory tract absorption. In the case of a developing fetus the route of uptake is primarily through the placental barrier via the blood stream of the mother. This raises many questions about the basic physiology of the placental barrier. Of particular interest in the developing fetus is the permeability of the placental barrier.

Until very recently it was assumed that the placental barrier was relatively impermeable to most chemical compounds that might harm the fetus. Unfortunately, it is now known that this assumption was in error. Current data indicate that most chemicals can cross the placenta, although the rate at which they cross is affected by a number of factors such as the molecular size of the chemical. Large molecular size slows the rate of transport across the barrier (Colburn and Clement 1992; Ginsberg, et al. 2002). This means that, in most cases, exposure of the mother to toxic chemicals leads to exposure of the fetus; the only issue is how quickly the exposure occurs.

In addition to the placental barrier, a barrier between the blood supply and brain tissue protects the central nervous system (CNS) from environmental contaminants. However, it is now known that the blood-brain barrier in early life is more permeable than it is for older children and adults. Thus, equal amounts of a toxin can produce higher chemical concentrations in the CNS in the prenatal and immediate postnatal periods than it would later in development (Daston, et al. 2004). Unfortunately, this is also the period of greatest CNS growth. Thus, greater permeability of the blood-brain barrier suggests a window of vulnerability of the CNS in very early life to environmental toxins.

A third set of variables that affect the risks of any particular agent on maternal or fetal physiology are referred to as toxicokinetic factors. These relate to the basic biochemical and physiological characteristics of the agent and its effect on the human body. Primary among the questions addressed at this level are rates and extent of absorption, distribution, metabolism and excretion (ADME) of a particular agent. There are many problems in characterizing these toxicokinetic effects for the fetus.

First, for ethical reasons, research on fetal toxicology must often be extrapolated from animal data. Sometimes data are available on adult humans and these data can be extrapolated. In either case, due to the singular characteristics of the fetal environment, these extrapolations may contain significant error. Further, assessment of ADME characteristics of a chemical must take into account large individual differences between mothers in such factors as rate of metabolism.

A fourth complication in determining toxic effects is that many toxins are stored in the body. Storage may be in fat, bone or muscle. An overweight mother, for example, may present more of a toxic environment for the fetus due to the increased volume of toxin-storing fat that the mother has accumulated throughout her life. The overall health of the mother may also play a role in fetal toxicity because many toxins are altered by the body and then eliminated via pulmonary gas exchange, in urine or in feces. If the mother suffers from renal difficulties (problems with kidney functioning), for example, this pathway for detoxification may not be as efficient, which may increase the exposure to the fetus.

Age-specific effects of many of these factors comprise a fifth concern. Absorption, distribution, metabolism and excretion of toxins vary enormously by the age of the fetus, due to the rapidity of the changes in physiology of the developing organism. For example, in very early life, metabolism is slowed. This may reduce the formation of toxic metabolites, but also slow the removal of the agent through the detoxification pathways. Supportive of this example is the finding that renal functioning is immature during the first weeks of life. This leads to a prolonged half-life of some pesticides (e.g., organochlorines) whose toxic effects are highly influenced by available fats in the body. These toxins may have reduced effects very early in fetal development, compared to the late perinatal period, due to low levels of fat at the early stages of development (Daston, et al. 2004).

A final set of considerations involves the developmental stages at which a particular organ system may be most vulnerable to toxic perturbation. It has been emphasized many times in this book that a variety of experts view the prenatal period as one of particular susceptibility due to the rapid changes in organ system development. Within the prenatal period, however, there are periods of more rapid development that seem to create particular windows of vulnerability for particular types of CNS tissue. With regard to the CNS, almost all systems originate during the first six weeks of life. However, some systems mature much sooner than others. For example, the spinal cord, medulla and pons are among the first to develop and are relatively complete within the first eight weeks of life. Other brain structures such as the hypothalamus, stratum, amygdala, limbic cortex and neocortex continue to develop through at least the 28th week of gestation, and some developmental processes continue until the second postnatal year (Faustman, et al. 2003).

Developing tissues and organs that influence many aspects of subsequent development participate in complex interactions during the prenatal period. As we have seen in Chapter 2 of this volume, these aspects include cell proliferation, migration, and apoptosis. Tissue populations that interact in this way during development share several characteristics as outlined by Daston, et al. (2004).

First, populations of cells interact, as opposed to individual cells. Second, the populations of interacting cells have differing developmental histories. Third, the populations of interacting cells are proximate to one another. Four, one population of cells transmits a message of importance for the development of a second population of cells and fifth, the second population of cells has the capability to receive the message. Thus, the development of any one organ and tissue system can be altered by pollutants by (a) altering the length of the period in which the cell populations communicate, (b) diminishing the amount of the chemical messenger that is transmitted between cell populations, (c) interference with reception of the chemical signal or (d) preventing the appropriate activity of the cell population receiving the message.

The nature of the interactions of cell types in human fetal development is incredibly complex and allows for a variety of actions of environmental toxins. Daston and his colleagues have described this vulnerability: "Because developing tissues and organs rely on such complex, temporally orchestrated interactions ... they are exquisitely sensitive to perturbations of their environment." (Daston, et al. 2004, pg. 252).

Given the paucity of (a) data on the basic toxicokinetics (absorption, distribution, metabolism and excretion) of any given chemical at any one time point in the developmental history of the children; (b) the large gaps in the knowledge of sensitive periods for specific tissues and systems of the CNS and (c) the number of environmental chemicals to which pregnant women and their fetuses are exposed is potentially large, the vast majority of research on fetal toxicology works backwards. That is, groups of children are identified who have a particular physiological or developmental anomaly (e.g., asthma, memory problems); and then the environments in which these children developed are examined to help determine a developmental pathway. In many cases the most difficult aspect of the environment to study is the prenatal environment, because the prenatal history is from three to 10 years old by the time the variables can be measured and isolated.

Other difficulties exist in researching environmental toxin pathways. For example, determining the presence of abnormal numbers of effects on women and their children is predicated on the assumption of uniform exposures. This is almost never the case.

Despite the difficulties of determining the risk of a given toxin during prenatal development, and the obvious shortcomings of research in this area, a great deal has been learned about the risks of a variety of chemical substances for human fetal development. This is the subject of Section E.

Chapter 12
Air and Water Pollution

The focus of this chapter is on air and water pollution and its effects on pregnancy and fetal development. With a few exceptions, this topic has been poorly researched with regard to long-term effects on child learning and behavior. However, there is a rapidly expanding literature on the extent of air and water pollution in the United States and around the world. Studies of these effects on offspring are beginning to appear in highly regarded scientific journals. It is the purpose of this chapter to make the reader aware of the nature and extent of air and water pollution, and to summarize some of the available studies that report outcomes for infants and children.

Air Pollution

Human beings have always existed in environments in which the air they breathed was at times unhealthy. Pollens, dust and smoke from grass and forest fires must have been problems for early man as they are today. However, each new technological development seems to be accompanied by some increased chance of pollutants. For example, since the discovery of fire and the advent of bringing fire into the home, human beings have been exposed to the products of combustion, including polluting gases and particulate matter contained in smoke. The industrial revolution brought human beings into contact with higher levels of combustion gases, as well as the chemicals that were developed to fuel machines (e.g., petrochemicals).

Raloff (2006) dates modern interest in the health effects of air pollution to a 1952 five-day smog in London that killed 12,000 people. Recent data shows that as many as 60,000 United States residents (usually the very young and the elderly) die each year from heart attacks and respiratory problems related to air pollutants (Raloff 2006). There is little research on the effects of prenatal exposures to air pollution, and no strong studies of long-term developmental effects related to prenatal exposures. However, researchers have repeatedly demonstrated neonatal effects of air pollution during the past two decades.

The Environmental Protection Agency (EPA) and similar groups around the world have studied the major pollutants of the air. Primary among them are carbon monoxide,

R.P. Martin and S.C. Dombrowski, *Prenatal Exposures: Psychological and Educational Consequences for Children.*
© Springer 2008

sulfur dioxide, nitrogen dioxide, ozone and particulate matter that is carried by the air. The following is a description of these pollutants and their general effects on health. This will be followed by a description of air pollution effects on the newborn.

Carbon Monoxide (CO)

CO is a gas that is undetectable by humans. It is odorless, colorless and tasteless. It results, primarily, from the combustion of fuels when some of the carbon is not completely burned. Vehicles burning fossil fuel account for 95 percent of the carbon monoxide that is detected in cities. Other sources include industrial exhaust from burning processes and wildfires.

Carbon monoxide levels vary by season. They are highest during cold weather, because vehicles and other equipment do not burn fuels as efficiently in cold weather as in warm weather. Also, homes heated by fuel combustion (wood, fuel oils) in the winter may contain high levels of carbon monoxide. Further, cold weather can cause temperature inversions. Normally, warm air near the surface of the earth rises to higher levels (warm air is lighter). This process carries pollutants away from the ground and dilutes them in the atmosphere. Cold air from mountains falls and, in some weather conditions, can remain at the surface of the earth particularly being trapped in valleys and low-lying areas in which humans often build cities. Thus, cities like Salt Lake City (built in a mountain valley) and Los Angeles (in a coastal area near mountains) are particularly susceptible to temperature inversions. Such inversions trap the polluted air in low-lying areas and greatly increase human exposure to pollution, including carbon monoxide, at relatively concentrated levels.

The negative effects of carbon monoxide are most often felt by persons with cardiovascular disease. Even among healthy persons, it can cause chest pains and other symptoms, particularly if the exposure occurs during exercise. According to the United States Environmental Protection Agency (*www.epa.gov/airnow/background.html*), very young children and fetuses (the gas crosses the placental barrier) may also be at risk from high carbon monoxide levels, although extensive data are not currently available.

Support for the adverse effects of carbon monoxide has been widely reported. For example, Yang, Chen, Yang and Ho (2004) studied the rate of hospital admissions for cardiovascular-related illnesses in Taiwan and possible associations with ambient levels of carbon monoxide, ozone and other pollutants. They found that, during the cold days of the year, all pollutants except ozone were significantly associated with increased hospital admissions. However, carbon monoxide levels had the strongest association with admissions for cardiovascular symptoms.

Sulfur dioxide (SO$_2$)

Sulfur dioxide is a gas produced by sulfur-containing fuels such as coal and oil. It is emitted in highest volume from power plants and some industrial boilers. Under normal conditions several physiological processes remove most SO$_2$ as it passes through nasal passages. However, under conditions of high oxygen use (e.g., exercise) it is inhaled deep into the lungs and can cause adverse health effects for persons with cardiovascular disease or chronic lung disease (e.g., asthma). Children and persons of advanced age seem most at risk. For example, Lin, et al. (2004) have documented a short-term association between levels of sulfur dioxide and hospital admissions of children with asthma symptoms.

Nitrogen dioxide (NO₂)

Nitrogen dioxide is a pollutant that is emitted by all combustion processes, such as the burning of fossil fuels in automobiles and the burning of coal in power plants. It plays a key role in the photochemically induced catalytic production of ozone that has a number of known negative effects on human health. Nitrogen dioxide in the air also results in increased levels of nitric acid deposits in soils and on plants. Recent studies (Richter, Burrows, Nuss, Granier and Niemeier 2005) based on satellite instrumentation measurements have shown that concentrations of nitrogen dioxide are decreasing in the United States and in Europe, but are greatly increasing in the industrial regions of China where increased fossil fuel use is taking place.

Lin, et al. (2004) have shown that there is an immediate effect of nitrogen dioxide, sulfur dioxide and other gaseous air pollutants (e.g., excluding particulate matter) on hospital admissions. Studying hospitalization of children ages six through 12 in Vancouver, they found a direct dose-response association between the number of asthma hospitalizations and levels of nitrogen dioxide and sulfur dioxide after controlling for ambient temperatures and relative humidity. Interestingly, the effects varied by socioeconomic classification, gender and type of pollutant. For nitrogen dioxide, significant positive associations were obtained for males in the low socioeconomic group, but not in the high socioeconomic group. For females, the same socioeconomic pattern was observed, when investigating sulfur dioxide. These differences may be the result of differing housing and play patterns of children in different socioeconomic groups. Children in lower socioeconomic groups may spend more time in outdoor play in areas that are proximate to sources of pollutants.

Ozone (O₃)

Ozone is a gas composed of three atoms of oxygen. Ozone occurs in the Earth's upper atmosphere and is helpful in reducing the level of ultraviolet energy (UV) that can be harmful to health. As the ozone hole over Antarctica increases in size, the risks of skin cancer due to the effects of UV increase. However, ozone also occurs at ground level. Ground level ozone is a pollutant and is harmful to health. It is created when pollutants emitted by vehicles, industrial plants, power plants and refineries react with sunlight. According to the Environmental Protection Agency (*www.epa.gov/airnow/background.html*) one in every three people in the United States is at risk of some health problem due to ground level ozone.

Ozone can have several effects, such as increasing susceptibility to respiratory infections and inflammation of the lining of the lungs. Chronic inflammation of the lungs can cause scarring of lung tissue. Ozone can have the immediate effect of irritating the respiratory system, causing coughing and throat irritation. It also aggravates asthma and other chronic lung conditions. For reasons that are unclear, there are known to be large individual differences in susceptibility to the negative effects of ozone. However, it is known to be most harmful to people who are active outdoors (children, athletes, outdoor workers) because physical activity causes the ozone to be pulled deep into the lungs, affecting more sensitive areas over a greater area of lung tissue.

Urch et al. (2005) studied the effects of ozone and particulate matter on cardiac and pulmonary functioning in a laboratory setting. They instructed volunteers to breath either filtered air or air that contained the amount of ozone and particulate matter typical for persons living or working in a heavily polluted city or in a traffic tunnel. The polluted air contained 150 micrograms of particles per cubic meter and 120 ozone molecules per billion air molecules. Those volunteers who were exposed to the polluted air experienced, on average, a 10 percent increase in diastolic blood pressure (the low pressure number). In the healthy young volunteers used in the study, this effect is short-term and caused no health problems. But in patients with subclinical high blood pressure (including some pregnant women), this small increase could push them into the clinical levels of hypertension.

Kim, Lee, Hong, Ahn and Kim (2004) documented that ozone has a direct effect on mortality and seems to operate as a threshold variable. They studied several models of the effect of ambient ozone on death rates in Seoul, Korea. They found a 2.6 percent increase in estimated relative risk in total mortality associated with a 21.5 ppb (parts per billion) increase of daily one hour maximum ozone lagged by one day using a linear model. Using a threshold model they found a 3.4 percent increase in estimated relative risk. There was also a seasonal effect. The relative risk of the threshold model was greatest in summer. These results indicated that mortality increased the day after a peak in ozone, but little effect was found at lower levels of ozone.

High ozone exposure has also been linked to immune system functioning in animal studies. Dohm, et al. (2005) studied cane toads in Hawaii. They found that micophages (a small cell that ingests and destroys bacteria and other foreign matter) from the amphibian's lungs were damaged, and failed to engulf foreign particles, one of the most important functions of this type of immune system cell. Nearly 40 percent of the cells harvested failed to carry out this function and many others had less than optimal responses.

From the point of view of potential damaging effects of air pollution on reproduction, increased levels of ambient ozone have been linked to sperm quality. Sokol et al. (2005) found that sperm counts were lower when the subjects lived in a high ozone area one to 14 or 70 to 90 days prior to semen donation to sperm banks. The research was noteworthy for the finding that other air pollutants were not associated with sperm quality and count.

Particulate Matter

Particulate matter (or particle pollution) includes mixtures of solid particles and liquid droplets that are suspended in the air. The damage imparted by particulate matter depends, to some extent, on the size of the particle. Particles greater than 10 micrometers (10 one-millionths of a meter) are thought to be less harmful to health than smaller particles. These larger particles do not remain suspended in the air for significant periods of time and are more easily visible so they can be avoided. Some sawdust particles, for example, would be of this size. On the other hand, particles less than 10 micrometers, a size smaller than the width of a human hair, have been shown to be harmful to health. Suspended material ranging from 10 micrometers to 2.5 micrometers is considered 'course' particulate matter. Examples include materials emitted from grinding operations in industrial settings and dust stirred up by vehicles on roads. The most harmful particulates are those less than 2.5 micrometers (called 'fine' particulate). They are so small that an electron microscope is required to detect their presence. These include particles from all types of combustion including motor vehicles, power plants, forest fires, agricultural burning and some industrial burning.

Particulate matter exposure causes health problems when particulate becomes lodged in the smallest recesses of lung tissue and, as a result, impedes the ability of this tissue to absorb oxygen. Once lodged in lung tissue, particulate matter not only increases respiratory effort, it can hamper cardiac function requiring the heart to work at higher rates to transport sufficient oxygen. Persons most affected by particulate matter pollution include people with heart and lung disease, older adults and children. The effect on children is correlated with age; the younger the child, the greater the effect since younger children have reduced lung capacity. Particulate concentration has been associated with cardiac arrhythmias and heart attacks. Persons with asthma or any chronic lung disease are particularly sensitive to high concentrations of particulate matter.

Somers, Yuak, White, Parfett and Quinn (2002) report evidence that microscopic particles cause heritable mutations by damaging the DNA of cells that produce sperm. The studies have been done with birds (herring gulls nesting near steel mills) and laboratory animals (mice). In their latest study Somers, McCarry, Malek and Quinn (2004) reported that when mice reared in an industrial setting breathed only filtered air, they experienced no more DNA damage than those raised in a rural setting. Those raised in the same industrial setting without filtered air had significantly more DNA damage to germ cells and a greater number of mutations. This research indicates that the causative agent was particulate matter that can be filtered, not the gases emitted from the industrial plant.

In a study of humans Peng, Dominick, Pastor-Barriuso, Zegler and Samet (2005) investigated the association between particulate matter concentrations in the largest 100 cities in the United States and deaths the following day, for each day from 1987 through 2000. They found that an increase of 10 micrograms per cubic meter of air of PM10 (particulate matter less than 10 micrometers) was associated with an average increase in deaths on the following day of 0.19 percent. These researchers also found large regional and seasonal differences in the association between particulate matter and mortality. For example, in the Northeast mortality rose in summer by almost 1 percent on any day after a 10 microgram per liter of air increase in PM10 particulates. The same increase only resulted in a 0.1 percent increase in deaths in mid-winter, perhaps because people spent less time outdoors. In Southern California, by contrast, a 10 microgram per cubic meter increase in particulate matter increased deaths by 0.5 percent year-round. This was attributed to the lack of seasonal variability in climate in Southern California and the activity patterns of persons in this region.

Combined Effects of Various Air Pollutants

The EPA produces a daily Air Quality Index (AQI) for 275 cities in the United States. This index is an aggregate of all five of the air pollutants described above and has a range from zero to 500. Calibrated on the basis of national air quality standards, a score of 100 or below is considered healthy air. Scores in the range of 101 to 150 are considered unhealthy for sensitive groups (e.g., the elderly, asthma patients), 151 to 200 is unhealthy for everyone, 201 to 300 is very unhealthy and 301 and above is considered hazardous. This index can be obtained for the monitored cities on the Internet (*www.epa.gov/airnow*).

The health risks from air pollution are partly attributable to the high correlation among concentrations of these different air pollutants. As they vary with time of day, season and region, all five of the pollutants typically vary together. Since many of these pollutants have common origins (e.g., vehicle emissions), it is not surprising that the pollutants associated with this source would increase during periods of high vehicle volume. Lee et al. (2003) reported the correlations among four different pollutants in Seoul, Korea measured at 20 different sites and calculated 24-hour averages across the region. The vast majority of the correlations were in the 0.68 to 0.86 range among sulfur dioxide, nitrogen dioxide and carbon monoxide particulate matter. One implication of this research is that individuals are exposed to multiple pollutants and the resulting effects are cumulative across pollutants and time.

Outcome Studies for Pregnant Women

The effect of air pollution has been most widely investigated with respect to its effect on birth weight. In general, studies conducted in several countries (China, Czech Republic, United States) have shown that there is an inverse relationship between air pollution and birth weight, with high levels of air pollution resulting in lower birth weight (Bobak 2000; Maisonet, Bush, Correa and Jaakkola 2001; Jedrychowski, et al. 2004; Perera, et al. 2004; Wang, Ding, Ryan and Xu 1997).

This relationship has practical significance since low birth weight has been shown to increase infant mortality and subsequent morbidity, including learning and behavior problems of children (see Chapter 3).

Berkowitz et al. (2003) studied a group of women in New York City who were pregnant at the time of the World Trade Center (WTC) collapse on September 11, 2001. The attack on the WTC and its subsequent collapse released high amounts of particulate matter including heavy metals and gases such as polycyclic aromatic hydrocarbons (PAH). Berkowitz and colleagues tested the assertion that high levels of PAH and particulate matter caused fetal growth retardation. To test this hypothesis, Berkowitz et al. found a matched control group of women who gave birth during the same period, but who did not live in the WTC neighborhood. They found that 8.2 percent of the babies in the WTC group were in the lowest 10 percent of birth weight for gestational age, compared to 3.8 percent of the control group. Because of the high levels of PAH and particulate matter released in the WTC collapse, the authors were unable to determine the specific contaminant that was most associated with growth retardation.

Perera et al. (2003) studied the effects of PAH on birth outcomes of a multiethnic population of African-American and Dominican women in New York. PAH was measured by personal air sampling devices. This study controlled for pesticide exposure through measurement of plasma metabolites of widely used pesticides, and limited the sample to women who did not smoke. They found that PAH was associated with decreased birth weight and birth length in these populations. In a subsequent report, Lederman et al. 2004 reported that women in the first trimester of pregnancy at the time of the WTC event had shorter gestations (-3.6 days) and infants with a smaller head circumference (-0.48 centimeters) than women in the later stages of pregnancy.

Similar findings have occurred in other countries for more typical levels of urban pollution. For example, Jedrychowski et al. (2004) studied exposure of 362 pregnant women in Poland to fine particulate matter (less than 2.5 micrometers in diameter) who gave birth between 34 and 43 weeks of gestation. These women were between 18 and 35 years of age, were non-smokers and had given birth to singletons. They found that, as fine particulate matter exposures increased, birth weight, birth length, and head circumference decreased.

Effects are not limited to low birth weight and other indicators of fetal size. Mendola (2005) studied births between 1997 and 2000 in seven Texas counties and the quality of the air in these counties. The focus of the study was on air quality early in pregnancy. These researchers found that women who had been exposed to high concentrations of carbon monoxide, sulfur dioxide or particulate matter were more likely than other women to have infants with heart defects. Similar effects have been found by other research groups (e.g., Ritz, et al. 2002).

In a recent systematic review of the literature on the association between air pollution and birth weight, Sram, Binkova, Dejmek and Bobak (2005) concluded that air pollution contributes to low birth weight and other indicators of fetal growth (length). Other effects of fetal health have not been sufficiently studied to make firm conclusions. Further, Sram et al. (2005) note that additional studies are needed to confirm the size of the effect and to clarify the most vulnerable periods during gestation for different pollutants.

Summary

Ozone, nitrogen dioxide, carbon monoxide, sulfur dioxide, and particulate matter are known to have negative effects on pulmonary functioning. These negative effects often result in increased stress to the cardiovascular system (high blood pressure, increased heart rate). The cardiovascular systems of pregnant women are already under stress due to increased blood volume, weight gain and circulatory problems associated with pregnancy. Further, the developing fetus depends entirely on the blood supply of the mother. Thus, factors that increases stress on the pulmonary or cardiovascular system of the mother may reduce oxygen levels or blood flow to the fetus. If the mother is healthy, such effects are likely to be marginal. However, if a pregnant mother has high blood pressure, heart disease or other health problems that reduce the efficiency of the pulmonary and cardiovascular systems (e.g., obesity), air pollution may have a significant effect on fetal growth and development.

Water Pollution

Water pollution has many sources. These include agricultural chemicals that run off into streams and rivers that are used as drinking water supply. Industrial waste also is found in drinking water. As is the case with agricultural chemicals, industrial pollutants can run off or be directly deposited into drinking water supplies. In addition, the chemicals that are used to purify water can have adverse health effects. Since water is one of nature's most effective solvents, a vast array of chemicals, both natural and man-made, can be carried by surface or subterranean water sources. Agricultural and industrial sources have been studied most often and will be given primary emphasis in this review. Finally, the research in relation to water purification will also be discussed.

A recent report by the United States Geological Survey on the water quality in streams and groundwater concluded that almost all of America's fresh water is tainted with low concentrations of chemical contaminants (Barnes et al. 2004). For example, more than 90 percent of all the water samples taken have detectable amounts of organic contaminants, including pharmaceuticals and hormones. Pesticides are found in water supplies in urban areas, as well as in farming areas where pesticides are applied to fields to reduce insect damage to crops. Although most surveys find that the majority of contaminants were well below Environmental Protection Agency standards for adverse effects on human health, such data point out that the human water supply is vulnerable to contamination by a wide range of agents.

Approximately 90 percent of households in America depend on public water supplies to provide tap water for drinking, bathing and household chores (*http:// www.epa.gov/safewater/creg.hjtml*). The remaining households have access to underground water supplies through wells or rely on water brought by truck and placed in cisterns. Because human beings are almost continually exposed to water through ingestion, inhalation and absorption, the quality of the water supply is of critical importance. Because water contamination is generally recognized as such an important public health issue, the federal government has enacted a number of legislative efforts to control water quality. The Safe Drinking Water Act is one of the most important of these policies. Through this act the Environmental Protection Agency has been designated to evaluate water quality.

Agricultural Pollutants

In 1962 Rachel Carson wrote the classic volume "Silent Spring," in which she documented the effects of organochlorine pesticides. These pesticides were frequently used at the time to control insects on farms and mosquitoes in populated areas. The most famous of these organochlorine compounds was DDT (dichlorodiphenyltrichloroethane). The appeal of DDT as an insecticide was that it had broad-spectrum potency and was resistant to breakdown (Raloff 2006). However, these same properties increased its potential as a toxin for other species, including humans. Organochlorines are now controlled in the United States and Europe, and to a lesser extent around the world.

Following the elimination or control of organochlorines, organophosphates became the most widely used agricultural and residential pesticide. Members of this group of pesticides included malathion and chlorpyrifos. As was the case for organochlorines, organophosphates were effective, but were found to have long lasting toxic effects on animals and humans. As a result of an accumulation of scientific evidence about toxic effects, this class of insecticide has been stringently controlled since the middle of the 1990s (Raloff 2006).

The organophosphorus pesticide chlorpyrifos (CPF) is a case in point. The use of this pesticide was halted in the United States in 2000. However, it remains in use through much of the world. The problem with CPF is that it has been shown to have damaging effects on fetal development below levels that would cause neurotoxic effects in the mother (Clegg and van Gemert 1999a, 1999b). Thus, its effects may go undetected during pregnancy and at the time of birth. CPF was originally thought to have adverse effects on brain development through inhibition of cholinesterase. However, there is now evidence that it disrupts neural cell replication and differentiation, axonogenesis and synaptogenesis and the functional development of neurotransmitter and neurotrophin systems (Aldridge, Meyer, Seidler and Slotkin 2005; Barone, Das, Lassiter and White 2000). There is evidence that the dopaminergic and serotonergic systems are particularly vulnerable. Aldridge et al. (2005) have found that, in rat models, the period of greatest vulnerability is the immediate perinatal period. Testing adult rats that had been exposed just prior to birth, and others that had been exposed at various times after birth, Aldridge et al. (2005) found that serotonin systems were affected over wide regions of the adult brain. Dopaminergic activity in the hippocampal region was strongly affected. These studies and others (e.g., Garcia, Seidler and Slotkin 2003) implicate prenatal and perinatal exposure to chlorpyrifos as having adverse outcomes on brain development in animal models.

Since the 1990s producers and users of insecticides have turned more often to products based on the observation that chrysanthemums produce a natural insecticide and can help prevent insect infestations in home gardens. The active ingredient in the chrysanthemum is a group of chemicals called pyrethrins. Manufacturers of insecticides have for some time produced synthetic versions of pyrethrins (called pyrethroids) and these have been marketed as natural and benign pesticides. As was the case with the classes of insecticides previously used in the United States, pyrethroids that leach into streams and rivers are now being shown to kill beneficial insects and crustaceans, and may be poisoning fish and other organisms. However, the data are yet too sparse to determine the effects on the food chain, on water supplies and on humans (Raloff 2006).

In addition to insecticides, herbicides used for commercial and residential purposes are known to have unintended consequences. For example, atrozine is a common herbicide in a group referred to as triazine herbicides. It is typically applied in the spring and remains in water supplies for months after application due to runoff during rains. Several research groups have reported reproductive effects on amphibians and mammals, particularly testicular deformities in frogs and feminizing hormonal changes in mammals. The mechanism for these effects is unknown, but may involve acceleration of the conversion of male hormones into estrogen.

Recent research indicates that atrozine in trace amounts is actually more damaging to some life forms than exposure to concentrated amounts. Storrs and Kiesecker (2004) model these effects by studying frogs. These researchers found that tadpoles exposed to atrozine in doses of three parts per billion (pbb) were more likely to die than controls living in pure water, and more likely to die than other tadpoles living in higher concentrations (25 or 65 pbb). The effects of trace amounts of atrozine are particularly important because the United States EPA allows 3 ppb in United States drinking water. Other herbicides, such as mecoprop and dicamba, also seem to have more damaging effects at similarly low concentrations than at high concentrations.

Atrozine has also been implicated in a number of human reproduction problems. Munger et al. (1997) surveyed 856 Iowa municipal drinking water supplies in the late 1980s. These researchers looked at the reproductive problems associated with one particular water supply that contained elevated levels of triazine herbicides. Low birth weight, prematurity and intrauterine growth retardation in singleton births by women living in 13 communities served by the water system were compared to other communities of similar size in the region. The communities served by the water system with high levels of triazines had an 80 percent increased risk of IUGR (relative risk = 1.8). Regression analysis revealed that the herbicides atrozine, metolachlor and cyanzinc were each significant predictors of IUGR, but the association was strongest for atrozine.

One of the major problems in doing research on the effects of pesticides (insectides, herbicides and fungicides) on pregnant women and their offspring is the large number of these compounds that are now in use. The United States EPA's Office of Pesticide Programs estimates that 891 active ingredients were registered as of 1997 and that almost 900 million pounds of pesticide active ingredients were used in the United States in 2001 (Colburn 2006). Approximately 80 percent of pesticides are used in agriculture, 10 percent in home and garden applications and the remaining 10 percent by governments or industry around buildings and industrial plants (Bradman and Whyatt 2005). In most agricultural applications several chemicals are combined with different formulations used by different manufacturers. Often insecticides, herbicides and fungicides are combined in the same formulation. Given the complexity of these formulations and the number of them, "it is impossible to determine the cumulative risk posed to wildlife and humans… " (Colborn 2006). The problem is exacerbated by the fact that most neurodevelopmental effects cannot be seen at birth or directly observed even later in life. They are expressed in terms of how an individual behaves. Further, exposures are very difficult to determine. This is particularly true of nonpersistent pesticides, those that have a biological half-life ranging from hours to days (Bradman and Whyatt 2005).

The problem of pesticide use in farming, and in lawn and garden care, is not limited to those who perform the application or to those proximal to its use. Colborn (2006) states, "It is fairly safe to say that every child conceived today in the Northern hemisphere is exposed to pesticides from conception through gestation and lactation regardless of where it is born." (pg 10).

We have focused our discussion to this point on the outdoor use of pesticides. However, new evidence indicates that indoor pesticides may be a significant problem in the United States. Adgate et al. (2000) found in a study of Minnesota households that 97 percent stored pesticide products, and 88 percent of the households had used pesticides within the past five months. Whyatt et al. (2002) reported in a study of minority women that 85 percent reported that pest control chemicals had been used in their homes during at least one pregnancy. Berkowitz et al. (2003) studied pesticide exposures in a large group of pregnant women who delivered babies at Mount Sinai Hospital in New York City. These researchers found that urinary metabolites of pesticides (e.g., phenoxybenzoic acid) were at higher levels in these women than in other studies of adults in the United States. Further, some metobolites had temporal variations corresponding to seasonal spraying with pyrethroid pesticides. All these studies indicate that indoor pesticide use may represent a particular risk to pregnant women.

Industrial Waste

Industrial processes that are responsible for the wide range of products enjoyed by people around the world also produce toxins in high numbers. Many man-made chemicals used in manufacturing have toxic effects. Among the most toxic are solvents used to dissolve other chemicals or to clean machinery.

Bove, Shim and Zeitz (2002) reviewed several studies in which the effects of chlorinated solvents were investigated on pregnancy outcomes. They found that use of these solvents was significantly associated with birth defects, including neural tube defects, cardiac defects and choanal artresia (a nasal defect resulting in blocking of the airway).

A range of solvents is used in the dry cleaning industry, sometimes exposing workers to high doses. In one documented case a cleaning solvent (tetracholorethylene) was found in the water supply at Camp LeJune, North Carolina between 1965 and 1985. Its source was traced to a dry cleaning establishment on base. Tetracholorethylene is a volatile organic compound that is known to cross the placental barrier. During the period of the study, variations in the concentration of tetracholorethylene were found to be associated with births of infants that were small-for-gestational-age (Sonnenfeld, Hertz-Piccioto and Kaye 2001). For mothers with a history of fetal death, or who were over the age of 35, there was a significant association with low birth weight. The reason for the age effect was unclear.

Public health officials have expressed increasing concern about environmental chemicals with estrogenic activity that are typically encountered in water. These chemicals mimic some of the effects of the hormone estrogen. The ability of estrogenic hormones to affect sexual differentiation of the brain during prenatal development has been understood for some time (Hutchinson 1997). Environmental chemicals that have some of the same effects as estrogen have been linked to altered sexual development in amphibians (e.g., frogs, alligators) (Guillette, Pickford, Crain, Rooney and Percival 1996), and have been theoretically linked to reduction in male semen quality in humans (Carlsen, Giwercman, Keiding and Skakkedaek 1992). Within the current chapter we have seen that the herbicide atrozine has been documented to have estrogenic effects on sexual differentiation in amphibians. In addition to reproductive phenomena, research has shown that estrogen interacts with the dopaminergic and serotonergic systems of the brain. This leads to the possibility that prenatal exposure to environmental chemicals that mimic the effects of estrogen could have long-term effects on the behavior of offspring. Adriani, Seta, Dessi-Fulgheri, Farabollini and Laviola (2003) have addressed this question in a recent study in which mother rats were orally administered a common environmental chemical (bisphenol A) that is known to have estrogenic effects. Bisphenol A is a widespread chemical that is released from plastics, the lining of food cans and from dental sealants. This chemical has been shown to alter the developmental and adult sexual behavior of male rodents and their offspring (Atanassova, et al. 2000). The mother rats in this study were administered levels of Bisphenol A that would be comparable to those encountered by humans. The offspring of both sexes were tested during the rat equivalent of adolescence for novelty preference. Novelty preference or novelty seeking was of particular interest because dopamine levels are positively associated with novelty seeking. Further, the serotonergic system is known to modulate impulsive responding. For female rats tested in adolescence, the effects of exposure to Bisphenol A were a decrease in novelty seeking. In adulthood both male and female rats exhibited less impulsive behavior. In a further test, restlessness was assessed. Exposed adult males exhibited a low level of restlessness and their behavior resembled the behavior of adult females in this regard. Finally, the response of the animals to amphetamines was studied, and it was found that the males exposed to bisphenol A had less response to amphetamines than did unexposed males. When all of these findings were taken together, the authors interpreted the results to indicate that low levels of environmental estrogenic chemicals altered the monoaminergic (dopamine and serotonin) functioning of the brain, and in particular produced males who responded more like females in terms of restlessness and impulsive behavior. The pollutant can also be interpreted to have resulted in increased novelty-induced stress and reduced readiness to react to environmental challenges.

Due to the widespread exposure of humans to estogenic chemicals in water, this kind of result raises important health and behavioral questions. Unfortunately, most studies currently published utilize animal models, and short- and long-term effects on humans remain to be determined.

Water Treatment

Some of the water contaminants considered to be most threatening to pregnant women and the developing fetus are by-products of chlorination disinfection (DBPs). Chlorination is the primary disinfectant used in public water supplies. Its primary function is to control the level of bacterial agents in the water that could cause harmful infections in humans. However, chlorine reacts with organic matter, such as dead leaves and grasses found in lakes and streams, and produces chemical by-products that are known to have teratogenic effects. The most common chemical by-product of this interaction that has negative health effects are trihalomethanes (Bove, Shim, and Zeitz 2002). The concentration of trihalomethanes and other DBPs in drinking water supplies depends on many factors, including the source of the water (groundwater, lake, river), the distance between the water treatment plant and the household, the temperature of the water (thus, the season of the year) and the pH of the water (Bove, et al. 2002).

Bove, et al. (2002) reviewed the extant studies on the effects of DPBs (and other chlorine-based water contaminants) on pregnancy outcomes. All the studies utilized archival data supplied by the EPA on water quality in a specific area, and databases in which pregnancy outcomes are collected (birth certificate databases, fetal death certificates, birth defect registries). Bove and colleagues found that there was a consistent finding that high levels of DBPs were significantly associated with small-for-gestational-age births, neural tube defects and spontaneous abortions. These effects were found not to be confounded by maternal illness or low socio-economic level.

Hwang, Magnus and Jaakkolal (2002) also studied DPB concentrations in Norway, as well as a wider range of by-products than many former studies. The by-products assessed were trihalomethanes, chlorophenols, chloral hydrate and haloacetonitriles. Water level concentrations from the years spanning 1993 to 1998 were obtained, and associations with birth defects during the same period were studied. Water supplies were classified based on water color, with darker color being associated with the presence of higher levels of organic matter. Results indicated that chlorinated water with high levels of organic matter resulted in significantly increased numbers of births with cardiac, respiratory and urinary tract problems. Ventral-septal defects (a birth defect of the heart) were the only statistically significant effects.

The most ambitious study of this type was recently carried out by Toledano et al. (2005) in three regions of the United Kingdom. These researchers measured the concentration of trihalomethanes in water supplies. This assessment was used as a proxy for the concentration of DBPs in general. The outcomes studied were stillbirths and low birth weight. Across all three regions there was a significant association between high concentrations of thihalomethanes and stillbirths. In one region, there was an additional association with low birth weight. However, the latter findings may have been produced by an association between water quality and socioeconomic deprivation.

A study by Infante-Rivard (2004) indicates that some fetuses are more susceptible than others to the negative effects of drinking water disinfection by-products. The study includes 493 cases of intrauterine growth restriction, defined as birth weight below the 10th percentile for gestational age and sex, and a set of matched controls. Data on disinfection by-products were obtained from municipal authorities in the locations in which the mothers resided. Exposure to any specific or to the total amount of trihalomethanes did not increase the risk of intrauterine growth restriction. However, mothers and newborns who had one polymorphism in the CYP2E1 gene (G1259C) were much more likely to experience intrauterine growth restriction if they lived in a community with high levels of trihalomethanes. This finding indicates that exposure to by-products of disinfection of drinking water can affect fetal growth, but only in genetically susceptible newborns.

Some researchers have commented on the shortcomings of water treatment body of research. The primary weaknesses include (a) a lack of measurement of the concentration of a range of DBPs in the water, (b) a lack of measurement of individual differences in water use habits and (c) use of infrequent assessment of water contamination which does not take into account season, location or weather-related variables known to affect concentrations of DBPs (King, et al. 2004). With regard to water use patterns, King et al. point out that a single shower can equal the exposure to water contamination through dermal absorption of drinking two liters of tap water.

Thus, if accurate measurements of water use are to be obtained, it is necessary to assess water use patterns in personal hygiene, household chores (e.g., washing dishes) and drinking.

Spot Sources of Pollution

Landfills are the repositories of refuse from homes, industry and, sometimes, farms. Materials in landfills contain many toxic chemicals that can be causes of air and water pollution. Several studies have shown that living near landfills increases risks to pregnant women and their fetuses. Dolk et al. (1998) studied infants born to women living within three kilometers of landfill sites in five European countries and found that there was a 33 percent increase in the risk of congenital abnormalities. Palmer et al. (2005) studied data on congenital anomalies in areas in which landfills had recently been started. These researchers found a significant increase in birth anomalies from the time prior to the presence of the landfill, and after the landfill had been opened, for women who were pregnant and lived within two kilometers of the landfill.

Wilhelm and Ritz (2003) studied effects of ambient air pollution on offspring of women who lived proximate to heavy traffic roadways in Los Angeles County between 1994 and 1996. Proximity was found to increase the incidence of preterm birth. Further, the risk was particularly high for women whose third trimester occurred during the fall/winter of the year, a period when the air in the Los Angeles basis is most polluted.

Summary: Water Pollution

There are very few long-range studies of children who were prenatally exposed to water pollutants. Of those studies that have been conducted, the data support the contention that many types of pesticides, industrial solvents and a few other by-products of industrial processes (Bisphenol A) have long-term effects on children when they are exposed during the prenatal period. Reviewing all the factors which produce toxicological effects of chemical compounds, there is a clear need to more accurately assess the dosage and toxicokinetics effects of each chemical compound. However, the number of potential pollutants that are, or could be, dissolved in water supplies is so large, that the projected cost of this research is enormous. This means that the public health research community will always be behind the production capabilities of the agricultural and industrial communities. The first line of defense is for clinicians in psychology, psychiatry, neonatology and pediatrics to carefully note epidemiological patterns of behavioral and emotional disturbances, with an eye toward potential prenatal effects.

Chapter 13
Heavy Metals and Household Chemicals

In Chapter 12 we discuss the relationship between air and water pollution and developmental problems during the fetal period and later in development. Most pollutants are delivered to humans either through the air or water. Some pollutants, however, have specific and well-known effects. This chapter focuses on the adverse effects of some of these specific pollutants, including heavy metals and chemicals found in most homes, and a few industrial by-products.

Heavy Metal Pollution

Mercury Poisoning

During the 1950s, tons of mercury were dumped in Minamata Bay in Japan producing a major disaster that affected the health of many persons living around the Bay. Children and adults in the area reported symptoms of loss of motor control, incoherent speech and psychiatric symptoms. Some became blind. Children born to mothers who were pregnant at the time had high rates of cerebral palsy and mental retardation. Research summarized by Newland and Rasmussen (2003) has also shown that symptoms associated with this mercury exposure became worse as the exposed population aged. By 1993, 2,256 children and adults had been diagnosed with what came to be called Minamata disease (Harada 1995). The symptoms all were traced to methyl-mercury contamination of fish that had been eaten by persons around the Bay. This event, more than any other single event, has focused the research community on the effects of heavy metal contaminants on neural development.

Mercury is a naturally occurring, ubiquitous metal that comes in metallic or elemental forms. When elemental mercury is emitted as a by-product of combustion it becomes methylated in the environment and accumulates in animal tissues, particularly in fish (McDowell, et al. 2004). In a nationally representative study, McDowell et al. (2004) assayed hair samples during the 1994 to 2000 period and found that mercury levels in hair samples were associated with the age of the

R.P. Martin and S.C. Dombrowski, *Prenatal Exposures: Psychological and Educational Consequences for Children.*
© Springer 2008

subject and the frequency with which fish was consumed. Older women and women who consume fish more frequently had higher levels of mercury in their hair. Women who consumed fish on a frequent basis had hair mercury levels that were three times higher than national levels. The level of mercury in maternal health samples is of particular importance since maternal hair mercury levels predict brain levels in the fetus (Cernichiari, et al. 1995).

A recent study by the Office of Prevention, Pesticides and Toxic Substances at the Environmental Protection Agency raises further concern. They found that at least 300,000 of the 4 million births in the United States in 2000 may have been exposed to too much dietary mercury. The researchers looked at dietary logs of 1,700 women and tested for blood levels of mercury. Women who had eaten fish and shellfish at least twice a week had blood mercury levels seven times higher than those who did not eat fish in the previous month (Weise, April 2004).

Methyl mercury accumulates in the tissues and cannot be removed by any practical cooking method. Approximately 95 percent of the methyl mercury ingested is absorbed. From the bloodstream it is absorbed by all tissues and is fully distributed within one to two days after a single dose. It is excreted predominantly in feces, but also in urine and sweat. Methyl mercury accumulates at greater concentrations in brain, muscle and kidney tissues than in other tissue types (Hightower and Moore 2003). Methyl mercury crosses from the mother to the fetus where it binds to red blood cells and other fetal tissues. At birth, cord blood has on average twice the level of methyl mercury than would be obtained from blood samples of the mother (Hightower and Moore 2003).

Large, long-living predator fish have the highest concentrations of methyl mercury. Predator fish that are consumed by humans include swordfish, shark, tuna and king mackerel, among others. The United States Environmental Protection Agency set the reference for safe levels of methyl mercury dosage at 0.1 micrograms/per kilogram/per day, or about one can of tuna per week for pregnant women (Hubbs-Tait, Nation, Krebs and Bellinger 2005).

Animal studies summarized by Newland and Rasmussen (2003) show that cognitive and memory task performance of offspring seem unaffected by mercury exposure to mothers during pregnancy. However, epidemiological studies on humans have found exposure to high concentrations of methyl mercury, such as occurred in Minamata Bay, to be related to mental retardation (Harada 1995) and other severe clinical abnormalities (Cox, et al. 1989). A few studies have demonstrated that low to moderate levels of exposure have been found to be associated with more subtle changes in language, attention and memory. These results indicate a classic dose-response relationship.

One of the strongest studies of the prenatal effects of moderate to low levels of mecury was done by Grandjean, Weihe, White and Debes (1998). They studied 1,022 consecutive births in the Faroe Islands. The population was chosen because of the high concentration of fish in the diet. The level of mercury in the hair of the mothers of these infants was studied. Of particular interest in this study were children of women who had concentrations of mercury in their hair that were marginally less than the levels thought sufficient to cause prenatal neurological damage. At age seven the cognitive and neurological performance of children in this moderate exposure group was compared to a control group of children whose mothers had very low concentrations of mercury. On six neuropsychological measures, the performance of the case group (the moderately exposed group) was lower than that of the controls, although the differences were not large. Motor skills were particularly affected. For example, on a finger tapping test the case group had a median score of 54 and the control group a score of 58, a statistically significant difference. Error scores on a hand-eye coordination measure were also lower for the case group. There was a significantly lower score for the case group on the block designs subtest of the Wechsler Intelligence Scale for Children-Revised, but not on the other subscales of this measure. Sizeable and significant differences were also noted on the Boston Naming Test, a measure of ability to provide verbal labels for line drawings of objects. These differences were obtained even when maternal cognitive ability was controlled. The results of this study seem to indicate that even low to moderate concentrations of mercury in mothers is sufficient to produce meaningful differences in the cognitive performance of children.

Lead Exposure

Lead was one of the first metals to be extracted in quantity by humans. It has a relatively low melting point and is soft, so it could be shaped with unsophisticated tools. Lead beads used for decoration have been found that date to 7000 B.C. and the process of lead production is described in the Bible (Jeremiah, 6: 29-30) (Pueschel, Linakis and Anderson 1996).

Lead has also been known to have negative effects on health for a very long time. Some reports indicate that lead poisoning occurred in many ancient peoples, including the Egyptians, Greeks and Romans (Pueschel, et al. 1996). Unfortunately, lead was also used for medicinal purposes by the ancient Chinese and in Europe during the Middle Ages. In Germany in the 17th Century and in other parts of Europe lead acetate was used to sweeten sour wines. In the Americas rum was often distilled in lead pipes. Benjamin Franklin became interested in the negative health effects of rum and correctly identified lead as the causative factor (Pueschel, et al. 1996).

The particularly harmful effects of lead on children were first diagnosed at the turn of the 20th Century. Gibson in Australia is said to be the first person to document the negative effects of lead paint on children in 1904. In the United States the first reports of lead poisoning were published in 1914, in which the link between central nervous system insult and environmental lead was clarified (Pueschel, et al. 1996). Despite known toxic effects, lead use in the United States increased to 1,500,000 tons by 1977. It was used in gasoline until 1980. Sources of lead in the environment include soil residues from leaded gasoline, some cans used in the storage of food, water pipes and lead-based paint in old buildings.

Pirkle and colleagues (Pirkle, et al. 1994) have analyzed blood lead levels of the United States population and selected population subgroups during two time periods: 1976 to 1980 (n=9,832) and 1988 to 1991 (n=12,119). From the time of the first analysis to the second, mean blood lead levels dropped from 0.66 to 0.15 micrograms/deciliter for non-Hispanic white children, and from 20.2 to 5.6 micrograms/deciliter for non-Hispanic black children. Note that the mean blood lead level for black children was 37 times higher than it was for white children, even though both groups dropped more than 70 percent during this period. The drop was attributed to the removal of lead from gasoline in the early 1980s, and the removal of lead from the solder in cans during this period.

More recent research shows that blood lead levels in preschool children have continued to drop. A national survey conducted between 1999 to 2002 revealed that United States preschool children had a mean blood lead level of 1.9 micrograms per deciliter, with only 1.6 percent of the children having a level above 10 micrograms (Center for Disease Control and Prevention 2005). Despite this reduction, 310,000 children have lead levels above recommended minimums (Hubbs-Tait, Nation, Krebs and Bellinger 2005).

Pirkle, et al. (1994) and others (e.g., Hubbs-Tait, et al. 2005) determined that the major factors associated with high blood lead levels were low income, non-Hispanic black race/ethnicity, younger age and male sex. Lee, Chun and Wong (2005) found that blood lead levels in women in the reproductive period correlated inversely with educational level. Blacks and Hispanics also had higher levels than whites. Other factors associated with blood lead levels were older age, living in an urban environment, alcohol consumption and cigarette smoking. Women who drank alcohol were more than five times as likely as those who did not to be in the highest decile for blood lead level; smokers were 4.5 times as likely. Women who had high intakes of vitamins (thiamin, ascorbic acid, folic acid) had lower blood lead levels. Schell, et al. (2003) found that women who ingested higher levels of iron and vitamin D during pregnancy had neonates with lower blood lead levels.

Peak blood lead levels occur in children when they are 18 to 30 months of age (Chen, Dietrich, Ware, Radcliffe and Rogan 2005). Blood lead levels in children are related to the seasons, with the highest levels occurring during the summer months (June to August). This may be due to the level of outside activity of children and their breathing of dust from streets and soil that contain lead. Yiin, Rhoads and Lioy (2000) implicate seasonal patterns in house dust lead levels, with a peak in winter. These researchers examined seasonal changes in residential dust lead content and its relationship to blood lead in preschool children. They collected dust samples from floors, windowsills and carpets. The geometric mean lead concentrations in children were 10.77 in the winter and 7.66 in the summer (mu g/dL). They found that the highest level of dust concentrations of lead paralleled the seasonal pattern in blood lead found in preschools.

Most of the literature on lead poisoning in children is on preschool and school-aged children, and the potential effects of prenatal exposure are, thus, obscured because it is not known when the exposure occurred. But there is a growing literature on effects of prenatal exposure to lead. It is known that lead readily crosses the placental barrier and begins to accumulate in organs from a very early period of fetal development (Dietrich 1996). Lead has been recognized as a poison for the fetus since the 1940s. The effects include the full range of reproductive causality, including spontaneous abortions, perinatal death, premature birth, low birth weight and minor physical anomalies (Dietrich 1996). High levels of lead exposure during the prenatal period have been implicated in a range of psychopathological conditions, from impaired attention and academic difficulties to severe mental illness.

In one important study Opler, et al. (2004) studied archived serum samples from a cohort of births in Oakland California in the late 1950s and early 1960s. They tracked those members of the cohort who had received a diagnosis of schizophrenia in the subsequent years. It was determined that persons who had been exposed to high levels of lead during the prenatal period had a 2.4 times greater probability of having a schizophrenia diagnosis later in life than those with a low lead exposure.

With regard to low-level exposure, Dietrich (1996) reviewed the outcome studies and concluded that in a number of studies from the United States and in other countries, the results have been much the same. There are initial measurable developmental delays, but these do not remain measurable in the early school years for IQ or academic achievement.

Much of the most provocative and rigorous studies of prenatal lead exposure comes from animal research. Several researchers have linked such exposures to aggressive behavior. For example, Delville (1999) found that when intruders were introduced into the home territory of male hamsters that were exposed to lead during gestation and lactation, the exposed animals were faster and more likely to attack and bite the intruder than controls. Similar results have been observed for predatory attacks with cats (Li, et al. 2003).

Prenatal lead exposure has also been linked to addictive behavior in animal models. For example, Nation, Cardon, Heard, Valles and Bratton (2003) found that adult rats that had been exposed to lead during the prenatal period and during lactation relapsed more quickly than controls to a behavior associated with cocaine use after the behavior had been extinguished. Rocha, Valles, Cardon, Bratton and Nation (2005) also found that rats who had been exposed to lead prenatally more rapidly learned behaviors that led to self-administered cocaine use than controls.

The pathway through which the fetus is exposed to lead during fetal development is clear. The lead that affects children during the prenatal period is taken from the blood supply of the mother. About half of the lead in blood is bound to hemoglobin (Anderson, Pueschel and Linakis 1996). Lead in the blood is known to bind to fetal hemoglobin with higher affinity than to adult hemoglobin. Approximately 1 to 10 percent of circulating lead binds to microligands in blood plasma. It is this type of lead that crosses cell membranes.

Unfortunately, not only current maternal lead exposure but also stored lead from post exposures affects the fetus. At any one exposure, 10 to 20 percent is deposited in soft tissue and 70 to 85 percent is deposited in bone as lead has a particular affinity for calcium. Lead stored in larger stronger bones has a half-life in the body up to 30 years (Anderson, et al. 1996). During the late stages of pregnancy a mother's bones sometimes dissolve slightly to provide enough calcium for the formation of the bones of the fetus. This process frees the lead that was in the bone matrix to contaminate the bones and other tissues of the fetus. Gulson, et al. (1997) found that pregnant women who did not take calcium supplements and got less than the daily recommend quantities of calcium through diet, had substantial lead mobilization beginning in the three- to six-month period of pregnancy. In a more recent study, Gulson, Mizon, Palmer, Taylor and Mahaffey (2005) gave pregnant women calcium supplements and found that lead concentrations in the blood did not begin to increase until six to eight months of pregnancy. Thus, the calcium supplements delayed lead mobilization, but did not eliminate it. Even more ominous was the finding that after delivery, blood lead levels increased due to the demand for calcium in breast milk, even in the calcium-supplemented women.

In animal models it has been determined that lead accumulates in mitochondria, capillary endothelial cells and in glial cells of the brain. The neonate and fetus appear to be particularly sensitive to lead poisoning because astrocytes (a star-shaped neuroglial cell) are incapable of removing endothelial lead, resulting in cell damage and death (Goldstein 1990). One hypothesis is that lead alters the processes of synaptogenesis that occur at high rates in the later stages of fetal development and up to the second year of life (Goldstein 1990). Prolonged lead exposure can also be associated with sustained neurotransmitter release, which results in poor control of neurological activity (Anderson, et al. 1996).

Cadmium

Cadmium is a white metal used in the manufacture of batteries, pigments and metal coatings. It is also found in trace amounts in cigarette smoke. Cadmium is also present in soil and, therefore, in some foods. In humans it accumulates in the kidneys, liver, lungs and prostate and is not readily excreted. Cadmium is known to cause a range of health problems in humans. These include lung cancer and kidney damage. Cadmium also affects the DNA repair mechanisms of cells. This seems to be the mechanism that links it to various forms of cancer, including lung cancer in smokers. Normally some cells die off naturally and others multiply. Errors commonly occur when cells multiple (replicate). DNA has mechanisms to repair these errors in cell replication, and is responsible for the control of tumor growth. Cadmium seems to interfere with this process.

Cadmium is a health problem primarily for industrial workers in industries in which the metal is used or is a by-product of industrial processes. However, prenatal exposure is possible through three additional sources: maternal smoking during pregnancy (or the smoke of others to which the mother is exposed), prenatal exposure to industrial waste and diet. Major sources of cadmium in diet are leafy vegetables, mollusks, cocoa, grains and animal organs (e.g. liver) (see Hubbs-Tait, et al. 2005, for a review).

A few studies have linked prenatal cadmium exposures to negative outcomes in animals. Newland, Ng, Baggs, Gentry, Weiss and Miller (1986), for example, exposed rat dams to various levels of cadmium and then tested the offspring as adults. The animals were trained on a fixed-ratio reinforcement schedule and then switched to another fixed-ratio schedule. The performance of prenatally exposed rats was generally poorer than controls.

Outcome studies of cadmium exposure during pregnancy of offspring behavior in humans are rare. However, Mokhtar, Hossny, El-Awady and Zekry (2002) studied umbilical cord blood samples of infants and found that there was a negative correlation between these cadmium levels and Apgar scores of newborns. Other researchers have studied children at older ages. Koger, Schettler and Weiss (2005) have summarized much of this literature and concluded that cadmium exposure is associated with learning disabilities, hyperactivity, hypoactivity, motor dysfunction and decreased IQ. Both Koger, et al. (2005) and Hubbs-Tait, et al. (2005) lament the lack of studies in this area, but view the literature as pointing to the need for further research. It is important to note that the large body of work on the negative effects of smoking on offspring behavior may be included in the cadmium literature, as this metal may be one of the important behavioral teratogens in cigarette smoke.

Various Chemical Exposures Found in Home Products

There is growing concern on the part of child psychologists, pediatricians and others about the effects of household chemicals on the development of the CNS of fetuses, infants and children. Currently human beings spend about 90 percent of their time indoors (Klepeis, et al. 2001). Therefore, it is particularly important to study the compounds that are part of the indoor environment.

In a recent book Winter and Koger (2004) emphasize that because a product is available in our home and garden store does not mean that it is safe. In fact, a large number of products contain chemicals that are unregulated and are not monitored by the Environmental Protection Agency because the chemicals are produced in small quantities. Thus, the effects of most chemicals on the developing neurology of the fetus or infant are unknown. Winter and Koger state that 78 percent of the 3,000 most highly produced chemicals in the United States have not been studied for neurotoxic effects. In addition, some chemicals that are known to be toxins (glycol ethers, phthalates) are not listed on product labels or are legally labeled in 'other' categories. These authors are particularly concerned that the use of household chemicals may be linked to increased reports of children with developmental disorders such as autism, Asperger's and attention-deficit disorders. This section reviews a small number of chemicals that are prevalent home products.

Polychlorinated biphenyls

Polychlorinated biphenyls (PCBs) are one of the best known and most often studied chemicals with regard to effects on human health and development. PCBs are a polycyclic, synthetic hydrocarbon once used in a wide range of industrial products including plastics, carbonless copy paper and electrical transformers. They have been banned in the United States since the 1970s and, subsequently, have been banned in all regions of the world. However, they are among the most persistent environmental contaminants with measurable quantities found in air, water and soil samples in most parts of the world. They can be found in tissue samples of most residents of industrialized countires (Jacobson and Jacobson 2000). Because PCBs have an affinity for dissolving in fat and are, thus, deposited in fat tissue, they are difficult for humans to eliminate from the body.

A number of research groups have shown prenatal exposure to PCBs results in detrimental health outcomes, particularly problems associated with less responsive immune systems. For example, Dallaire, et al. (2004) have shown that prenatal exposure to PCBs in the Inuit populations in Canada result in infants who have a higher number of hospitalizations for infections during the first year of life. Infections included upper and lower respiratory tract infections, otitis media (middle ear infections) and gastrointestinal infections. Most of these infants were exposed to PCBs in utero due to the consumption by their mothers of contaminated fish. Reduced immunological capacity can have a variety of adverse developmental outcomes due to reduced energy and vigor, reduction of opportunities for play and an increased number of days of school that are missed.

Few studies of the long-term effects of PCBs have been done. However, since the 1980s Jacobson and Jacobson (2000) have been following a group of 313 children who were prenatally exposed to PCBs. It was one of the first efforts to study long-term moderate exposure of mothers and infants. Exposure was the result of maternal consumption of PCB-contaminated Lake Michigan sports fish. PCB contamination of the fetuses was indexed by analysis of PCB levels in umbilical cord serum at the time of delivery. At birth the PCB-exposed babies were smaller than controls, weighing about 200 grams less than non-exposed controls. This size difference persisted through the assessment at the fourth postpartum year (Jacobson and Jacobson 1997). In the cognitive realm, the exposed infants, when tested at seven months of age, were found to spend about half the time looking at novel stimuli as the control group. This is interpreted as a memory deficit in the context of the Fagan test, a test of perceptual inhibition in infants. Follow-up studies at age four continued to find short-term memory deficits as assessed by the McCarthy Scales of Children's Abilities and other measures. The most highly exposed group in the study was three times as likely to have low average IQ and twice as likely to be at least two years behind in reading (Jacobson and Jacobson 2000) as control subjects.

In a similar study Lai, et al. (2002) studied 118 children born between 1978 and 1985 in Taiwan in a region that had been exposed to contaminated cooking oil in

1978. These children were tested in 1992 through 1995 at age seven through adolescence. Compared to matched controls, the PCB-exposed children had a three-point IQ decrement. In addition, the total score on the Achenbach Child Behavior Checklist was three points higher than controls. Further, the Rutter Child Behavior Scale was six points higher for the exposed group than for controls. The higher score for the exposed group on the Achenbach Child Behavior Checklist and the Rutter Child Behavior Scale indicate higher levels of behavior problems.

In 1989 the World Health Organization published data indicating that contamination of breast milk with PCBs and dioxins was higher in the Netherlands, Belgium, Germany and the United Kingdom than in most other areas of the world. As a result, the Dutch government launched a longitudinal prospective study known as the Dutch PCB/Dioxin Study to study the effects of these contaminants on children's health. The Dutch cohort included approximately 400 healthy pregnant women, half of whom intended to breast-feed their infants, and half of whom intended to bottle-feed their infants. Maternal exposure to PCBs was assessed from maternal blood during the last month of pregnancy, from umbilical cord blood at the time of delivery and, for the breast-fed group, in breast milk. Dioxins were measured in breast milk only. Neuro-developmental measurements were obtained at three, seven, 18, 42 and 84 months of age. The sample was limited to white first- or second-born full-term infants delivered vaginally without the use of forceps or vacuum extraction procedures. Half of the women were recruited from the highly industrialized region of the Netherlands in the vicinity of Rotterdam. The other half lived in Groningen or surrounding rural regions in the northern part of the Netherlands. The PCB and dioxin levels obtained from the sample were comparable to those obtained in other highly industrialized regions of the world.

Total PCB levels and dioxin levels in breast milk were found to be negatively related to a measure of neurological functioning obtained at 10 to 21 days after birth (Huisman, et al. 1995a). The measure was primarily of postural tone and reflexes. Cord blood levels of PCBs were associated with measurable deficits in neurological functioning at 18 months, based on scores of motor developmental milestones (e.g., walking, grasping, sitting) (Huisman, et al. 1995b). No associations were found with scores on the Bayley scales administered at three, seven and 18 months of age. At 42 months the Kaufman Assessment Battery for Children (K-ABC) was administered to all offspring of the cohort. Prenatal PCB exposure was associated with significantly lower scores on all three scales of the Kaufman measure (Sequential Processing, Simultaneous Processing and Overall Cognitive Score). The most highly exposed children scored six to eight points lower than the least exposed children on the K-ABC (Lanting, et al. 1998; Patandin, et al. 1999). For the Rotterdam sample, cognitive development was assessed with the McCarthy Scales of Children's Abilities at 84 months. No significant main effects were obtained for PCBs or dioxins measured through any source (cord blood, breast milk, maternal blood). However, an important interaction with family background was obtained. Prenatal PCB exposure was associated with significantly poorer cognitive and memory performance in the children born to younger mothers, to parents with lower verbal IQ and to parents with less education. As Schantz,

Widholm and Rice (2003) point out in a review of this and other studies of PCB and dioxin effects, these results point to the subtle mediating effects of PCB and environmental variables. No other study of prenatal PCB exposure has followed children as long as the Dutch study, nor have any other studies provided the same complexity of measurements both of these pollutants or of psychological outcomes.

One smaller recent study is, however, noteworthy in the finding of long-term effects of PCBs. Steward, et al. (2005) followed up on a sample of children (n = 202) who had known prenatal exposure to PCBs. PCB exposure was assessed through the analysis of umbilical cord blood obtained immediately after birth. Subjects were placed in five groups, depending on the levels of PCBs found in the samples. Children were tested using the Continuous Performance Test at age eight, and the Extended Continuous Performance Tests at 9½. After controlling statistically for many covariates (e.g., maternal IQ, maternal sustained attention), it was determined that the PCB-exposed groups at age eight had higher levels of impulsive responding on the CPT. Further at age 9½, there was further evidence that the impulsive responding was related to impaired response inhibition, and not to impaired sustained attention. This research is noteworthy for a more detailed measurement of psychological processes related to attention than is typical of studies on the effects of toxic substance exposure.

As the review by Schantz, et al. (2003) indicates, the body of evidence for PCB effects on neurodevelopment of children is growing. Studies in the United States, Europe, the Faroe Islands and Taiwan all indicate a negative relationship with developmental phenomena, although all measures of toxic load (e.g. in breast milk, umbilical cord blood) do not show this relationship for all measures. There has been only one study that has failed to find an association (Gladen and Rogan 1991)

The mechanism for the effects of PCBs is currently not known. A good deal of attention has been placed on the potential of PCBs to disrupt the functioning of the endocrine system. Also, as noted above, adverse effects on the immune system have been noted. With regard to the CNS, PCB may interfere with the thyroid hormone, which is necessary to stimulate neuronal and glial proliferation and differentiation during late gestation and the early postnatal periods. For example, PCB exposure has been associated with fetal brain concentrations of thyroid hormones in a prenatally exposed Dutch sample (Koopman-Esseboom, et al. 1994).

Fluorine-based Coatings

One class of products penetration in the home are those products that are designed to withstand both water and oil penetration. These include stain resistant coatings and floor polishes. These products utilize fluorine-based compounds as the primary active ingredient. Many of these compounds break down in the environment to the compound perfluorooctane sulfonate (PFOS).

Unfortunately this compound is persistent and has been found in the blood of people. Lau, et al. (2003) have shown that this pollutant has negative developmental effects in mice and rats. Rats exposed to high levels of PFOS (about the level of humans working in factories that make the fluorine-based precursors of PFOS) had higher rates of cleft palate and other developmental problems than controls. They also were smaller for gestational age. In addition, within a few hours of birth, rats exposed to moderate to high dosages began to die at high rates. The compound seems to have altered other processes that are necessary for appropriate lung development. Further, of those that did survive, some brain enzymes were found to be impaired, particularly choline acetyltransferase.

Pthalates

Pthalates are used in cosmetics, deodorants and many plastics. The most common consumer products containing phthalates are soaps, shampoos, perfumes, hairsprays, nail polishes, insect repellents, carpet backing, paints and glues. They are also found in some medical products. In rodents, pthalates have been shown to be associated with abnormalities of the genitals of males (e.g., reduced testis weight) and other influences on the secondary sexual characteristics of the male (e.g., retention of thoracic nipples) (Gray, et al. 2000; Foster, Mylchreest, Gaido and Sar 2001).

Recently Silva, et al. (2004) has shown that most of the United States population is exposed to phthalates. Further, Duty, et al. (2003) have shown that these exposures may be affecting the reproductive capabilities of human males. In a study of 168 men who were one member of the subfertile couples participating in a study, it was determined that there was a dose-response relationship between one type of phthalate (mono-butyl phthalate) and sperm motility and sperm concentration. Sperm concentration was also associated with a second type of phthalate (monobenzyl phthalate). In all cases, sperm parameters were lower with increasing concentrations of phthalate, supporting the dose-response relationship expected in toxic substances. These findings may help shed light on the pattern of increasing sperm abnormalities in men that has occurred over the past 50 years. Specifically, lower sperms counts, reduced sperm motility and higher percentages of malformed sperm have been reported in recent decades (Sharpe and Skakkebaek 1993). No published studies are available that link these sperm abnormalities to pathologies of offspring.

Latini, et al. (2003), working in Perrino Hospital in Brindisi, Italy, has shown that pthalates levels in infants are associated with negative outcomes. These researchers tested blood from 84 newborns' umbilical cords for the presence of di- (2-ethylhexyl)- phthalate and mono-ethyhexyl-phthalate (MEHP). The body converts the former into the MEHP. Of the 84 newborns in the study, 65 had detectable levels of MEHP. The 65 with some level of the phthalate had an average gestational length of 38.2 weeks, while those with no detectable concentration had an average gestational length of 39.2 weeks.

Flame-Retardant Chemicals

Polybrominated diphenyl ether (PBDE) is a chemical used in many household products as a flame-retardant. It works well, saves many lives and prevents a large number of injuries each year. However, since the late 1990s, findings have been reported at scientific meetings suggesting that PBDE may pose particular risks to fetuses and young children (Raloff 2003). In 1999 Swedish scientists reported to a meeting of chemists that they had studied breast milk samples that had been stored over the past 25 years. They found PBDE in the earliest samples. Further, the concentrations of PBDE in these samples increased over the period of sample collection. At an Environmental Protection Agency conference in 2002 Hites summarized a review of PBDE concentrations in humans (typically in samples of human fat or blood). The review indicated that the concentrations in the United States are 10 to 20 times that in Europe, and the concentrations in Europe are twice those found in Japan (Raloff 2003). In August of 2003 Raloff reports that, at a meeting of toxicologists and related professionals, 84 papers were on brominated flame retardants.

From the point of view of offspring effects, some of the most troubling reports were from animal researchers who demonstrated that fairly low exposures to PBDEs in the uterine environment could damage the reproductive and nervous system of fetuses. In one study by Talsness (reviewed by Raloff 2003), pregnant females rats were exposed to one form of PBDE on the sixth day of their pregnancies. This exposure resulted in an increase in miscarriages, compared to controls. However, what was more worrisome was that, in a follow-up study, researchers mated offspring of PBDE-treated mothers to an unexposed partner. In the offspring of this mating, high levels of birth defects were noted, including missing vertebrate or skull bones. Also, the offspring of exposed mothers were less fertile. Other researchers have reported memory and learning impairments in animal models after prenatal exposure to PBDE (see review by Raloff 2003).

Work on PBDE is very new and is only slowly becoming available. No studies are currently available on outcomes for humans whose mothers were exposed during pregnancy. However, the evidence is clear enough from animal models that such major companies as Sony and Toshiba have voluntarily phased out brominated fire retardants from their electronic products.

Acrylamide

Another known environmental toxin that humans are widely exposed to is acrylamide. Acrylamide has recently become the subject of mass media publications, as well as scientific publications, because it has been determined that this toxin is produced when some starchy foods are cooked at high temperatures. Among the foods most widely tested that produced acrylamides were French fries and potato chips.

Acrylamide is also used in the production of polyacrylamide that, in turn, is used in water treatment, pulp and paper production and mineral processing. Polyacrylamide is also used in dyes, adhesives, contact lenses, soil conditioners, cosmetics and skin creams, food packaging materials and permanent press fabrics. Acrylamide has been shown to induce neurotoxicity in highly exposed occupational groups. Further, laboratory animals that are exposed have been shown to have higher rates of cancer, genetic damage to sperm and adverse effects on development. Unfortunately, there is no research to indicate the effects on the fetus if a pregnant woman is exposed. Safe levels of exposure are the subject of continued debate.

Volatile Organic Compounds

Volatile organic compounds (VOCs) are another category of pollutant that has been studied in both the indoor and outdoor context. Some VOCs present indoors are p-dichlorobenzene (moth cakes, room air fresheners, toilet bowl deodorizers), chloroform (chlorinated water) and the fragrances alpha and beta pinene and delta limonene (cleaning products, room fresheners). Adgate, et al. (2004) studied the exposures to these compounds in multiple locations for children in Minneapolis. They found that the home environment provided the largest exposure to these compounds, with exposure rates that were several orders of magnitude greater than the outdoor environment. Median exposure levels were well above health benchmarks for several VOCs. This study and others by this research group indicate that estimates of outdoor air pollution probably underestimate exposures to some pollutants, in particular to VOCs.

Summary

Heavy metals have been known for some time to have toxic effects on children, particularly those children who are exposed during the prenatal and immediate postnatal environment. The strongest research linking prenatal exposure to heavy metals to negative outcomes during childhood and adolescence is for maternal ingestion of mercury and lead during pregnancy. Research has linked both learning and behavior problems to heavy metal exposure.

This chapter also presented provocative, but less rigorous and extensive evidence, linking some chemicals found in the home to negative outcomes for offspring. Most of the studies presented use animal models. Polychlorinated biphenyls, volatile organic chemicals, pthalates, acrylamides and flame retardants made with polybrominated diphenyl ether are among the chemicals most likely to be toxic to the fetus. The strongest evidence is for polychlorinated biphenyls, and these chemicals have now been banned in most countries of the world. Unfortunately, soil residues have a long half-life, and many infants continue to be exposed through dust and other means.

    This chapter presented a small sampling of substances that are found in home products that seem to be potentially harmful to the human fetus. One of the complications in understanding and researching the prenatal effects of these chemicals is that they are used in small quantities, in many combinations, in a range of products. The products vary in the amount contained, the speed with which the products degrade to release harmful chemicals and the probability that they would end up in the bloodstream of a pregnant women. The task for the research community is daunting.

    Some countries have become more proactive in their social policies regarding household and industrial chemicals than is the case in the United States. For example, proposed legislation before the European Parliament (Registration, Evaluation and Authorization of Chemicals) would require that a chemical be proven safe before it is sold. In the United States, all chemicals are legal unless there are proven to be unsafe under the Toxic Substances Control Act. Proving that a chemical is toxic can take decades, particularly if its effects do not produce easily observed teratology, leaving the population at risk while the evidence accumulates. Some European countries have extensive biomonitoring programs in which human blood, urine and breast milk are tested for environmental toxins and stored for later analyses when new, more sensitive tests are made available. The United States lags behind its European peers in these biomonitoring efforts.

Section F
Historical Perspective and the Future

History

Scattered throughout this book we have provided historical and literary references to document how human beings have viewed certain prenatal exposures and attempted to understand physical and behavioral abnormalities of their children that present at birth. This understanding allows for the placement of the current state of our knowledge within an historical context.

Prescientific Understanding of Teratology

Depictions of abnormalities of infants in cave paintings and petrogylphs suggest that, since the dawn of recorded history, humans have contemplated babies born with deformities. In Mesopatamia the *Summa izbu* was circulated which chronicled types of deformities that had been observed and the interpretation given to these deformities by religious leaders. This body of knowledge was circulated throughout the Ancient Near East with deformity being interpreted as messages from the divine. In particular, it was substantially relied upon to predict the future success of a monarch's reign. The Greek and Roman civilizations produced works based upon birth defects that continued to be referenced until the 17th Century. These sources allowed the reader to look up a particular birth defect and read the interpretation of that defect, which was typically viewed as a judgment from God.

Although there was a natural tendency to believe that malformed infants were the result of divine intervention, during the earliest records of human history there are references to environmental causes for gestational malformation or behavioral predispositions. In the Old Testament there are admonitions against the use of alcohol during pregnancy (Judges 13:7). Carthage and Sparta prohibited newlyweds from consuming alcohol, perhaps to protect against the possibility of alcohol-related birth defects. Aristotle recognized that drunken women conceive children with developmental problems saying that "foolish, drunken, or hare-brain women, for the most part, bring forth children like unto themselves" (as cited in Mattson and Riley 1998).

Thus, the folklore of many cultures, from the beginnings of written history through the 19th Century, revealed the observations of its citizens regarding factors occurring during pregnancy that altered the behavior of the infant and child. Some of this folklore was encoded in literatue of the culture. For example, a pregnant Queen Elizabeth in Shakespeare's "King Henry VI," on learning of the imprisonment of her husband, says that she must stop her tears so that she doesn't damage the heir to the English crown (Part 3, Act IV, Scene IV; reported by DePietro 1998, pg. 71).

The Emergence of Scientific Thought

Slowly, over the past 300 years, the study of birth defects has moved away from folklore and theology toward a more scientific set of explanations for gestational malformations and gestationally based behavioral predispositions. William Prefect in the late 1700s observed that there was a greater prevalence of "insanity" among those persons who were exposed prenatally to a particularly virulent influenza epidemic. At the turn of the 20th Century Kraeplin (1919), one of the fathers of modern psychiatry, commented that "infections in the years of development might have a causal significance" for dementia praecox (p. 240). A similar observation was made by Karl Menninger after the 1919 influenza pandemic.

In addition to early epidemiological studies, experimental studies began to shed light on the biological explanations for adverse pregnancy outcomes. These studies used animal models of human pathology. For example, in 1877, Dareste exposed pregnant fowl to non-lethal heat and found that the heat produced congenital anomalies in offspring (Warkany 1986).

Some of the most important scientific breakthroughs came in the 1940s and 50s. In 1941, Gregg discovered that mothers who contracted rubella during pregnancy had offspring with severe eye cataracts and other physical deformities. In addition to Gregg's discovery, two highly publized events grabbed the attention of the general public and medical officials around the world. Perhaps the most important was the thalidomide tragedy. Prior to the late 1950s most medical authorities believed that the developing fetus had a special protected status provided by the placental barrier. However, the clear link between births of children with malformed arms and legs subsequent to the use during pregnancy of a drug designed to control pregnancy-related nausea (thalidomide) conclusively demonstrated that the placental barrier was not as impermeable as had been thought. The thalidomide event also clearly demonstrated the central issues in fetal teratogenesis. The timing of the exposure is critical. In the case of thalidomide, only when the drug was taken during a one- to two-week period of pregnancy was an effect on the fetus observed. This event, more than any other, produced a cognitive shift in thinking about the vulnerability of the prenatal period.

The second major event that occurred during the 1950s that altered the scientific view of the vulnerability of the fetus was the mercury poisoning disaster in Minamata Bay in Japan. During the 1950s tons of mercury were dumped in this bay. Soon, children and adults in the area reported symptoms of loss of motor control, incoherent speech and psychiatric symptoms. Children born to mothers who were pregnant at the time had high rates of cerebral palsy and mental retardation. Research on these effects began to appear in the late 1950s. One of the important leasons learned from this incident was the long-term effects of the poisoning during gestation, even for persons who had no observable malformation at the time of birth. By the 1990s it was clear that the effects of this mercury exposure became worse as the exposed population aged. By 1993, 2,256 children and adults had been diagnosed with what came to be called Minamata disease (Harada 1995).

In 1968 in France and then 1973 in the United States, alcohol became recognized as a teratogen when fetal alcohol syndrome entered mainstream parlance, with recognition that gestational alcohol exposure had deleterious effects on the cognitive, behavioral and physical development. Soon after recognition of the harmful effects of alcohol, gestational smoking research accelerated. The first reported relationship was with low birth weight, but since that time hundreds of studies have reported an association between gestational cigarette smoke and numerous behavioral, educational, cognitive, social-emotional and physical outcomes.

In the area of behavioral teratology, another event that occurred during the 1950s had a seminal effect on thinking about prenatal perturbations of fetal development, although the effects were not documented for three decades. In 1988 Mednick, Machon, Huttunen and Bonnett (1988) reported that the population of Finland exposed to the 1957 influenza pandemic had an increased rate of schizophrenia, when compared to other years in which rates of influenza were lower. Stimulated by this finding, many researchers attempted to replicate this finding with the majority supporting this association. This study, perhaps more than others, re-energized the efforts of researchers in psychiatry and related fields to investigate links between infection cycles and other environmental events occurring during gestation and psychiatric illness.

The Current State of Knowledge

So, what have we learned from the data that has accumulated during the past 60 years? Stated another way: What are the broad generalizations that can be made from all the findings reviewed in this book?

First, we have learned that a broad range of substances have toxic affects during the prenatal period that can result in long-term medical, cognitive and behavioral problems. Such substances include chemicals ingested by mothers in food (e.g., heavy metals), in the air (e.g., particulate matter) and water (e.g., agricultural chemicals), and mood-altering substances used for recreational purposes (e.g., alcohol, components of cigarette smoke and other recreational drugs). The list of maternally ingested substances that have been demonstrated to be harmful to the fetus is much larger than would have been expected 25 years ago.

Second, we have also learned that a broad range of maternal health conditions can have adverse affects on fetal health and development. These include, primarily, factors that have an impact on cardiac output, pulmonary efficiency and metabolism of sugars (e.g., diabetes). The range of maternal health conditions that has been implicated also includes conditions that influence these factors, such as maternal obesity.

Third, much of the data reviewed in this book makes clear that maternally ingested substances and maternal health conditions often manifest during the perinatal period in the form of preterm birth and low birth weight. They can also alter the ability of the placenta to provide oxygen to the fetus, resulting in hypoxia. Further, each of these perinatal effects (low birth weight, preterm birth, hypoxia/ anoxia) can result in additional damage to the fetus, especially to the rapidly developing central nervous system.

Fourth, in many instances a dose-response relationship has been established between prenatal events and the abnormality of the behavior that is observed during development. Thus, the more the mother smokes or the more alcohol she drinks during pregnancy, the greater the risk of abnormal cognitive and behavioral outcomes. Also, the more severe the medical condition of the mother the worse the outcome. For example, untreated and severe prenatal diabetes has more negative effects than mild or well controlled maternal diabetes.

The fifth generalization that can be gleaned from current data is that the timing of the prenatal perturbation is of critical importance in determining the type and extent of damage to the developmental process. For some substances the data indicate a brief window in which toxic affects are most likely to occur. For others, the substance may have affects throughout pregnancy (or at least at more than one time), but the effects may be different, depending on the timing of exposure or the ingestion of the substance.

Sixth, much has been learned about fetal development, particularly of the central nervous system, during the past 50 years. This knowledge has opened the door to the incredible complexity of central nervous system development. Specifically, it is clear that the developing central nervous system has a protracted period of vulnerability which extends beyond organogenesis (e.g., beginning of the first trimester). This includes the developmental processes that occur throughout the fetal and neonatal period and into infancy, including neurogenesis, neuronal differentiation, neuronal migration, arborization and synaptogenesis, synaptic organization, myelination, neuronal apoptosis and gliogenesis, glial migration and differentiation.

The seventh generalization that can be gleaned from the research reviewed in this book is that there is little cognitive or behavioral specificity in the type of behavior or learning problem that is likely to result from any set of prenatal toxic events. In general, attention, memory and emotional and behavioral regulation are adversely affected by a broad range of maternal health conditions, as well as by a broad range of maternally ingested substances. This principle indicates that it will be fruitless to try to find a behavioral profile that will identify the prenatal events that contributed to the profile. It indicates also that, given our current diagnostic schemes in psychology and psychiatry, there is likely to be a great deal of comorbidity.

An additional generalization from this body of knowledge is, perhaps, the most optimistic. Most children who are exposed to pollutants, maternally ingested drugs or subjected to maternal illness during the prenatal period seem to develop normally. Even some children who are exposed to high levels of toxins are indistinquishable from their unexposed peers. This seems to occur for two primarily reasons. First, there are large individual differences in the susceptibility of individuals to toxic substances or events. Second, many children who are exposed to an adverse prenatal experience are exposed to several. Thus, those who are affected may be the result of accumulated risks.

A ninth generalization based on the data reviewed in this volume is that adverse prenatal events often set off a cascade of events, each one of which adds further risks of abnormal development. For example, Miller, et al. (2002) studied 90 infants who had indications of having suffered asphyxia (e.g., Apgar score <= 5). These infants varied in the amount of seizure activity they experienced, from none to severe recurrent seizures. At an average age of six days, the infants were given MRIs to study the amount of brain injury that had occurred. Miller and colleagues found that seizure scores predicted several indicators of neonatal brain injury. They conclude that severity of seizures in human newborns with perinatal asphyxia is independently associated with brain injury. Thus, in this case asphyxia increased the risks of seizures which further increased the risks of brain injury. A second example of this type of cascade of risks is in babies of diabetic mothers. Maternal diabetes increases the rate of a wide range of pregnancy complications. It also leads to abnormally large fetuses. These large fetuses are subject to further risks. There may be difficulties in vaginal delivery related to asphyxia, subdural hemorrhage (hemorrhage within the brain), facial palsy and fracture of the clavical.

Finally, prenatal risks interact with other environmental risks. The Asbury, et al. (2006) study exemplifies this interaction particularly well. They studied differences in behavior of monozygotic twins, and correlated these differences with birth weight. They found that anxiety, hyperactivity, conduct problems, peer problems and academic achievement correlated significantly with monozygotic differences in birth weight. But they also found that these differences in birth weight were more strongly related to differences in birth weight in families that exhibited greater family risks. (For more discussion of this study, see Chapter 3)

Future Directions

Although the research reviewed in this book indicates that a great deal has been learned, it seems most appropriate to describe the field of behavioral teratology as in the early stages of development. To use the developmental terminology of our subject matter, the field has come through the fetal period and infancy, but is perhaps best characterized as in its toddlerhood. It has taken its first steps, but is not walking steadily yet.

Progress in the future will come through (a) studying an increasing number of toxins and maternal health conditions; (b) conducting more long-term follow-up of children exposed during the prenatal period to events and conditions that perturb development; (c) paying more attention to the interactions among toxins, and between toxins and maternal health conditions; (d) beginning to study gene-environment interactions in the context of prenatal perturbations; (e) attending more closely to the interactions between social and psychological conditions of the mother during pregnancy, and the toxic effects of ingested substances, or adverse maternal health conditions, (f) and doing a better job of measurement of the dose of the developmental perturbing event. The following discussion will expand on each of these points.

One of the most remarkable ways in which somatic and behavioral teratology have made progress during the past 50 years is simply by documenting a broader and broader range of factors that perturb fetal development. The field has come a long way from the view that the fetus is protected from all but a handful of toxins and conditions. Particularly with regard to pollutants, a surprising range of chemical compounds have been implicated. Given the rate at which new man-made chemicals are being produced, there is an urgent need to expand the range of substances studied. Even using animal models for much of this research, it appears impossible to study each of the thousands of new compounds. Basic science must lead in establishing what groups of compounds are most likely to perturb prenatal development. The cost of both the basic sciences and the human application will be high.

In addition to expanding the range of chemicals studied, the greatest need is for more long-term follow-up studies. When we set out to summarize the literature for this book, we thought that it would be possible to find a substantial body of research documenting long-term effects of most of the broad classes of known teratogenes. We have found, instead, that long-term follow-up studies are rare. However, such studies are the foundation on which behavioral teratology is based, since most of the behaviors of interest cannot be observed in the neonate. Further, the structural and physiological processes that set the stage for these behaviors can be so subtle that it is unlikely that they will be observable in infancy. Longitudinal research is difficult and expensive. However, huge amounts of data are collected each year and discarded or left unanalyzed due to a lack of understanding of its utility. Perhaps greater use of such data will facilitate progress in behavioral teratology (more about this later).

One of the most important generalizations about the research that we have summarized is that many infants and children seem to develop normally despite exposure to pollutants, maternally ingested chemicals, poor maternal nutrition or poor maternal health during pregnancy. Why are some individuals more susceptible to adverse prenatal events than others? One possibility is that some of the children that are most affected have experienced more than one adverse event. Women who live in poverty may not obtain good prenatal care, may not as a result obtain appropriate prenatal vitamins and may also live in residential areas with high levels of air and water pollution. Pregnant women who suffer from mental illness may self-medicate abusing several drugs. Fetuses of migrant workers may have more contact with agricultural chemicals and may experience high levels of maternal stress due to being in a foreign country and living in crowded conditions. Very little is known at this point about the effects of accumulated prenatal risks, or the interaction among risks.

Prenatal risks should also be strongly influenced by the genetic makeup of the fetus. Would a gene-environment interaction of this type help explain the very high rates of preterm delivery and low birth weight babies among African-American women? Further, children come into the world with genetic-based cognitive and behavior predisposition. How do specific adverse prenatal experiences interact with these predispositions to influence the risks toward abnormal behavior? At this stage of the development of the field, the answer is that we have no idea other than such interactions seem likely.

Finally, there is an obvious need to do a better job in behavioral teratology research of measuring the timing and extent of fetal exposure to toxins, substances or adverse events. Infection during pregnancy is an example. The field would be substantially moved forward if there were seriological measurements of antibodies indicating that the mother had been exposed to a particular virus. Clinical diagnosis can also be useful, but fetal development may be perturbed by exposure to pathogens for which there are no clinical manifestations. Repeated assessments of stress during pregnancy with measurement of cortisol would greatly improve the understanding of the effects of the level and duration of stress during pregnancy. Better assessment of exercise patterns and outdoor activity of pregnant women living in an environment in which they are exposed to air pollutants would be helpful.

An even more fundamental problem than the accuracy of the measurement is the issue of what to measure. For instance, in the case of the influenza virus, which has been linked to schizophrenia in progeny, several by-products of infection including circulating cytokines, response to fetal and maternal antibodies and maternal fever, have been implicated as the agent of teratogenesis. With regard to stress, is the effect on the fetus due to circulating biochemical product of the HPA axis, or is it due to the coping mechanisms used by women who are highly stressed? Perhaps they gain excessive weight, abuse street drugs or do not eat properly. While research has begun to investigate a range of possible factors associated some exposures such as influenza, this is the exception rather than the rule.

It is relatively easy to determine the shortcomings of this body of knowledge. It is much more difficult to say how these problems can be addressed in the world of limited funding, and sensitive and ethical care of research participants. The essential elements of behavioral teratology research are careful measurement of exposure, and longitudinal follow-up with careful measurement of outcomes. Such research requires multidisciplinary teams. The technical aspects of seriological analysis or other biochemical assays require highly specialized laboratory skills. The appropriate assessment of cognitive and psychological outcomes requires specialized workers. There are also specialized skills involved in subject recruitment, tracking and retention in longitudinal work. Thus, many longitudinal projects of sizeable samples now have price tags of hundreds of thousands of dollars per year or even higher. Careful, prospective research of this kind is needed, but the resource limitations will always mean that there will be few such studies.

Some types of research can be accomplished, however, with data that has been collected for other purposes. Millions of dollars are spent each year by hospitals recording data related to pregnancy and delivery. Birth records of every birth in the United States are available from the Centers for Disease Control. Every child in school in the United States is repeatedly assessed for educational attainment, and children who have special problems in schools have repeated and detailed assessments of their behavior. Hospitals keep records of admissions and some countries (e.g., those in the Nordic countries) keep lifelong health records of every hospitalization. Computerization of these data sets has occurred in most sectors so birth, medical, educational and criminal data are available for large segments of the population.

Currently there are many impediments to the appropriate study of these data. A primary concern is the informed consent of persons who have been assessed to use the information that is available. Incompatible computer systems, poor data quality, missing data and many other problems impede progress in this realm. However, these problems seem small in comparison to the resource issues that are encountered in implementing large-scale prospective longitudinal research which requires individualized assessment over long periods of time. If credit card companies, advertisers, retail firms and others can access extensive individualized data for the purposes of commerce, then perhaps the technical and political will can be found to utilize similar systems for the improved health and psychological well-being of children.

Appendix: Brief Medical Dictionary Related to Pregnancy

(Many definitions were based on definitions in Tabers Cyclopedic Medical Dictionary, 15th edition, Philadelphia: Davis. Other definitions were obtained from the National Center for Health Statistics.)

abruptio placenta	Premature separation of a normally implanted placenta from the uterus
abortion	Expulsion of the product of conception before the fetus has attained viability; see induced abortion
adactyly	A congenital anomaly consisting of absence of fingers or toes
albuminuria	The presence of readily detectable amounts of serum protein (especially serum albumin) in the urine. It is usually a sign of kidney impairment. This condition can occur as a result of pregnancy
alveoli	Small hollow sacs or cavities, particularly the small air sacs in the lungs
amniocentesis	A procedure consisting of puncture of the amniotic cavity

1. to aspirate fluid for amniotic fluid analysis
2. to inject radiopague substance for amniography
3. to determine pressure changes of amniotic fluid which permit the continuous monitoring of uterine contractibility
4. to monitor the fetal heart rate
5. to detect possible genetic disorder antenatally

amnion	The membrane around fetus on the innermost aspect of the placental sac
amniotic fluid	The fluid contained in the amniotic sac
amygdala	A mass of grey matter in the anterior portion of the temporal lobe. Part of the limbic system controlling arousal and emotion

ancephalus	A congenital anomaly the main feature of which is the absence of cerebral hemispheres
anemia	A hemoglobin level of less than 13.0 g/dL or a hematocrit of less than 39 percent
antibody	A protein substance produced by the immune system that is developed in response to, and interacting with, an antigen. This forms the basis for acquired immunity. Examples include bacteria, viruses and toxins. Some antigens are formed by the body itself
antigen	A substance that induces the formation of antibodies by the immune system. May result in agglutination, precipitation, neutralization, complement-fixation or increased susceptibility to phagocytosis
anencephaly	Congenital absence of brain and spinal cord
anoxia	Without oxygen
Apgar Score	A clinical rating of five areas of functioning of the fetus; ratings are done by the physician at one and five minutes after birth. The Apgar score is a useful measure of the need for resuscitation and a predictor of the infant's chances of surviving the first year of life. It is a summary measure of the infant's condition based on heart rate, respiratory effort, muscle tone, reflex irritability, and color. Each of these factors is given a score of zero, one or two, thus the score ranges from zero (near death) to 10 (optimal)
apoptosis	Disintegration of cells into membrane-bound particles that are then destroyed by other cells
asthma	Spasmatic disruption of breathing accompanied by wheezing caused by a spasm of the bronchial tubes or by swelling of their mucous membrane
asphyxia	Physiological condition caused by insufficient intake of oxygen, as when there is interference in placental circulation or from premature separation of placenta
attitude, obstetric	The intrauterine position of the fetus
autonomic nervous system	The part of the nervous system that is concerned with control of involuntary bodily functions, such as glands, smooth muscle tissue and heart
Braxton-Hicks contractions	Painless contractions of the uterus throughout gestation; sometimes known as false labor

breech presentation	At the time of birth, the fetus presents with buttocks or foot instead of the face or head
	a. complete breech - thighs flexed on abdomen and legs flexed upon thighs b. footling ¥ the foot presents c. frank breech¥ legs extended over ventral body surface d. knee ¥ the knee presents
biphasic temperature curve	Referring to the two general temperature levels in the menstrual cycle
	a. the lower temperature level, known as the estrogenic phase, extends from the onset of menstruation to a short period after ovuwlation b. the higher temperature level follows ovulation
blighted ovum	An impregnated ovum which has ceased to grow within the first trimester
cerebral palsy	A bilateral symmetrical nonprogressive paralysis resulting from developmental defects in the brain or trauma at the time of birth
cerebellum	A portion of the brain forming the largest portion of the rhombenephalon. It lies dorsal to the pons and medulla oblongata, overhanging the latter. It is involved in control of skeletal muscles
Cesarean section	The removal of the fetus through an incision into the uterus:
	a. classic–incision into the corpus uteri b. lower uterine segment - incision into the lower portions of the corpus uteri
cephalopelvic disproportion	The relationship of the size, presentation and position of the fetal head to the maternal pelvis prevents dilation of the cervix and/or descent of the fetal head
cleft lip	An anomaly resulting from failure of facial processes of the embryo to fuse. In the case of cleft lip, it is a congenital cleft or separation of the upper lip. May be associated with cleft palate
cleft palate	A congenital fissure or separation in the roof of the mouth forming a communicating passageway between mouth and nasal cavities. May be unilateral or bilateral, and complete or incomplete
club foot	Deformities of the foot in which the foot is twisted out of shape or position; it does not result from trauma and is congenital

chorion	The outer envelope around the fetus; the inner envelope is the amnion
circulatory/respiratory	A general category of infant or fetal anomaly used by the National Center for Health Statistics to indicate any anomaly of these systems
colostrum	The yellowish fluid secreted by the mammary gland during the pregnancy and for the first two or three days post-delivery
contraception	The voluntary prevention of pregnancy
cord prolapse	The premature explusion of the umbilical cord in labor before the fetus is delivered
corpus callosum	The great body of brain tissue that connects the cerebral hemispheres
corticotrophin releasing factor	A substance present in the hypothalamus that controls secretions of adrenocorticotrophin
cytoarchitecture	Pertaining to the structure and arrangement of cells
cytokines	Proteins produced by the body in response to infection and trauma. Important mediators of an individual's immunological defense. Specific cytokines produced in response to infection are hypothesized to adversely impact brain development.
cytomegalovirus	One of a group of herpesviruses. In humans it inhabits the salivary glands
Diabetes mellitus	A disorder of carbohydrate metabolism, characterized by hyperglycemia and glycosuria, and resulting from inadequate production or utilization of insulin. The most common clinical symptom is frequent urination
dilation of the cervix	The gradual opening of the cervix to permit passage of the fetus
Down's syndrome	Also known as trisomy 21; a chromosomal abnormality that results in a child with sloping forehead, small ear canals, presence of epicanthal folds causing an Oriental appearance, gray or very light yellow spots at periphery of the iris, short broad hand with single palmar crease (simian crease), a flat nose or absent bridge, low-set ears and generally dwarfed physique
dysfunctional labor	Labor which does not progress in a normal pattern

eclampsia	Coma and convulsive seizures occurring in pregnant women from the 20th week of pregnancy through the first week postpartum. Symptoms include edema of legs and feet, puffiness of face, hypertension, severe headaches, rapid pulse
ectopic pregnancy	Fertilized ovum implanted outside of uterine cavity; in the fallopian tube, ovary or some area of the abdomen
effacement	The process of shortening and thinning of the cervix
embryo	The product of conception, especially during the first three months of life
encephocele	The protrusion of the brain through a cranial fissure
engagement	The descent of the fetal head through the pelvic inlet
enzyme	An organic catalyst produced by living cells. They are complex proteins
erythocytes	A mature red blood cell or corpuscle. Each is a non-nucleated, biconcave disk averaging 7.7 microns in diameter
esophageal atresia	The congenital absence or closure of the esophagus
esophageal fistula	An abnormal passage between the trachea and the esophagus
episiotomy	An incision of perineum to facilitate delivery and prevent perineal laceration; perineum is that tissue lying at the base of the pelvic floor, between the vagina and the anus
face presentation	At the time of delivery or soon before, the baby is head down in the birth canal a. brow presentation: the forehead presents b. sinciput presentation: the large fontanel presents c. vertex presentation: the upper and back part of the head presents; this is the most common and preferred presentation; see breech presentation
fetal distress	A life-threatening condition due to fetal anoxia, hemolytic disease or other causes; indicative of fetal hypoxia
fetal hemolytic disease	A blood disorder caused by antibody antigen reaction in Abo, Rh or other blood group incompatibility. Maternal antibodies cross the placenta, agglutinate fetal blood cells and destroy them. Fetal anemia develops

fetal monitoring	The continuous recording of fetal heart rate patterns from a direct fetal electrocardiogram electrode and uterine contractions using a transcervical catheter
fetotoxicity	The toxic effects of maternal medication on fetus and neonate
fetus	The unborn child after the first three months of development
free radical	An atom or group of atoms that has an unpaired electron and, thus, is not bound to another chemical compound and they are highly reactive
fontanel, fontanelle	The junction point of cranial sutures which remains widely open in the newborn
gastroschisis	A congenital fissure that remains open in the wall of the abdomen
genital herpes	Infection of the skin of the genital area by the herpes simplex virus
gestation	A synonym for pregnancy, although it often refers to the fetus, while pregnancy refers to the mother. As in the statement, "the fetus was delivered at 26 months gestation"
glial cells	Neuroglia cells, including astrocytes, oliogodendroglia and microglia
glycosuria	The presence of glucose in the urine
Goodell's sign	The softening of the uterine cervix, indicative of pregnancy
gravida	A pregnant woman, or the state of being pregnant. A mother may be described as a gravida 2, meaning this is her second pregnancy
gyri	The convolutions of the cerebral hemisphere of the brain. Gyri are separated by shallow grooves (sulci) or deep grooves (fissures)
heart malformations	A term used by the National Center for Health Statistics to indicate any congenital anomaly of the heart
hernia, diaphragmatic	The protrusion or projection of an organ or part of an organ through the wall of the cavity that normally contains it. In this case, the protrusion of abdominal contents through the diaphragm

hematocrit	The volume of erythrocytes packed by centri fugation in a given volume of blood. The hematocrit is expressed as the percentage of total blood volume that consists of erythrocytes or as the volume in cubic centimeters of erythrocytes packed by centrifugation of blood. Normal values at sea levels: mean, 47 percent; women, 42 percent
hemoglobin	A protein consisting of a colored iron containing portion (hematin) and a simple protein (globin). It combines readily with oxygen to form an unstable compound (oxyhemoglogin). It is carried on erythrocytes (red blood cells)
hemoglobinopathy	A group of diseases, including sickle cell disease, caused by or associated with the presence of one of several forms of abnormal hemoglobin in the blood
hemorrhage	Excessive blood loss that in pregnancy and delivery is often indicated by timing such as antepartum (before birth), intrapartum (during delivery) or postpartum (after delivery) hemorrhage
hippocampus	A structure on the floor of the inferior horn of the lateral ventricle of the brain. Implicated in short-term memory
hyaline membrane	Hyaline is a crystalline, translucent substance on the surface of lung tissue that is present in the fetus, but begins to break down prior to the time of birth to facilitate the fetus being able to assimilate oxygen by breathing air
hyaline membrane disease	A disorder primarily of prematurity, manifested clinically by respiratory distress (see RDS) and pathologically by pulmonary hyaline membranes and incomplete expansion of the lungs at birth
hydramnios	A condition in which there are excessive amounts of amniotic fluid
hydrocephalus	The increased accumulation of cerebrospinal fluid within the ventricles of the brain. Results from the interference with normal circulation and with absorption of the fluid that results from destruction of the foramina of Magendie and Luska
hyperemesis gravidarum	Severe nausea and vomiting during pregnancy
hyperglyemia	Increase of blood sugar as occurs in diabetes mellitus. This condition increases susceptibility to infection and often precedes diabetic coma

hypertension	Blood pressure persistently greater than 140/90 diagnosed prior to onset of pregnancy or before the 20th week of gestation
hypertensive disorders of pregnancy	High blood pressure of 140/90 or greater developing during gestation or in early puerperium, typically restricted to the onset after the 20th week of gestation; proteinuria, edema, convulsions and coma may be present
hypothalamus	The portion of the diencephalons comprising the ventral wall of the third ventricle. It lies beneath the thalamus. It contains neuroscretions that are important in control of metabolic activities, such as maintenance of water balance, sugar and fat metabolism and regulation of body temperature
hypoxia	A deficiency in amount of oxygen reaching tissues
hypoglycemia	The deficiency of sugar in the blood
hypoxia	Insufficient oxygenation of the blood
incompetent cervix	A condition characterized by painless dilation of the cervix in the second trimester or early in the third trimester of pregnancy, with prolapse of membranes through the cervix and ballooning of the membranes into the vagina, followed by rupture of the membranes and subsequent expulsion of the fetus
induction of labor	The initiation of uterine contractions before the spontaneous onset of labor by medical and/or surgical means for the purpose of delivery
involution of uterus	The postpartum return of uterus to its former shape and size
induced abortion	The voluntary expulsion of fetus, brought about by mechanical means or drugs
IUGR	Referring to the interuterine growth retardation of the fetus
ischemia	The local and temporary deficiency of blood supply to a body part due to obstruction of the circulation to that part
labor	Normal uterine contractions which result in the delivery of the fetus
	1. missed labor: a few contractions at full-term, then cessation of labor and fetal retention, usually due to death of fetus in utero or extrauterine pregnancy

	2. precipitate labor: hasty labor
	3. premature labor: labor before full-term
	4. protracted labor: prolonged labor
labor stages	There are typically three stages of labor:

1. cervical dilatation: first stage begins with uterine contractions, terminates with complete cervical dilatation
2. expulsion: second stage, from complete dilatation of the cervix to the birth of the baby
3. placental separation and expulsion: third stage, from
4. delivery of neonate to expulsion of the placenta

| lactic acid | A colorless syrupy liquid formed in milk and other foods, and also formed during muscular activity by the breakdown of glycogen |

| leukocyte | Whtie blood corpuscle. There are two types: granulocytes (those with granules in their cytoplasm) and agranulocytes (lacking granuales) |

| limbic system | A group of brain structures including the hippocampus, amygdale, dentate gyrus, cingulated gyrus, gyrus fornicatus, as well as other structures. This system is involved in motivation and arousal, thus in emotion |

| Magendie's foramen | The median of three openings in the roof of the fourth ventricle. It is in front of the cerebellus and behind the pons varolii. Is often closed in cases of congenital hydrocephalus |

| malformed genitalia | Congenital anomalies of the reproductive organs; a rough category of anomalies used by the National Center for Health Statistics |

| meconium | The first feces of the newborn, or fecal material of the fetus; it is composed of salts, amniotic fluid, mucus, bile and epithelial cells; is greenish-black to light brown, almost odorless, and tarry in consistency |

| meconium aspiration syndrome | Aspiration of meconium by the fetus or newborn, which adversely affects the lower respiratory system |

| meninges | The membranes covering the spinal cord and brain; consists of three lays; the dura mater (external), the arachnoid (middle) and the pia mater (internal) |

meningocele	A congenital anomaly in which the meninges protrude through an opening of the skull or spinal column
microcephalus	A head that is significantly small; typically congenital, often results in mental retardation
multipara	A woman who has given birth to two or more children; see primipara
natural childbirth	A loosely defined term indicating childbirth without anesthetic
NCHS	The National Center for Health Statistics
neural tube	Tube formed from the fusion of the neural folds from which the brain and spinal cord arise
NICU	An acronym for a neonatal intensive care unit
Oligodendroglial cells	Adventitial (on outermost covering) cells found in central nervous system with characteristic vine-like processes
oligohydamnios	A deficiency in the amount of amniotic fluid
omphalocele	A congenital hernia of the navel
parturient	A woman in labor
pelvis	The bony ring adapted to childbearing in females. It is composed of the sacrum, coccyx and hipbones
PEM	An acronym for protein-energy malnutrition
perinatology	The study of the infant before, during and after birth
periventricular regions	The region of the brain around the ventricals
pH	Stands for potential of hydrogen. The degree of acidity or alkalinity of a substance. The neutral point is pH 7. Acidity is indicated by lower numbers and alkalinity by higher numbers
placenta	Vascular structure which provides nutrition for the fetus and which develops from the fertilized ovum
placenta abruptio	A condition in which the placenta prematurely detaches from the uterine wall generally causing severe hemorrhage; also referred as placenta ablatio
placenta accreta	An adherent placenta which remains attached to uterus after delivery
placenta previa	A condition in which the placenta is implanted in lower segment of uterine wall. There are three types:

	a. marginal insertion: placenta comes to the ostium uteri (opening of the uterus), but does not cover it
	b. partial placenta previa: placenta incompletely covers the ostium uteri
	c. complete or central placenta previa: placenta covers the ostium uteri
polycythemia	An excess of red blood cells (syn: erythrocytosis)
polydactyly	A condition of having more than the normal number of fingers and toes
precipitous labor	Refers to extremely rapid labor and delivery lasting less than three hours
preeclampsia	A toxemia of pregnancy characterized by increasing hypertension, headaches, albuminuria and edema of the lower extremities
premature birth	Births occurring at less than 37 weeks gestation, measured from date of last menstrual period
premature rupture of membranes	The rupture of the membranes holding the amniotic fluid at any time during pregnancy, and more than 12 hours before the onset of labor
presentation or lie	The relation which the long axis of the fetus bears to that of the mother. A distinction is made between longitudinal and transverse presentations; longitudinal presentations occur in 99.5 percent of cases and includes the following varieties:

A. breech: presentation of the fetal buttock

1. complete breech: thighs flexed on abdomen and legs flexed upon thighs
2. footing: the foot or feet presents
3. frank breech: legs extended over ventral body surface
4. knee: the knee presents

B. face presentation¾ presentation of the fetal head

1. brow: the forehead presents
2. sinciput: the large fontanel presents
3. vertex: the upper and back part of the head presents; this is most common and preferred

primipara	A woman who has delivered her first child after the period of viability
puerperium	The period of 42 days following childbirth and expulsion of the placenta and membranes

puerperal hematoma	Escape of blood into the mucosa or subcutaneous tissues of the external genitalia forming painful vaginal or vulvar hematomas (blood tumors)
puerperal infection	Infection during the puerperium
puerperal septicemia	Presence of pathogenic bacteria in the blood during the puerperium
Puerperal sepsis	Infection of the genital tract occurring within the postpartum period; also known as childbed fever
Respiratory Distress Syndrome (RDS)	A disease the clinical signs of which include delayed onset of respiration and low Apgar scores. Caused by delivery of an infant who has not matured to the point where the lungs can manufacture the lecithin-rich pulmonary surfactant
rectal atresia	A congenital absence or closure of a normal body opening or tubular structure; in this case the rectum
rectal stenosis	A constriction or narrowing of a passage or orifice; in this case the rectum
renal disease	Pertaining to diseases of the kidney
Rh sensitization	The process or state of becoming sensitized to the Rh factor as when an Rh-negative woman is pregnant with an Rh-positive fetus
seizures, general	A recurrent paroxysmal disorder of cerebral function characterized by sudden, brief attacks of altered consciousness, motor activity or sensory phenomena. Also referred to as epilepsy
seizures, petit mal	An epilepsy attack in which there is a brief, less than 30-second, loss of consciousness but there is no fall. The eyes flutter and the patient stops all other activity
seizures, grand mal	A generalized epileptic seizure which effects the entire brain. A seizure proceeds with loss of consciousness, falling and tonic then clonic contractions of the muscles. Urinary and fecal incontinence may occur. The attack usually lasts two to five minutes
SIDS	Stands for sudden infant death syndrome. The completely unexpected and unexplained death of an apparently well baby. Occurrs more frequently in the third and fourth months of life, and premature infants, in males and in infants living in poverty. Occurs more often in the winter than the summer months
SGA	A term which indicates that the fetus is small for gestational age; refers to the size of the fetus

spina bifida	A congenital defect in the wall of the spinal canal caused by lack of union between the laminae of the vertebrae; lumbar portion is the section chiefly affected
stimulation of labor	The augmentation of previously established labor by use of oxytocin
sulci	The shallow grooves separating gyri in the cerebral cortex
surfactant, pulmonary	A phosphlipid substance important in controlling the surface tension of air-liquid emulsion that is present in the lungs. Abnormalities in this surfactant have been noted in prematurity, and hyaline membrane disease
syndactyly	A fusion of two or more toes or fingers
subinvolution	Failure of the uterus to reduce to its normal size after delivery
teratogens	Noxious agents (mechanical, infectious, chemical, nutritional) capable of disrupting normal gestation with subsequent antenatal death or the birth of a misshapen, deformed neonate
teratology	The study of disfiguring malformation due to arrested embryonic growth and fetal development of organs or structures
thalamus	The largest subdivision of the diencephalon, consisting primarily of the ovoid gray mass in the laternal wall of the third venticricle. All sensory stimuli, except olfactory, are received by the thalamus
tocolysis	The use of medications to inhibit preterm uterine contractions for the purpose of extending the length of pregnancy and avoiding a preterm birth
trophoblast	A layer of ectoderm which attaches the conceptus to the uterine wall, nourishes the embryo and has invasive propensities, thus malignant potentials
ultrasound	A procedure used for the visualization of the fetus and placenta by means of ultrasonic sound waves
umbilical cord	The cord that connects the circulatory system of the fetus to the placenta
vacuum extraction	The instrumental delivery of infant with a vacuum extractor
version	The process of turning the fetus in the uterus

1. cephalic version¾ the head is made the presenting part
2. podalic version¾ the breech is made the presenting part

vulva   That portion of the female external genitalia lying posterior to the mons veneris consisting of the labia majora, labia minora, clitoris, vestibule of the vagina, vaginal opening and bulbs of the vestibule

References

Section A: Introduction

Dirckx, J. H. (Ed.) (1997). *Stedman's concise medical dictionary for the health professions. 3rd edition*. Baltimore: Williams and Wilkins.

Johnson, S. (2006). *The ghost map*. New York: Riverside Books.

Kraeplin, E. (1919). *Dementia praecox and paraphrenia*. Edinburgh, Scotland: E and S Livingston.

Warkany, J. (1986). Teratogen update: Hyperthermia. *Teratology, 33*, 365-371.

Dombrowski, S. C. and Martin, R. P. (2007). Perinatal exposure in later psychological and behavioral disabilities. *School Psychology Quarterly, 22*, 1-7.

Chapter 1

Allen, M. C., Donohue, P. K., and Dusman, A. E. (1993). The limit of viability—Neonatal outcome of infant born at 22 to 25 weeks gestation. *New England Journal of Medicine, 329*, 1597-1601.

American Psychiatric Association (1994). *Diagnostic and statistical manual of mental disorders: 4th edition*. Washington, DC: American Psychiatric Association.

Anderson, A. C., Pueschel, S. M., and Linakis, J. G. (1996). Pathophysiology of lead-poisoning. In S. M. Pueschel, J. G. Linakis, and A. C. Anderson (Eds.), *Lead poisoning in childhood* (pp. 75-96). Baltimore, Maryland: Brookes.

Angold, A., Costello, E. J., and Erbani, A. (1999). Comorbidity. *Journal of Child Psychology and Psychiatry and Allied Disciplines, 40*, 57-87.

Aylward, G. P. (1997). *Infant and early childhood neuropsychology*. New York: Plenum.

Bellinger, D. (1996). Learning and behavioral sequelae of lead poisoning. In S. M. Pueschel, J. G. Linakis, and A. C. Anderson (Eds.), *Lead poisoning in childhood* (pp. 97-116). Baltimore, Maryland: Brookes.

Bromet, E. J., and Fennig, S. (1999). Epidemiology and natural history of schizophrenia. *Biological Psychiatry, 46*, 871-881.

Capaldi, D. M., and Patterson, G. R. (1994). Interrelated influences of contextual factors on antisocial behavior in childhood and adolescence for males. In D. C. Fowles, P. Sutker, and S. H. Goodman (Eds.), *Progress in experimental personality and psychopathology research* (pp. 165-198). New York: Springer.

Coie, J. D., and Dodge, K. A. (1998). Aggression and antisocial behavior. In W. Damon (Series Ed.) and N. Eisenbert (Vol. Ed.), *Handbook of child psychology. Social, emotional, and personality development* (5th ed., pp. 779-862). New York: Wiley.

Costello, E. J., Angold, A., Burns, B. J., Stangl, D. K., Tweed, D. L., Erkanli, A., and Worthman, C. M. (1996). The Great Smoky Mountains Study of youth: Goals, design, methods, and the prevalence of DSM-IIIR disorders. *Archives of General Psychiatry, 53*, 1129-1136.

DeFries, J. C., and Fulker, D. W. (1985). Multiple regression analysis of twin data. *Behavior Genetics, 15*, 467-478.

Dobbing, J., and Smart, J. L. (1974). Vulnerability of developing brain and behavior. *British Medical Bulletin, 30*, 164-168.

Downey, G., and Coyne, J. (1990). Children of depressed parents: An integrative review. *Psychological Bulletin, 108*, 50-76.

Field, T. (1992). Infants of depressed mothers. *Development and Psychopathology, 4*, 49-66.

Gershon, A. A., Gold, E., Nankesis, G. A. (1997). Cytomegalovirus. In A. S. Evans, R. A. Kaslow (eds.), *Viral infections of humans. Epidemiology and control* (pp. 229-251). New York: Plenum.

Greenbaum, P. E. Prange, M. E. Friedman, R. M., and Silver, S. E. (1991). Substance abuse prevalence and comorbidity with other psychiatric disorders among adolescents with severe emotional disturbances. *Journal of the American Academy of Child and Adolescent Psychiatry, 30*, 575-583.

Gortmaker, S. L., Walker, P. K., Weitzman, M., and Sobol, A. M. (1990). Chronic conditions, socioeconomic risks, and behavioral problems in children and adolescents. *Pediatrics, 85*, 267-276.

Hack, M., and Fanaroff, A. A. (1999). Outcomes of children of extremely low birthweight and gestational age in the 1990's. *Early Human Development, 3*, 193-218.

Hodapp, R. M., and Dykens, E. M. (2003). Mental retardation (intellectual disabilities). In E. J. Mash and R. A. Barkley (Eds.), *Child psychopathology* (pp. 486-519). New York: Guilford.

Johnson, D. E. (2000). Medical and developmental sequelae of early childhood institutionalization in eastern European adoptees. In C. A. Nelson (Ed.), *The effects of early adversity on neurobehavioral development: The Minnesota symposia on child psychology, Vol. 31* (pp. 113-162). Mahwah, N.J.: Erlbaum.

Khoury, M. J. (1997). Genetic epidemiology and the future of disease prevention and public health. *EpidemiologicReviews, 19*, 175-180.

Lyon, G. R., Fletcher, J. M., and Barnes, M. C. (2003). Learning disabilities. In E. J. Mash and R. A. Barkley (Eds.), *Child psychopathology* (pp. 520-586). New York: Guilford.

Merikangas, K. R. (2000). Familial and genetic factors and psychopathology. In C. A. Nelson (Ed.), *The effects of early adversity on neurobehavioral development: The Minnesota symposia on child psychology, Vol. 31* (pp. 281-316). Mahwah, N.J.: Erlbaum.

Mash, E. J., and Barkley, R. A. (2003). *Child psychopathology, 2nd edition*. New York: Guilford.

Moore, K. L., and Persaud, T. V. N. (1993). *Before we are born*. Philadelphia: W. B. Saunders.

Norman, M. G., and Armstrong, D. D. (1998). Disturbances of brain development. In C. E. Coffey, and R. A. Brumback (eds.), *Textbook of pediatric neuropsychiatry* (pp. 43-64). Washington, DC: American Psychiatric Association.

Patterson, G. R. (1982). *Coercive family process*. Eugene, OR: Castalia.

Pennington, B. F. (1999). Dyslexia as a neurodevelopmental disorder. In H. Tager-Flusberg (Ed.), *Neurodevelopmental disorders* (pp. 307-330). Cambridge, MA: MIT Press.

Ruggeri, M., Leese, M., Thornicroft, G., Bisoffi, G., and Tansella, M. (2000). Definition and prevalence of severe and persistent mental illness. *British Journal of Psychiatry, 177*, 149-155.

Rutter, M. (1989). Isle of Wight revisited: Twenty-five years of child psychiatric epidemiology. *Journal of the American Academy of Child and Adolescent Psychiatry, 28*, 633-653.

Seligman, L. D., and Ollendick, T. H. (1998). Comorbidity of anxiety and depression in children and adolescents: an integrative review. *Clinical Child and Family Psychology Review, 1*, 125-144.

Shannon, M. W. (1996). Etiology of childhood lead poisoning.. In S. M. Pueschel, J. G. Linakis, and A. C. Anderson (Eds.), *Lead poisoning in childhood* (pp. 37-58). Baltimore, Maryland: Brookes.

Sroufe, L. A. (1997). Psychopathology as an outcome of development. *Development and Psychopathology, 9*, 251-268.

Szatmari, P. (1992). The epidemiology of attention-deficit hyperactivity disorders. *Child and adolescent psychiatry clinics of North America, 1*, 361-372.

Willcutt, E. G., and Pennington, B. F. (2000). Psychiatric comorbidiy in children and adolescents with reading disability. *Journal of Child Psychology and Psychiatry, 41*, 1039-1048.

Chapter 2

Altman, J. and Bayer, S. A. (1980). Development of the brain stem in the rat. II. Thymidine-radiographic study of the time of origin of neurons of the upper medulla, excluding the vestibular and auditory nuclei. *Journal of Comparative Neurology, 194*, 37-56.

Aylward, G. P. (1997). *Infant and early childhood neuropsychology*. Plenum Press: New York.

Bayer, S.A., Altman, J., Russo, R.J., and Zhang, X. (1993). Timetables of neurogenesis in the human brain based on experimentally determined patterns in the rat. *Neurotoxicology. 14*: 83-144

Bayer, S.A., Yackel, J.W., and Puri, P.S. (1982). Neurons in the rat dentate gyrus granular layer substantially increase during juvenile and adult life. *Science. 216(4548)*: 890-892

Capone, G. (1996). *Human brain development*. Baltimore: Brookes.

Caviness, V.S Jr., Goto, T., Tarui, T., Takahashi, T., Bhide P.G., and Nowakowski, R.S. (2003). Cell output, cell cycle duration and neuronal specification: a model of integrated mechanisms of the neocortical proliferative process. *Cerebral Cortex, 13*, 592-598

Crossman, A. R. and Neary, D. (2000). Neuroanatomy: An illustrated colour text (2nd Edition). New York: Churchill Livingstone.

Dobbing J. and Sands J. 1979. Comparative aspects of the brain growth spurt. *Early Human Development 3*(1): 79-83.

Dombrowski, S. C., Noonan, K., and Martin, R. P. (2007). Low birth weight and cognitive outcomes: Evidence for a gradient relationship in an urban, poor African-American birth cohort. *School Psychology Quarterly, 22*, 26-43.

Fatemi, S. H., Emamian, E. S., Kist, D., Sidwell, R., Nkajima, N., Akhter, P., et al. (1999). Defective corticogenesis and reduction in reelin immunoreactivity in cortex and hippocampus of prenatally infected neonatal mice. *Molecular Psychiatry, 4*, 145-154.

Hatten, M. E. (1999). Central nervous system neuronal migration. *Annual Reviews of Neuroscience, 22*, 511-539.

Hatten, M. E., and Mason, C.A. (1990). Mechanism of glial-guided neuronal migration in vitro and in vivo. *Experientia, 46*, 907-916.

Hynd, G. W. and Willis, W. G. (1988). *Pediatric Neuropsychology*. Philadelphia: W.B. Saunders.

Kolb, B and Fanite, B. (1989). Development of the child's brain and behavior. In C. R.. Reynolds, C. R. and E. Fletcher-Janzen (Eds.), *Handbook of clinical child neuropsychology. Critical issues in neuropsychology* (pp. 17-39). New York, NY: Plenum Press.

Kolb, B. and Gibb, R. (1999). Neuroplasticity and recovery of function after brain injury. In D. T. Stuss (Eds.), *Cognitive neurorehabilitation* (pp. 9-25). New York, NY: Cambridge University Press.

Kuida, K., Zheng, T.S., Na, S., Kuan, C., Yang, D., Karasuyama, H., et al. (1996). Decreased apoptosis in the brain and premature lethality in CPP32-deficient mice. *Nature. 384(6607)*: 368-72.

Kuzniecky, R.I. (1994). Magnetic resonance imaging in developmental disorders of the cerebral cortex. *Epilepsia. 35 Suppl 6: S44-56.*

Layde, P.M, Edmonds, L.D, and Erickson, J.D. (1980). Maternal fever and neural tube defects. *Teratology, 21*: 105-108.

Lynberg, M.C., Khoury, M.J., Lu X., and Cocian T. (1994). Maternal flu, fever, and the risk of neural tube defects: A population based case-control study. *American Journal of Epidemiology 140*: 244-255.

Mednick, S. A., Machon, R. A., Huttunen, M. O., and Bonnett, D. (1988). Adult schizophrenia follow-ing prenatal exposure to an influenza epidemic. *Archives of General Psychiatry*, 45, 189-192.

Montgomery, D. L. (1994). Astrocytes: Form, functions, and roles in disease. *Veterinary Pathology, 31*, 145-167.

Milunsky, A, Ulcickas, M., Rothman, K.J., Willet, W., Jick, S., and Jick, H. (1992). Maternal heat exposure and neural tube defects. *Journal of the American Medical Association* 268: 882-885.

Nowakowski, R. S. (1987). Basic concepts of CNS development. *Child Development, 58*, 568-595.

Nowakowski, R.S., Caviness, V.S Jr., Takahashi, T., and Hayes, N.L. (2002). Population dynamics during cell proliferation and neuronogenesis in the developing murine neocortex. *Results and Problems in Cell Differentiation, 39*, 1-25.

Nowakowski, R.S., Hayes, N.L. (1999). CNS development: an overview. *Development and Psychopathology, 11*, 395-417.

Nowakowski, R. S. and Rakic, P. (1981). The site of origin and route and rate of migration of neurons to the hippocampal region of the rhesus monkey. *Journal of Comparative Neurology, 196*, 129-154.

Oppenheim, R. W. (1991). Cell death during development of the nervous system. *Annual Review of Neuroscience, 14*, 453-501.

Rakic, P. (1972). Mode of cell migration to the superficial layes of fetal monkey neocortex. *Journal of Comparative Neurology, 145*, 61-84.

Rakic, P. (1978). Neuronal migration and contact guidance in the primate telencephalon. *Post Graduate Medical Journal, 54*, 25-40.

Rakic, P. (1992). Early developmental events: Cell lineages, acquisition of neuronal positions, and areal and laminar development. *Neurosciences Research Program Bulletin, 20*, 439-452.

Rakic, P., Bourgeois, J-P., Eckenhoff, Zecevic, and Goldman-Rakic, P.S. (1986). Concurrent over-production of synapses in diverse regions of the primate cerebral cortex. *Science, 232*, 232-235

Rakic, P., and Singer, W. (1988). *Neurobiology of the neocortex*. New York: Wiley.

Schore, A.N. (2001). Effects of a secure attachment relationship on right brain development, affect regulation, and infant mental health. *Infant Mental Health Journal 22*, 7-66.

Shiota, K. (1982). Neural tube defects and maternal hyperthermia in early pregnancy: Epidemiology in a human embryonic population. *American Journal of Medical Genetics, 12*, 281-288.

Sidman, R. L. and Rakic, P. (1973). Neuronal migration with special reference to developing human brain: A review. *Brain Research, 62*, 1-35.

Sidman, R.L. and Rakic, P. (1982). Development of the human central nervous system. In W. Haymaker and R. D. Adams (Eds.) *Histology and Histopathology of the Nervous System.* (pp. 3-145). Springfield Ill.; Thomas.

Takahashi, T., Nowakowski, R. S., and Cavines, V. S. (1995). Early ontogeny of the secondary population of the embryonic murine cerebral wall. *Journal of Neuroscience, 15*, 6058-6068.

Zaidi, A.U., D'Sa-Eipper, C., Brenner, J., Kuida, K, Zheng, T.S., Flavell, RA., et al. (2001). Bcl-X(L)-caspase-9 interactions in the developing nervous system: evidence for multiple death pathways. *Journal of Neuroscience, 2*, 169-175.

Section B: Perinatal Mediators and Markers of Disturbances of Fetal Development: Introduction

Barker, D. J. P., (1998). In utero programming of chronic disease. *Clinical Science, 95*, 115-128.

Lewit, E. M., Baker, L. S., Corman, H., and Shiono, P. H. (1995). The direct cost of low birth weight. *The Future of Children, 5*, 35-56.

Chapter 3

Allen, M. C., Donohue, P.K., and Dusman, A. E. (1993). The Limit of Viability – Neonatal Outcome of Infants Born at 22 to 25 Weeks' Gestation. *New England Journal of Medicine, 329*, 1597-1601.

Asbury, K., Dunn, J. F., and Plomin, R. (2006). Birthweight-discordance and differences in early parenting related to monozygotic twin differences in behaviour problems and academic achievement at age 7. *Developmental Science, 9*, 1-22.

Benton, A. L. (1940). Mental development of prematurely born children. *American Journal of Orthopsychiatry, 10*, 719-746.

Bhutta, A. T., Cleves, M. A., Casey, P. H., Cradock, M. M., and Anand, K. J. S. (2002). Cognitive and behavioral outcomes of school-aged children who were born preterm: A meta-analysis. *Journal of the American Medical Association, 288*, 728-737.

Breslau, N., Paneth, N. S., and Lucia, V. C. (2004). The lingering academic deficits of low birth weight children. *Pediatrics, 114*, 1035-1040.

Carran, D. T., Scott, K. G., Shaw, K., and Beydoun, S. (1989). The relative risk of educational handicaps in two birth cohorts of normal and low birthweight disadvantaged children. *Topics in Early Childhood Special Education, 9*, 887-892.

Forfar, J. O., Hume, R., McPhail, F. M., Maxwell, S. M., Wilkinson, E. M., Lin, J. P. et al. (1994). Low birthweight: a 10-year outcome study of the continuum of reproductive casualty. *Developmental Medicine and Child Neurology, 36*, 1037-1048.

Grant, E. G. (1986). Sonography of the premature brain: Intracranial hemorrhage and periventricular leukomalacia. *Neuroradiology, 28*, 476-490.

Hack, M., Breslau, N., Aram, D., Weissman, B., Klein, N., and Borawski-Clark, E. (1992). The effect of very low birth weight and social risk on neurocognitive abilities at school age. *Journal of Developmental Behavioral Pediatrics, 13*, 412-420.

Hack, M., Breslau, N., Weissman, B., Aram, D., Klein, N., Borawski, E. (1991). Effect of very low birth weight and subnormal head size on cognitive abilities at school age. *New England Journal of Medicine, 325*, 231-237.

Hack, M., Flannery, D. J., Schluchter, M., Cartar, L., Borawski, E., and Klein, N. (2002). Outcomes in young adulthood for very-low-birth-weight infants. *New England Journal of Medicine, 346*, 149-157.

Hack, M., Klein, N., and Taylor, G. (1995). Long-term developmental outcomes of low birth weight infants. *The Future of Children, 5*, 176-196.

Hack, M., Taylor, G., Klein, N., and Eiben, R. (1994). Outcome of <750 gm birthweight children at school age. *New England Journal of Medicine, 331*, 753-759.

Hall, A., McLeod, A., Counsell, C., Thomson, L., and Mutch, L. (1995). School attainment, cognitive ability, and motor function in a total Scottish very-low birthweight population at eight years: A controlled study. *Developmental Medicine and Child Neurology, 37*, 1037-1050.

Horwood, L. J., Mogridge, N., and Darlow, B. A. (1998). Cognitive, educational, and behavioural outcomes at 7 to 8 years in a national very low birthweight cohort. *Archives of Disability in Child Fetal and Neonatal Education, 79*, 12-20.

Hoy, E. A., Sykes, D. H., and Bill, J. M.(1992). The social competence of very-low-birthweight children: Teacher, peer, and self-perceptions. *Journal of Abnormal Child Psychology, 20*, 123-150.

Hunt, J. V., Tooley, W. H., and Harvin, D. (1982). Learning disabilities in children with birthweights <= 1500 grams. *Seminars in Perinatology, 6*, 280-287.

Johnson, E. O. and Breslau, N. (2000). Increased risk of learning disabilities in low birth weight boys at age 11 years. *Social and Biological Psychiatry, 7*, 490-500.

Lubchenco, L. O., Horner, F. A., Reed, L. H., Hix, I. W., Jr., Metcalf, D., Cohig, R. et al., (1963). Sequelae of premature birth: Evaluation of premature infants of low birth weights at ten years of age. *American Journal of Diseases of Children, 106*, 101-115.

McCormick, M. C., Brooks-Gunn, J., Workman-Daniels, K., Turner, J.and Peckham, G. J. (1992). The health and developmental status of very low birth weight children at school age. *Journal of the American Medical Association, 267*, 2204-2208.

McCormick, M. C., Gortmaker, S. L., and Sobol, A. M. (1992). Very low birth weight children: Behavior problems and school difficulty in a national sample. *Journal of Pediatrics, 117*, 687-693.

McNutt, S. J. (1885a). Double infantile spastic hemiplegia with the report of a case. *American Journal of Medical Sciences, 89*, 58-79.

Paneth, N., Rudelli, R., Kazam, E., and Monte, W. (1994). *Brain Damage in the Preterm Infant.* London: Mac Keith Press.

Picard, E. M., Del Dotto, J. E., and Breslau, N. (2000). Prematurity and low birth weight. In K. O. Yeates, M. D. Ris, and G. H. Taylor (Eds)., *Pediatric Neuropsychology: Research, Theory, and Practice.* New York: The Guilford Press.

Rose, S. A., and Feldman, J. F. (2000). The relation of very low birth weight to basic cognitive skills in infancy and childhood. In C. A. Nelson (Ed.), *The effects of early adversity on neurobehavioral development: The Minnesota symposia on child psychology, vol. 31* (pp. 31-60). Mahwah, N. J.: Erlbaum.

Saigal, S., Rosenbaum, P., Stoskopf, B., Hoult, L., Furlong, W., Feeny, D. et al. (2005). Development, reliability and validity of a new measure of overall health for pre-school children.. *Quality of LifeResearch, 14*, 243-252.

Saigal, S., Szatmari, P., Rosenbaum, P., Campbell, D., and King, S. (1991). Cognitive abilities and school performance of extremely low birth weight children and matched term controls at age 8 years: A regional study. *Journal of Pediatrics, 118*, 751-760.

Schreuder, A. M., Veen, S., Ens-Dokkum, M. H., Verloove-Vanhorick, S. P., Brand, R., and Ruys, J. H. (1992). Standardized method of follow-up assessment of preterm infants at the age of 5 years: use of the WHO classification of impairments, disabilities, and handicaps. *Pediatric Perinatal Epidemiology, 6*, 363-380.

Shenkin, S. D., Starr, J. M., and Deary, I. J. (2004). Birth weight and cognitive ability in childhood: a systematic review. Birth weight and cognitive ability in childhood: a systematic review. *Psychological Bulletin, 130*, 989-1013.

Sommerfelt, K., Ellertsen, B., and Markestad, T. (1993). Personality and behaviour in eight-year-old, non-handicapped children with birth weight under 1500g. *Acta Paediatrica, 82*, 723-728.

Sommerfelt, K., Ellertsen, B., and Markestad, T. (1996). Low birthweight and neuromotor development.: A population based, controlled study. *Acta Paediatrica, 85*, 604-610.

Stjernqvist, K., and Svenningsen, N. W. (1999). Ten-year follow-up of children born before 29 gestational weeks: health, cognitive development, behavior and school achievement. *Acta Paediatrica, 88*, 557-562.

Taylor, H. G., Klein, N., and Hack, M. (2000). School-age consequences of birth weight less than 750g: A review and update. *Developmental Neuropsychology, 17*, 289-321.

Taylor, H. G., Klein, N., Minich, N. M., and Hack, M. (2000). Middle-school age outcomes in children with very low birthweight. *Child Development, 71*, 1495-1511.

Teplin S., Burchinal M., Johnson-Martin N., Humphrey R.A., and Kraybill E.N. (1991). Neurodevelopmental, health, and growth status at age 6 years of children with birth weights less than 1001 grams. *Pediatrics, 118*, 768-777.

WHO. Division of Family Health. The incidence of low birth weight. A critical review of available information. *World Health Statistics Quarterly, 1980, 33*, 197-224.

Chapter 4

Amor, L. B., Grizenko, N., Schwartz, G., Lageix, P., Chantal, B., Ter-Stepanian, M., et al. (2005). Perinatal complications in children with attention-deficit hyperactivity disorder and their unaffected siblings. *Journal of Psychiatry and Neuroscience, 30*, 120-126.

Andrews, W. W., Hauth, J. C., Goldenberg, R. L., Gomez, R., Romero, R., and Cassell, G. H. (1995). Amniotic fluid interleukin-6 correlations with upper genital tract microbial colonization and gestational age in women delivered after spontaneous labor versus indicated delivery. *American Journal of Obstetrics and Gynecology, 173*, 606-612.

Azzopardi, D., Guarino, I., Brayshaw, C., Cowan, F., Price-Williams, D., Edwards, A. D. et al. (1999). Prediction of neurological outcome after birth asphyxia from early continuous two-channel electroencephalography. *Early Human Development, 55*, 113-123.

Barker, D. J. P., (1998). In utero programming of chronic disease. *Clinical Science, 95*, 115-128.

Berg, A. T. (1989). Indices of fetal growth-retardation, perinatal hypoxia-related factors and childhood neurological morbidity. *Early Human Development, 19*, 271-283.

Brake, W. G., Sullivan, R. M., and Gratton, A. (2000). Perinatal distress leads to lateralized medial prefrontal cortical dopamine hypofunction in adult rats. *Journal of Neuroscience, 20*, 5538-5543.

Burke, C. J., and Tannenberg, A. E.(1995). Prenatal braindemage and placental infarction: an autopsy study. *Developmental Medicine and Child Neurology, 37*, 555-562.

Caslin, A., Heath, D. and Smith, P. (1991). Influence of hypobaric hypoxia in infancy on the subsequent development of vasoconstrictive pulmonary vascular disease in the Wistar albino rat. *Journal of Pathology, 163*, 133-141.

Davis, H. P., Tribuna, J., Pulsinelli, W. A., and Volpe, R. T. (1986). Reference and working memory of rats following hippocampal damage induced by transient forebrain ischemia. *Physiology and Behavior, 37*, 387-392.

Gunn, A. J. Parer, J. T., Mallard, E. C., Williams, C. E., and Gluckman, P. D. (1992). Cerebral histological and electrophysiological changes after asphyxia in fetal sheep. *Pediatric Research, 31, 486-491.*

Handley-Derry, M., Low, J. A., Burke, S. O., Waurick, M., Killen, H., and Derrick, E. J., (1997). Intrapartum fetal asphyxia and the occurrence of minor deficits in 4- to 8-year-old children. *Developmental Medicine and Child Neurology, 39*, 508-514.

Higgins, R. D., Raju, T. N., Perlman, J., Azzopardi, D. V., Blackmon, L. R., Clarke, R. H et al. (2006). Hypothermia and perinatal asphyxia: executive summary of the National Institute of Child Health and Human Development workshop. *Journal of Pediatrics, 148*, 170-183.

Holmes, G. L., and Ben-Ari, Y. (2001). The neurobiology and consequences of epilepsy in the developing brain. *Pediatric Research, 49*, 320-325.

Jiang, Z. D. (1995). Long-term effect of perinatal and postnatal asphyxia on developing human auditory brainstem responses: peripheral hearing loss. *International Journal of Pediatric Otorhinolaryngology, 33*, 225-238.

Jobe, A. H., and Bancolari, E. (2001). Bronchopulmonary dysplasia. *American Journal of Respiratory Critical Care Medicine, 163*, 1723-1729.

Miller, S. P., Weiss, J., Barnwell, A., Ferriero, D. M., Latal-Hajnal, B., Ferrer-Rogers, A. et al. (1972). Seizure-associated brain injury in term newborns with perinatal asphyxia. *Neurology, 58*, 542-548.

Myers, R. E. (1972). Two patterns of perinatala brain damage and their conditions of occurrence. *American Journal of Obstetrics and Gynecology, 112*, 246-276.

Rose, S. A., and Feldman, J. F. (2000). The relation of very low birth weight to basic cognitive skills in infancy and childhood. In C. A. Nelson (Ed.), *The effects of early adversity on neurobehavioral development: The Minnesota symposia on child psychology, vol. 31* (pp. 31-60). Mahwah, N. J.: Erlbaum.

Shankaran, S., Laptook, R. A., Ehrenkranz, R. A., Tyson, J. E., McDonald, S. A., Donovan, E. F. et al., (2004). Whole-body hypothermia for neonates with hypoxic-ischemic encephalopathy. *New England Jorunal of Medicine, 353*, 1574-1584.

Sartori, C., Alleman, Y., Trueb, L., Delabays, A., Nicod, P., and Scherrer, U. (1999). Augmented vasoreactivity in adult life associated with perinatal vascular insult. *Lancet, 353*, 2205-2207.

Tang, J.R., le Cras, T. D., Morris, K. G., and Abman, S. H. (2000). Brief perinatal hypoxia increases severity of pulmonary hypertension after reexposure to hypoxia in infant rats. *American Journal of Physiology: Lung Cellular and Molecular Physiology, 278*, l356-l364.

Volpe, J. J. (2001). Perinatal brain injury: from pathogenesis to neuroprotection. *Mental Retardation and Developmental Disabilities Research, 7*, 56-64.

Wienerroither, H., Steiner, H., Tomaselli, J., Lobendanz, M., and Thun-Hohenstein, L. (2001). Intrauterine blood flow and long-term intellectual, neurologic, and social development. *Obstetrics and Gynecology, 97*, 449-453.

Section C: Maternal Illness: Introduction

Cox, S. M. Werner, C. L., Hoffman, B. L., and Cunningham, F. G. (2005). *Williams Obstetrics 22nd edition.* Norwalk: Appleton and Lange.

Chapter 5

Acs, N., Banhidy, F., Puho, E., and Czeizel, A. E. (2005). Maternal influenza during pregnancy and risk of congenital abnormalities in offspring. *Birth Defects Research: A Clinical Molecular Teratology, 73*, 989-996.

Adams, W., Kendell, R. E., Hare, E. H., and Munk-Jorgensen, P. (1993). Epidemiological evidence that maternal influenza contributes to the aetiology of schizophrenia– An analysis of Scottish, English, and Danish data. *British Journal of Psychiatry, 163*, 522-534.

Akbarian, S., Bunney, W. E., Potkin, S. G., Wigal, S. B., Hagman, J. O., Sandman, C. A., and Jones, E. G. (1993). Altered distribution of nicotinamide-adenine-dinucleotide-phosphate-diaphorase cells in the frontal lobe of schizophrenics implies disturbances or cortical development. *Archives of General Psychiatry, 50*, 168-177.

Alford, C. A., Stagno, S., Pass, R. F., and Britt, W. J. (1990). Congenital and perinatal cytomegalovirus infections. *Reviews of Infectious Diseases, 12*, S745-S753.

Arajujo, D. M., and Cotman, C. W. (1995). Differential effects of interleukin-1b and interleukin-2 on glia and hippocampal neurons in culture. *International Journal of Developmental Neuroscience, 13*, 201-212.

Avgil, M., and Ornoy, A. (2006). Herpes simplex virus and epstein-barr virus infections in pregnancy: Consequences of neonatal or intrauterine infection. *Reproductive Toxicology, 21*, 436-45.

Baldwin, S., and Whitley, R. J. (1989). Intrauterine herpes simplex virus infection. *Teratology, 39*, 1-10.

Barr, C. E., Mednick, S. A., and Munk-Jorgensen, P. (1990). Exposure to influenza epidemics during gestation and adult schizophrenia. *Archives of General Psychiatry, 47*, 869-874.

Barron, S. D., and Pass, R. F. (1995). Infectious causes of hydrops fetalis. *Seminar Perinatology, 19*, 493-501.

Bates, P. R., Hawkins, A., Mahadik, S. P., and McGrath J. J. (1996). Heat stress lipids and schizophrenia. *Prostaglandins Leukotrienes and Essential Fatty Acids, 55*, 101-7.

Benveniste, E. N. (1992). Inflammatory cytokines within the central nervous system: sources, function, and mechanism of action. *American Journal of Physiology, 263*, C1-16.

Bologonese, R. J., Corson, S. L., Fuccillo, D. A., Sever, J. L., and Traube, R. (1973). Evaluation of possible transplacental infection with rubella vaccination during pregnancy. *American Journal of Obstetrics and Gynecology, 117*, 939-941.

Bonthius, D.J. and Karacay, B. (2003). Sydenham's chorea: not gone and not forgotten. *Seminars in Pediatric Neurology, 10*, 11-9.

Boyd, J. H., Pulver, A. E., and Stewart, W. (1986). Season of birth: Schizophrenia and bipolar disorder. *Schizophrenia Bulletin, 12*, 173-186.

Bradbury, T. N., and Miller, G. A. (1985). Season of birth in schizophrenia: A review of evidence, methodology, and etiology. *Psychological Bulletin, 98*, 569-594.

Brown, A. S., Begg, M. D., Gravenstein, S., Schaefer, C. A., Wyatt, R. J., Bresnahan, M., et al. (2004). Serologic evidence for prenatal influenza in the etiology of schizophrenia. *Archives of General Psychiatry, 61*, 774-780.

Brown, A. S., Cohen, P., Greenwald, S., and Susser, E. S. (2000). Non-affective psychosis after prenatal exposure to rubella. *American Journal of Psychiatry, 157*, 438-443.

Brown, A. S., Cohen, P., Harkavy-Friedman, J., Babulas, V., Malaspina, D., Gorman, J. M. et al. (2001). Prenatal rubella, premorbid abnormalities, and adult schizophrenia. *Biological Psychiatry, 49*, 473-486.

Brown, A. S., Schaefer, C. A., Quesenberry, C. P. Jr., Liu, L., Babulas, V. P., and Susser, E. S. (2005). Maternal exposure to toxoplasmosis and risk of schizophrenia in adult offspring. *American Journal of Psychiatry, 162*, 767-773.

Buka, S. L., Tsuang, M. T., Torrey, E. F., Klebanoff, M. A., Bernstein, D., and Yolken, R. H. (2001). Maternal infections and subsequent psychosis among offspring. *Archives of General Psychiatry, 58*, 1032-1037.

Burny, W., Liesnard, C., Donner, C., and Marchant, A. (2004). Epidemiology, pathogenesis and prevention of congenital cytomegalovirus infection. *Expert Review of Antiinfective Therapy, 2*, 881-94.

Cannon, M., Cotter, D., Sham, P. C., Larkin, C., Murray, R. M., Coffey, V. P., and O'Callaghan, E. (1994). Schizophrenia in an Irish sample following prenatal exposure to the 1957 influenza epidemic: a case-controlled, prospective follow-up study. *Schizophrenia Research, 11*, 95-106.

Cannon, M., Cotter, D., Coffey, V. P., Sham, P. C., Takei, N., Larkin, C., Murray, R. M., and O'Callaghan, E. (1996). Prenatal exposure to the 1957 influenza epidemic and adult schizophrenia: A follow-up study. *British Journal of Psychiatry, 168*, 368-371.

Chao, C.C., and Hu, S. (1994). Tumor necrosis factor-alpha potentiates glutamate neurotoxicity in human fetal brain cultures. *Developmental Neuroscience, 16*, 171-179.

Chess, S. (1977). Follow-up report on autism in congenital rubella. *Journal of Autism and Child Schizophrenia 7*, 69–81.

Chess, S., Korn, S., and Fernandez, P. (1971). *Psychiatric disorders of children with congenital rubella syndrome.* New York: Brunner/Mazel.

Chiba, M. E., Saito, M., Suzuki, N., Honda, Y., and Yaegashi, N. (2003). Measles infection in pregnancy. *Journal of Infection, 47*, 40-44.

Coffey, V. P., and Jessop, W. J. (1959). Maternal influenza and congenital deformities: a prospective study. *Lancet, 2*, 935-938.

Cordero, J. F. (2003). A new look at behavioral outcomes and teratogens: A commentary. Birth Defects Research (Part A). *Clinical and Molecular Teratology, 67*, 900-902.

Crow, T. J. (1983). Is schizophrenia an infectious disease? *Lancet*, 173-175.

Crow, T. J., and Done, D. J. (1992). Prenatal exposure to influenza does not cause schizophrenia. *British Journal of Psychiatry, 161*, 390-393.

Dalod, M., Salazar-Mather, T. P., Malmgaard, L., Lewis, C., Asselin-Paturel, C., Briere, F., Trinchieri, G., and Biron, C. A. (2002). Interferon α/β and interleukin 12 responses to viral infections: pathways regulating dendritic cell cytokine expression in vivo. *Journal of Experimental Medicine, 195*, 517-528.

Dassa, D., Takei, N., Sham, P. C., and Murray, R. M. (1995). No association between prenatal exposure to influenza and autism. *Acta Psychiatrica Scandinavica, 92*, 145-149.

DeLong, G. R., Bean, S. C., and Brown, F. R. III (1981). Acquired reversible autistic syndrome in acute encephalopathic illness in children. *Archives of Neurology, 38*, 191-194.

Desmonts, G., and Couvreur, J. (1974). Congenital toxoplasmosis: A prospective study of 378 pregnancies. *New England Journal of Medicine, 290*, 1110-1116.

Deykin E. Y., and MacMahon, B. (1979).Viral exposure and autism. *American Journal Epidemiology, 109*, 628–638.

Dombrowski, S. C., Martin, R. P., and Huttunen, M. O. (2003). Association between maternal fever and psychological/behavioral outcomes: An hypothesis. *Birth Defects Research (Part A): Clinical and Molecular Teratology, 67*, 905-910.

Edwards, M. J. (2006). Review: Hyperthermia and fever during pregnancy. *Birth Defects Research (Part A), 76*, 507-516.

Edwards, M. J., Walsh, D. A., and Li, Z. (1997). Hyperthermia, teratogenesis and the heat shock response in mammalian embryos in culture. *International Journal of Developmental Biology, 41*, 345-358.

Elbou Ould, M. A., Luton, D., Yadini, M., Pedron, B., Aujard, Y., Jacoz-Aigrain, E. et al. (2004). Cellular immune response of fetuses to cytomegalovirus. *Pediatric Research, 55*, 280–286.

Erlenmeyer-Kimling, L., Folnegovic, B. S., Hrabak-Zerjavic, V., Borcic, B., Folnegovic-Smalc, V., and Susser, E. (1994). Schizophrenia and prenatal exposure to the 1957 A2 influenza epidemic in Croatia. *American Journal of Psychiatry, 151*, 1496-1498.

Fahy, T. A., Jones, P. B., Sham, P. C., Takei, N., and Murray, R. M. (1993). Schizophrenia in Afro-Caribbeans in the UK following prenatal exposure to the 1957 A2 influenza epidemic. *Schizophrenia Research, 6*, 98-99.

Fowler, K. B., and Boppana, S. B. (2006).Congenital cytomegalovirus (CMV) infection and hearing deficit. *Journal of Clinical Virology, 35*, 226-31.

Fowler, K. B., McCollister, F. P., Dahle, A., J., Boppano, S., Britt, W. J., and Pass, R. F.. (1997). Progressive and fluctuating sessorineural hearing loss in children with asymptomatic congenital cytomegalovirus infection. *Journal of Pediatrics, 130*, 624-630.

Freij, B. J., South, M. A., and Sever, J. L. (1988). Maternal rubella and the congenital rubella syndrome. *Clinical Perinatology, 15*, 247-257.

Fuccillo, D. A. (1988). Congenital Varicella. In J. L. Sever and R. L. Brent (Eds.), *Teratogen update: Environmentally induced birth defect risks* (pp. 101-105). New York: Alan R. Liss.

Ghaziuddin, M., Tsai, L. Y., Eilers, L., and Ghaziuddin, N. (1992). Brief report: autism and herpes simplex encephalitis. *Journal of Autism and Developmental Disorders, 22*, 107-113.

Gilberg, C. (1986). Onset at age 14 of a typical autistic syndrome. A case report of a girl with herpes simplex encephalitis. *Journal of Autism and Developmental Disorders, 16*, 369-375.

Gilmore, J. H., and Jarskog, L. F. (1997). Exposure to infection and brain development: cytokines in the pathogenesis of schizophrenia. *Schizophrenia Research, 24*, 365-67.

Giulian,D., Li, J., Li, X., George, J., and Rutecki, P. A. (1994). The impact of microglia-derived cytokines upon gliosis in the CNS. *Developmental Neuroscience, 16*, 128-36.

Goodall, E. (1932). The exciting cause of certain states, at present classified under schizophrenia by psychiatrists, may be infection. *Journal of Mental Science, 78*, 746-755.

Gomez, R., Romero, R., Ghezzi, F., Yoon, B. H., Mazor, M., and Berry, S. M. (1998). The fetal inflammatory response syndrome. *American Journal of Obstetrics and Gynecology, 179*, 194-202.

Granata, T. (2003). Rasmussen's syndrome. *Neurological Sciences, 24* (Suppl. 4) S239-4.

Greer, M. K., Lyons-Crews, M., Mauldin, L. B., and Brown, F. R. III (1989). A case study of the cognitive and behavioral deficits of temporal lobe damage in herpes simplex encephalitis. *Journal of Autism and Developmental Disorders, 19*, 317-326.

Gregg, N. (1941). Congenital cataract following German measles in the mother. *Transactions of the American Ophthalmological Society, 3*, 35-45.

Grillner, L., Forsgren, M., Barr, B., Bottiger, M., Danielsson, L., and De Verdier, C. (1983). Outcome of rubella during pregnancy with special reference to the 17th-24th weeks of gestation. *Scandinavian Journal of Infectious Diseases, 15*(4), 321-325.

Grossman, J. H. (1986). Congenital syphilis. In J. L. Sever and R. L. Brent (Eds.), *Teratogen update: Environmentally induced birth defect risks* (pp. 113-117). New York: Liss..

Hakosalo, J., and Saxen, L. (1971). Influenza epidemic and congenital defects. *Lancet, 2*, 1346-1347.

Hanshaw, J. B., and Dudgeon, J. A. (1978). *Viral diseases of the fetus and newborn*. Philadelphia: W.B. Saunders Company.

Hardy, J. B., Azarowicz, E. N., Mannini, A., Medearis, D. N., and Cooke, R. E. (1961). The effect of Asian influenza on the outcome of pregnancy. *American Journal of Public Health, 51*, 1182-1188.

Hedrick, J. (1996). The effects of human parvovirus B19 and cytomegalovirus during pregnancy. *Journal of Perinatal Neonatal Nursing, 10*(2), 30-39.

Hesse, K., Hock, C., and Otten, U. (1998). Inflammatory signals induce neurotrophin expression in human microglia cells. *Journal of Neurochemistry, 70*, 69-707.

Hollier, L. M., and Grissom, M. D. (2005). Human herpes viruses in pregnancy: Cytomegalovirus, epstein-barr virus, and varicella zoster virus. *Clinics in Perinatology, 32*, 671-696.

Hunter, A. G. (1984). Neural tube defects in eastern Ontario and western Quebec: Demography and family data. *American Journal of Medical Genetics, 19*, 45-63.

Hutto, C., Willett, L., Yeager, A., and Whitely, R. (1985). Congenital herpes simplex virus (HSV) infection: Early vs. late gestational acquisition. *Pediatric Research, 19*, 296.

Ingalls, T. H. (1960). Prenatal human ecology. *American Journal of Public Health, 50*, 50-54.

Ivarsson, S. A., Bjerre, I., Vegfors, P., and Ahlfors, K. (1990). Autism as one of several disabilities in two children with congenital cytomegalovirus infection. *Neuropediatrics, 21*, 102-103.

Ivarsson, S. A., Lernmark B., and Svanberg L. (1997). Ten-year clinical, developmental, and intellectual follow-up of children with congenital cytomegalovirus infection without neurologic symptoms at one year of age. *Pediatrics, 99*(6), 800-803.

Jarskog, L. F., Xiao, H., Wilkie, M. B., Lauder, J. M., and Gilmore, J. H. (1997). Cytokine regulation of fetal dopaminergic and serotonergic neuron survival in vitro. *International Journal of Developmental Neuroscience, 15*, 711-716.

Jones, K. L., Johnson, K. A., and Chambers, C. D. (1994). Offspring of women infected with varicella during pregnancy: a prospective study. *Teratology, 49*, 29-32.

Jorgensen, O. S., Goldschmidt, V. V., and Vestergaard, B. F. (1982). Herpes simplex virus (HSV) antibodies in child psychiatric patients and normal children. *Acta Psychiatrica Scandinavica, 66*, 42-49.

Kashden, J., Frison, S., Fowler, K., Pass, R. F., and Boll, T. J. (1998). Intellectual assessment of children with asymptomatic congenital cytomegalovirus infection. *Journal of Developmental and Behavioral Pediatrics, 19*, 254-259.

Kendell, R. E., and Kemp, I. W. (1989). Maternal influenza in the etiology of schizophrenia. *Archives of General Psychiatry, 46*, 878-882.

Kilidireas, K., Latov, N., Strauss, D. H., Gorig, A. D., Hashim, G. A., Gorman, J. M.., et al. (1992). Antibodies to the human 60 kDa heat-shock protein in patients with schizophrenia. *Lancet, 340*(8819), 569-72.

Kluger, M.J., Wieslaw, K., and Mayfield, K. P. (2001). Fever and immunity. In R. A. Ader, D. L. Felten, and N. Cohen (Eds.), *Psychoneuroimmunology* (3rd ed., pp. 687-702). New York: Academic Press.

Knobloch, H. and Pasamanick, B. (1975). Some etiologic and prognostic factors in early infantile autism and psychosis. *Pediatrics, 55*, 182-191.

Korones, S. B., Todaro, J., Roane, J. A., and Sever, J. L. (1970). Maternal virus infection after the first trimester of pregnancy and status of offspring to 4 years of age in a predominantly Negro population. *Journal of Pediatrics, 77*, 245-251.

Kraeplin, E. (1919). Dementia Praecox and Paraphrenia. E and S Livingstone: Edinburgh.

Kumar, M. L., and Prokay, S. L. (1983). Experimental primary cytomegalovirus infection in pregnancy: timing and fetal outcomes. *American Journal of Obstetrics and Gynecology, 145*, 56-60.

Kumar, M. L., Nankervis, G. A., Jacobs, I. B., and Emhart, C. B. (1984). Congenital and postnatally acquired cytomegalovirus infection: long-term follow-up study. *Journal of Pediatrics, 104*, 674–679.

Kunugi, H., Nanko, S., Takei, N., Saito, K., Hayashi, N. and Kazamatsuri, H. (1995). Schizophrenia following in utero exposure to the 1957 influenza epidemics in Japan. *The American Journal of Psychiatry, 152*, 450-452.

Larsen, J. W. (1986). Congenital toxoplasmosis. In J. L. Sever and R. L. Brent (Eds.), *Teratogen update: Environmentally induced birth defect risks* (pp. 97-100). New York: Liss.

Limosin, F., Rouillon, F., Payan, C., Cohen, J. M., and Strub, N. (2003). Prenatal exposure to influenza as a risk factor for adult schizophrenia. *Acta Psychiatrica Scandinavica, 107*, 331-335.

Lindquist, S. (1986). The heat shock proteins. *Annual Review of Biochemistry, 55*, 1151-1191.

Lotspeich L. J, and Ciaranello, R. D. (1993). The neurobiology and genetics of infantile autism. In R. Bradley (Ed.), *International Review of Neurobiology*, (pp. 87-129). San Diego: Academic.

Lynberg, M. C., Khoury, M. J., Lu, X., and Cocian, T. (1994). Maternal flu, fever, and the risk of neural tube defects: A population-based case-control study. *American Journal of Epidemiology, 140*(3), 244-255.

Machon, R. A., Huttunen, M. O., Mednick, S. A., Sinivuo, J., Tanskanen, A., Bunn Watson, J., Henriksson, M. and Pyhala, R. (2002). Adult schizotypal personality characteristics and prenatal influenza in a Finnish birth cohort. *Schizophrenia Research, 54*, 7-16.

Machon, R. A., Mednick, S. A., and O'Huttunen, M. O. (1997). Adult major affective disorder after prenatal exposure to an influenza epidemic. *Archives of General Psychiatry, 54*, 322-328.

Maier, S. F., Watkins, L.R. and Nance, D. M. (2001). Multiple routes of action of interleukin-1 on the nervous system. In R. A. Ader, D. L. Felten, and N. Cohen (Eds.), *Psychoneuroimmunology* (3rd ed., pp. 563-583). New York: Academic Press.

Malek-Ahmadi, P. (2001). Cytokines and etiopathogenesis of pervasive developmental disorders. *Medical Hypotheses, 56*, 321-4.

Markowitz, P. I. (1983). Autism in a child with congenital cytomegalovirus infection. *Journal of Autism and Developmental Disorders, 13*, 249-253.

Mattson, S. N., Jones, K. L., Gramling, L. J., Schonfield, A. M., Riley, E. P., and Harris, J. A.. (2003). Neurodevelopmental Follow-up of Children of Women Infected with Varicella During Pregnancy: A Prospective Study. *Pediatric Infectious Disease Journal, 22*, 819-823.

McGrath, J. and Castle, D. (1995). Does influenza cause schizophrenia? A five year review. *Australian and New Zealand Journal of Psychiatry, 29*, 23-31.

McGrath, J., Pemberton, M, Welham, J. L., and Murray, R. M. (1994). Schizophrenia and the influenza epidemics of 1954, 1957 and 1959: A southern hemisphere study. *Schizophrenia Research, 14*, 1-8.

Mednick, S. A., Machon, R. A., Huttunen, M. O., and Bonnett, D. (1988). Adult schizophrenia following prenatal exposure to an influenza epidemic. *Archives of General Psychiatry, 45*, 189-192.

Mednick, S., Huttunen, M. O., and Machon, R. A. (1994). Prenatal influenza infections and adult schizophrenia. *Schizophrenia Bulletin, 20*(2), 263-267.

Mehler, M. F., and Kessler, J. A. (1999). Cytokines in brain development and function. *Advances in Protein Chemistry, 52*, 223-251.

Menninger, K. A. (1928). The schizophrenic syndromes as a product of acute infectious disease. *Archives of Neurology and Psychiatry, 20*, 464-481.

Menser, M. A., Dods, L., and Harley, J. D. (1967). A twenty-five year follow-up of congenital rubella. *Lancet, 2*, 1347-1350.

Miller, E., Cradock-Watson, J. E., and Pollock, T. M. (1982). Consequences of confirmed maternal rubella at successive stages of pregnancy. *Lancet, 2*, 781-784.

Milunsky, A., Ulcickas, M., Rothman, K. J., Willet, W., Jick, S. S., and Jick, H. (1992). Maternal heat exposure and neural tube defects. *Journal of the American Medical Association, 268*, 882-885.

Mino, Y., Oshima, I., Tsuda, T., and Okagami, K. (2000). No relationship between schizophrenic birth and influenza epidemics in Japan. *Journal of Psychiatric Research, 34*, 133-8.

Mittleman, B. B. (1997). Cytokine networks in Sydenham's chorea and PANDAS. *Advances in Experimental Medicine and Biology, 418*, 933-5.

Mittleman, B. B., Castellanos, F. X., Jacobsen, L. K., Rapoport, J. L. Swedo S. E., and Shearer, G. M. (1997). Cerebrospinal fluid cytokines in pediatric neuropsychiatric disease. *Journal of Immunology, 159*, 2994-9.

Morgan, V., Castle, D., Page, A., Fazio, S., Gurrin, L., Burton, P. et al., (1997).Influenza epidemics and incidence of schizophrenia, affective disorders and mental retardation in Western Australia: no evidence of a major effect. *Schizophrenia Research, 26,* 25-39.

Muller, N., Riedel, M., Ackenheil, M., and Schwarz, M. J. (1999). The role of immune function in schizophrenia: An overview. *European Archives of Psychiatry and Clinical Neuroscience, 249,* 62-68.

Nawa, H., Takahashi, M., and Patterson P. H. (2000). Cytokine and growth factor involvement in schizophrenia–support for the developmental model. *Molecular Psychiatry, 5,* 594-603.

Nelson, C. T., and Demmler, G. J. (1997). Cytomegalovirus infection in the pregnant mother, fetus, and newborn infant. *Clinics in Perinatology, 24,* 151-160.

Ni, J., Bowles, N. E., Kim, Y. H., Demmler, G., Kearney, D., Bricker, J. T., and Towbin, J. A. (1997). Viral infection of the myocardium in endocardial fibroelastosis. Molecular evidence for the role of mumps virus as an etiologic agent. *Circulation, 95,* 133–139.

O'Callaghan, E., Sham, P. C., Takei, N., Murray, G. and Murray, R. M. (1991). Schizoprenia after prenatal expos to 1957 A2 influenza epidemic. *Lancet, 337,* 1248-1250.

O'Callaghan, E., Sham, P. C., Takei, N., Murray, G., Glover, G., Hare, E. H., and Murray, R. M. (1994). The relationship of schizophrenic births to 16 infectious diseases. *British Journal of Psychiatry, 165,* 353-356.

Pass, R. F., Fowler, K. B., Boppana, S. B., Britt, W. J., and Stagno, S. (2006). Congenital cytomegalovirus infection following first trimester maternal infection: symptoms at birth and outcome. *Journal of Clinical Virology, 35,* 216-20.

Patterson, P. H. (2002). Maternal infection: Window on neuroimmune interactions in fetal brain development and mental illness. *Current Opinion in Neurobiology, 12,* 115-118.

Pearl, K. N., Preece, P. M., Ades, A., and Peckham, C. S. (1986). Neurodevelopmental assessment after congenital cytomegalovirus infection. *Archives of Disabled Child, 61,* 323–326.

Persaud, T. V. (1985). Causes of developmental defects. In T. V. Persaud, A. E. Chudley, and R. G. Skalko (Eds.), *Basic Concepts in Teratology* (pp. 69-102). New York: Liss.

Petersen, N. S. (1990). Effects of heat and chemical stress on development; *Adv. Genet.* **28** 275–296

Preece, P. M., Blount, J. M., Glover, J., Fletcher, G. M., Peckham, C. S., and Griffiths, P. D. (1983). The consequences of primary cytomegalovirus infection in pregnancy, *Archives of Disabled Child, 58,* 970-975.

Rogers, S. W., Twyman, R. E., and Gahring, L. C. (1996). The role of autoimmunity to glutamate receptors in neurological disease. *Molecular Medicine Today, 2,* 76-81.

Ross, S. A. and Boppana, S. B. (2005). Congenital cytomegalovirus infection: outcome and diagnosis. *Seminars in Pediatric Infectious Diseases, 16,* 44-49.

Rothwell, N. J., Giamal, L., and Toulmond, S. (1996). Cytokines and their receptors in the central nervous system: Physiology, pharmacology, and pathology. *Pharmacology, 69,* 85-95.

Rothwell, N. J., and Hopkins, S. J. (1995). Cytokines and the nervous system II: Actions and mechanisms of action. *Trends in Neurosciences, 18,* 130-136.

Sarnat, H. B. (1995). Ependymal reactions to injury: A review. *Journal of Neuropathology and Experimental Neurology, 54,* 1-15.

Selten, J. P., Brown, A. S., Moons, K. G., Slaets, J. P., Susser, E. S., and Kahn, R. S. (1999). Prenatal exposure to the 1957 influenza pandemic and non-affective psychosis in The Netherlands. *Schizophrenia Research, 38,* 85-91.

Selten, J. and Slaets, J. (1994). Evidence against maternal influenza as a risk factor for schizophrenia. *British Journal of Psychiatry, 164,* 674-676.

Selten, J, and Slaets, J. (1994b). Second trimester exposure to 1957 A2 influenza is not a risk factor for schizophrenia: The Dutch national register. *British Journal of Psychiatry, 164,* 674-676.

Selten, J., and Slaets, J. (1998). Prenatal exposure to influenza and schizophrenia in Surinamese and Dutch Antillean immigrants to The Netherlands. *Schizophrenia Research, 30,* 101-103.

Sever, J. L. (1986). Perinatal infection and damage to the central nervous system. In M. Lewis, *Learning disabilities and prenatal risk* (pp.194-209). Chicago: University of Illinois Press.

Sham, P. C., O'Callaghan, E., Takei, N., and Murray, G. K. (1992). Maternal viral infection and schizophrenia. *British Journal of Psychiatry, 161*, 273-274.

Sham, P. C., O'Callaghan, E., Takei, N., Murray, G. K., Hare, E., and Murray, R. M. (1992). Schizophrenia following pre-natal exposure to influenza epidemics between 1939 and 1960. *British Journal of Psychiatry, 160*, 461-466.

Shepard TH. Catalog of Teratogenic Agents.pp1867 9th ed.Baltimore,MD: Johns Hopkins University Press, 1998

Shiota, K. (1982). Neural tube defects and maternal hyperthermia in early pregnancy: Epidemiology in a human embryonic population. *American Journal of Medical Genetics, 12*, 281-288.

Siegel, M. (1973). Congenital malformations following chickenpox, measles, mumps, and hepatitis. Results of a cohort study. *Journal of American Medical Association, 226*, 1521-1524.

Siegel, M., Fuerst, H. T., and Peress, N. S. (1966). Comparative fetal mortaltiy in matenal virus diseases: a prospective study on rubella, measles, mumps, chickenpox, and hepatitis. *New England Journal of Medicine, 274*, 768.

Singh, V. K., and Jensen, R. L. (2003). Elevated levels of measles antibodies in children with autism. *Pediatric Neurology, 28*, 292–294.

Singh, V. K., Lin, S. X., Newell, E., and Nelson, C. (2002). Abnormal measles-mumps-rubella antibodies and CNS autoimmunity in children with autism. *Journal of Biomedical Science, 9*, 359–364.

Singh, V. K., Lin, S. X., and Yang, V. C. (1998). Serological association of measles virus and human herpesvirus-6 with brain autoantibodies in autism. *Clinical Immunology and Immunopathology, 89*, 105–108.

Sinha, A. A., Lopez, M. R., and McDevitt, H. O. (1990). Autoimmune diseases: The failure Of self-tolerance. *Science, 248*, 1380-1388.

South, M., and Sever, J. (1985). Teratogen update: The congenital rubella syndrome. *Teratology, 31*, 297-307.

South, M. A., Thompkins, W. A., Morris, C. R., and Rawls, W. E. (1969). Congenital malformations of the central nervous system associated with genital type (type 2) herpes virus. *Journal of Pediatrics, 75*, 13-18.

Strauss, D. H. (1999). Heat shock proteins and autoimmune mechanisms of disease in schizophrenia. In A. E. Susser, A. S. Brown, and J. M. Gorman (Eds.), *Prenatal Exposures in Schizophrenia* (pp. 215-239). Washington, DC: American Psychiatric Press.

Stubbs, E. G. (1978). Autistic symptoms in a child with congenital cytomegalovirus infection. *Journal of Autism and Childhood Schizophrenia, 8*, 37-43.

Susser, E., Lin, S. P., Brown, A. S., Lumey, L. H., and Erlenmeyer-Kimling, L. (1994). No relation between risk of schizophrenia and prenatal exposure to influenza in Holland. *American Journal of Psychiatry, 151*, 922-924.

Sweeten, T. L., Posey, D. J., and McDougle, C. J. (2004). Autistic disorder in three children with cytomegalovirus infection. *Journal of Autism and Developmental Disorders, 34*, 583-586.

Taber, L. H. (1982). Evaluation and management of syphilis in pregnant women and newborn infants. *Pediatric Infectious Disease, 1*, 224-227.

Takei, N., Mortensen, P. B., Klaening, U., Murray, R. M., Sham, P. C., O'Callaghan, E, et al. (1996). Relationship between in utero exposure to influenza epidemics and risk of schizophrenia in Denmark. *Biological Psychiatry, 40*, 817-824.

Takei, N., Sham, P., O'Callaghan, E., Glover, G., and Murray, R. M. (1993). Does prenatal influenza diverts susceptible females from later affective psychosis to schizophrenia? *Acta Psychiatrica Scandinavica, 88*, 328-336.

Takei, N., Sham, P., O'Callaghan, E., Glover, G., and Murray, R. M. (1994). Prenatal influenza and schizophrenia: Is the effect confined to females? *American Journal of Psychiatry, 151*, 117-119.

Takei, N., Van Os, J., and Murray, R. M. (1995). Maternal exposure to influenza and risk of schizophrenia: A 22-year study from the Netherlands. *Journal of Psychiatric Research, 29*, 435-445.

Temple, R. O., Pass, R. F., and Boll, T. J. (2000). Neuropsychological functioning in patients with asymptomatic congenital cytomegalovirus infection. *Journal of Developmental and Behavioral Pediatrics, 21*, 417-422.

Torrey, E. F. and Peterson, M. R.(1973). Slow and latent viruses in schizophrenia. *Lancet, ii*, 22-24.

Torrey, E. F., Rawlings, R., and Waldman, I. N. (1988). Schizophrenic births and viral diseases in two states. *Schizophrenia Research, 1*, 73-77.

Torrey, E. F., and Yolken, R. H. (1995). Could schizophrenia be a viral zoonosis transmitted from house cats? *Schizophrenia Bulletin, 21*, 167-171.

Uhlmann, V., Martin, C. M., O'Sheils, L., Pilkington, I., Silva, F., Killalea, B., et al., (2002). Potential viral pathogenic mechanism for new variant inflammatory bowel disease. *Molecular Pathology, 55*, 84-90.

Urakubo, A., Jarskog, L. F., Lieberman, J. A., and Gilmore, J. H. (2001). Prenatal exposure to maternal infection alters cytokine expression in the placenta, amniotic fluid, and fetal brain. *Schizophrenia Research, 47*(1), 27-36.

Venables, P. H. (1996). Schizotypy and maternal exposure to influenza and to cold temperature: The Mauritius study. *Journal of Abnormal Psychology, 105*, 53-60.

Waddington, J. L., O'Callaghan, E., Youssef, H. A., Buckley, P., Lane, A., Cotter, D., and Larkin, C. (1999). Schizophrenia: Evidence for a "cascade" process with neurodevelopmental origins. In E. S. Susser, A. S. Brown, and J. M. Gorman (Eds.), *Prenatal exposure in schizophrenia* (pp. 3-34). Washington, DC: American Psychiatric Press.

Warkany, J. (1986). Teratogen update: Hyperthermia. *Teratology, 33*, 365-371.

Westergaard, T., Mortensen, P. B., Pedersen, C. B., Wohlfahrt, J., and Melbye, M. (1999). Exposure to prenatal and childhood infections and the risk of schizophrenia: suggestions from a study of sibship characteristics and influenza prevalence. *Archives of General Psychiatry, 56*, 993-998.

Williamson, W. D., Desmond, M. M., LaFevers, N., Taber, L. H., Catlin, F. I., and Weaver, T. G. (1982). Symptomatic congenital cytomegalovirus. Disorders of language, learning, and hearing. *American Journal of Diseases in Children, 136*, 902-905.

Wilson, M. G., Heins, H. L., Imagawa, D. T., and Adams, J. M. (1959). Teratogenic effects of Asian influenza. *Journal of the American Medical Association, 171*, 116-119.

Wong, A., Tan, K. H., Tee, C. S., and Yeo, G. S. H. (2000). Seroprevalence of cytomegalovirus, toxoplasma and parvovirus in pregnancy. *Singapore Medical Journal, 41*, 151-155.

Wright, P., and Murray, R. M. (1996). Prenatal influenza, immunogenes and schizophrenia: A hypothesis and some recent findings. In J. L. Waddington, and P. F. Buckley (Eds.), *The neurodevelopmental basis of schizophrenia*. New York: R. G. Landes Company.

Wright, P., Takei, M. D., Rifkin, L., and Murray, R. M. (1995). Maternal influenza, obstetric complications, and schizophrenia. *American Journal of Psychiatry, 152*, 1714-1720.

Yolken, R. (2004). Viruses and schizophrenia: a focus on herpes simplex virus. *Herpes. 11* (Suppl. 2), 83A-88A.

Zgorniak-Nowosielska, I., Zawilinska, B., and Szostek, S. (1996). Rubella infection during pregnancy in the 1985-86 epidemic: Follow-up after seven years. *European Journal of Epidemiology, 12*, 303-308.

Zhao, B., and Schwartz, J. P. (1998). Involvement of cytokines in normal CNS development and neurological diseases: Recent progress and perspectives. *Journal of Neuroscience Research, 52*, 7-16.

Chapter 6

Aerts, L., Pijnenborg, R., Verhaeghe, J., Holemans, K., and Assche, F. (1996). Fetal growth and development. In A. Dornhorst and D. R. Hadden (Eds.), *Diabetes and pregnancy, an international approach to diagnosis and management* (pp. 77-98). London: Wiley.

Al Ghafli, M. H., Padmanadhan, R., Kataya, H. H., and Berg, B. (2004). Effects of a-lipoic acid supplementation on maternal diabetes-induced growth retardation and congenital anomalies in rat fetuses. *Molecular and Cellular Biochemistry, 261*, 123-135.

Ananth, C. V., Peedicayil, A., and Savitz, D. A. (1995). Effect of hypertensive diseases in pregnancy on birthweight, gestational duration, and small-for-gestational-age births. *Epidemiology, 6*, 391-395.

Anderson, J. L., Kim, W. D., Canfield, M. A., Shaw, G. M., Watkins, M. L., and Werler, M. M. (2005). Maternal obesity, gestational diabetes, and central nervous system birth defects. *Epidemiology, 16*, 87-92.

American Diabetic Association (2004). Diabetes information: All about diabetes. (retrieved 2004). *http://www.diabetes.org/about-diabetes.jsp*

Bracken, M. B., Triche, E. W., Belanger, K., Saftlas, A., Beckett, W. S., and Leaderer, B. P. (2003). Asthma symptoms, severity, and drug therapy: a prospective study of effects of 2204 pregnancies. *Obstetrics and Gynecology, 102*, 739-752.

Barrett, C. T. (1987). Management of infants of diabetic mothers. In B. S. Nuwayhid, C. R. Brinkman, and S. M. Lieb (Eds.), *Management of the diabetic pregnancy* (pp. 120-127). New York: Elsevier.

Basso, O., Christensen, K., and Olsen, J. (2001). Higher risk of pre-eclampsia after change of partner: an effect of longer interpregnancy intervals? *Epidemiology, 12*, 624-629.

Brody, J. E. (June, 2004). Beginning a pregnancy already overweight. New York Times, June 29, 2004. pg D7.

Cogswell, M. E., Perry, G. S., Schieve, L. A., and Dietz, W. H. (2001). Obesity in women of childbearing age: risks, prevention, and treatment. *Primary Care Update: Obstetrics and Gynecology, 8*, 89-105.

Dombrowski, M. P., Schatz, M., Wise, R., Momirova, V., Landon, M., Mabie W., et al., (2004). Asthma during pregnancy. *Obstetrics and Gynecology, 103*, 5-12.

Dunn, F., Brydon, P., Smith, K., and Gee, H. (2003). Pregnancy in women with type 2 diabetes: 12 years outcome data 1990-2002. *Diabetic Medicine, 20*, 734-738.

Epidemiology and Statistical Unit, CDC (2001). Trends in asthma morbidity and mortality. Washington: Center for Health Statistics.

Evers, I. M., de Valk, H. W., and Visser, G. H. A. (2004). Risk of complications of pregnancy in women with type 1 diabetes: nationwide prospective study in the Netherlands. *British Medical Journal, 328, 915-921. (doi:10.1136/bmj.38043.583160.EE)*

Hampton, T. (2004). Maternal diabetes and obesity may have lifelong impact on health of offspring. *Journal of the American Medical Association, 292*, 789-790.

Hameed, A., Karaalp, H. S., Tummala, P. P., Wani, O. R., Canetti, M., Akhter, M. W. et al. (2001). The effect of valvular heart disease on maternal and fetal outcome of pregnancy. *Journal of the American College of Cardiology, 37*, 893-899.

Kallen, B., Rydhstroem, H., and Aberg, A. (2000). Asthma during pregnancy—a population-based study. *European Journal of Epidemiology, 16*, 167-171.

Klonoff-Cohen, H. S., Havitz, D. A., Cefalo, R. C., and McCann, M. F. (1989). An epidemiologic study of contraception and preeclampsia. *Journal of the American Medical Association, 262*, 3143-3147.

Lauenborg, J., Hansen, T., Jensen, D. M., Vestergaard, H., Molsted-Pedersen, L., Hornnes, P., et al. (2004). Increasing incidence of diabetes after gestational diabetes: a long-term follow-up in a Danish population. *Diabetes Care, 27*, 1194-1199.

Li, D. K., and Wi, S. (2000). Changing paternity and the risk of preeclampsia/eclampsia in the subsequent pregnancy. *American Journal of Epidemiology, 151*, 57-62.

Lupton, M., Oteng-Ntim, E., Ayida, G., and Steer, P. J. (2002). Cardiac disease in pregnancy. *Obstetrics and Gynecology, 14*, 137-143.

Von Mutius, E. (2001). Paediatric origins of adult lung disease. *Thorax, 56*, 153-157.

Mineribi-Codish, I., Fraser, D., Avnun, L., Glezerman, M., and Heimer,D. (1998). Influence of asthma in pregnancy on labor and the newborn. *Respiration, 65*, 130-135.

National Center for Chronic Disease Prevention and Health Promotion of the Centers for Disease Control (2005). Frequently asked questions. *(http://www.cdc.gov/diabetes.faq/basics.htm)*.

Peat, J. K., Gray, E. J., Mellis, C.M., Leeder, S. R., and Woolcock, A. J. (1994). Differences in airway hyperresponsiveness between children and adults living in the same environment: an epidemiological study in two regions of New South Wales. *European Respiratory Journal, 7*, 1326-1329.

Pederson, and Molstead-Pederson, L. (1981). Early growth delay detected by ultrasound marks increased risk of congenital malformation in diabetic pregnancy. *British Medical Journal, 283*, 269-271.

Perlow, J. H., Montgomery, D., Morgan, M. A., Towers, C. V., and Porto, M. (1992). Severity of asthma and perinatal outcome. *American Journal of Obstetrics and Gynecology, 167*, 963-967.

Roberts, J. M. (1998). Pregnancy related hypertention. In R. K. Creasy, R. Resnik (Eds), *Maternal fetal medicine (4th ed.)* (pp 833-872).. Philadelphia: Saunders.

Roberts, J. M., Pearson, G., Cutler, J., and Lindheimer, M. (2003). Summary of the NHLBI working group on research on hypertension during pregnancy. *Hypertension, 41*, 437-445.

Robillard, P.Y, and Hulsey, T. C. (1994). Association of pregnancy-induced hypertension with duration of sexual cohabitation before conception. *Lancet, 344*, 973-976.

Saftlas, A. F., Levine, R. J., Klebanoff, M. A., Martz, K. L., Ewell, M. G., Morris, C. D., et al. (2003). Abortion, changed paternity, and risk of preeclampsia in nulliparous women. *American Journal of Epidemiology, 157*, 1108-1114.

Sibai, B. M. (2006). Treatment of hypertension in pregnant women. *New England Journal of Medicine, 335*, 257-265.

Sui, S. C., and Colman, J. M. (2001). Heart disease and pregnancy. *Heart, 85*, 710-715.

Sui, S. C., Sermer, M., Colman, J. M., Alvarez, A. N., Mercier, L. A., Morton, B. C. et al. (2001). Prospective multi-center study of pregnancy outcomes in women with heart disease. *Circulation, 96*, 515-521.

Svare, J. A., Hansen, B. B., and Molsted-Pedersen, L. (2001). Perinatal complication in women with gestational diabetes mellitus. *Acta Obstetricia et Gynecologica Scandinavica, 80*, 899-904.

Thilen, U., and Olsson, S. B. (1997). Pregnancy and heart diseases: a review. *European Journal of Obstetrics and Gyneocology and Reproduction Biology, 75*, 43-50.

Vahratian, A., Zhang, J., Troendle,, J. F., Savitz, D. A., and Siega-Riz, A. M. (2004). Maternal prepregnancy overweight and obesity and the pattern of labor progression in term nulliparous women. *Obstetrics and Gynecology, 104*, 943-951.

Zimmet, P., Alberti, K.G. M. M., and Shaw, J. (2001). Global and societal implications of The diabetes epidemic. *Nature, 414*, 782-787.

Chapter 7

Azaois-Braesco, V., and Pascal, G. (2000). Vitamin A in pregnancy: requirements and safety limits. *American Journal of Clinical Nutrition, 71*, 1325S-1133S.

Butterworth, R. F. (1990). Vitamin deficiencies and brain development. In N. M. Van Gelder, R. F. Butterworth, and B. Drujan, (Eds)., *(Mal)Nutrition and the infant brain* (pp. 207-224). New York: Wiley-Liss.

Cannon, M., Kendell, R., Susser, E., and Jones, P. (2003). Prenatal and perinatal risk factors for schizophrenia. In Murray, R. M., Jones, P. B., Susser, E., van Os, J., Cannon, M. (eds). *The epidemiology of schizophrenia* (pp. 74-99). Cambridge, England: Cambridge University Press.

Chen, Q., Connor, J. R., and Beard, J. L. (1995). Brain iron, transferring and ferritin concentrations are altered in developing iron-deficient rats. *Journal of Nutrition, 125*, 1529-1535.

Cheng, S., Tylavksy, F., Kroger, H., Karkkainen, A., Lyytikainen, A., Koistinen, A., et al. (2003). Association of low 25-hydroxyvitamin D concentrations with elevated parathyroid hormone concentrations and low cortical bone density in early pubertal and prepubertal Finnish girls. *American Journal of Clinical Nutrition, 78*, 485-492.

Davies, G., Welham, J., Torrey, E. F., McGrath, J. (2000). Season of birth and latitude: a systematic review and meta-analysis of northern hemisphere studies. *Schizophrenia Research, 41*, 63.

deMaeyer, E., and Adiels-Tegman, M. (1985). The prevalence of anaemia in the world. *World Health Statistics Quarterly, 38*, 302-316.

Devereaux, G., Turner, S. W., Craig, L. C., McNeill, G., Martindale, S., Harbour, P. J., Helms, P. J., and Seaton A. (2006). Low maternal vitamin E intake during pregnancy is associated with asthma in 5-year-old children. *American Journal of Respiratory Critical Care medicine, 174*, 499-507.

Eyles, D., Brown, J., Mackay-Sim, A., McGrath, J., and Feron, F. (2003). Vitamin D3 and brain development. *Neuroscience, 118*, 641-653.

Feleke, Y., Abdulkadir, J., Mshana R., Mekbib, T. A., Brunvand, L., Berg, J. P. et al. (1999). Low levels of serum calcidiol in an African population compared with a North European population. *European Journal of Endocrinology, 141*, 358-360.

Felt, B. T., and Lozoff, B. (1996). Brain iron and behavior or rats are not normalized by treatment of iron deficiency anemia during early development. *Journal of Nutrition, 126*, 693-701.

Georgieff, M. K., Landon, M. B., Mills, M. M., Hedlund, B. E., Faassen, A. E., Schmidt, R. L., et al., (1990). Abnormal iron distribution in infants of diabetic mothers: spectrum and maternal antecedents. *Journal of Pediatrics, 117*, 455-461.

Gilliland, F. D., Berhane, K. T., Li, Y. F., Gauderman, J., McConnell, R., and Peters, J. (2003). Children's lung function and antioxidant vitamin, fruit, juice and vegetable intake. *American Journal of Epidemiology, 158*, 576-584.

Goldenberg, R. L., Tamura, T, Cliver, S. P., Cutter, G. R., Hoffman, H. J., and Cooper, R. L. (1992). Serum folate and fetal growth retardation: A matter of compliance? *Obstetrics and Gynecology, 79*, 791.

Gombart, A. F., Borregaard, N., and Koeffler, P. (2005). Human cathelicidin antimicrobial peptide (CAMP) gene is a direct target of the vitamin D receptor and is strongly up-regulated in myeloid cells by 1,25-dihydroxyvitamin D$_3$. *The FASEB Journal, 19*, 1067-1077.

Gottleib, D. J., Biasini, F. J., and Bray, N. W. (1988). Visual recognition memory in UIGR and normal birth weight infants. *Infant Behavior and Development, 11*, 223-228.

Groner, J. A., Holtzman, N. A., Charney, E., and Millitts, E. (1986). A randomized trial of oral iron on tests of short-term memory and attention span in young pregnant women. *Journal of Adolescent Health Care, 7*, 44-48.

Grover, S. R., and Morley, R. (2001). Vitamin D deficiency in veiled or dark-skinned pregnant women. *Medical Journal of Australia, 175*, 251-252.

Hack, M., Breslau, N., Weissman, B., Aram, D., Klein, N., and Borawski, E. (1991). Effect of very low birth weight and subnormal head size on cognitive abilities at school age. *New England Journal of Medicine, 325*, 231-237.

Harik-Khan, R. I., Muller, D. C., and Wise, R. A. (2004). Serum vitamin levels and the risk of asthma in children. *American Journal of Epidemiology, 159*, 351-357.

Hilman, L. S., and Haddad, J. G. (1976). Perinatal vitamin D metabolism. III. Factors influencing late gestational human serum 25-hydroxyvitamin D. *American Journal of Obstetrics and Gynecology, 125*, 196-200.

Looker, A., C., Dallman, P. R., Carroll, M. D., Gunter, D. W., and Johnson, C. L. (1997). Prevalence of iron deficiency in the United States. *Journal of the American Medical Association, 277*, 973-976.

Lozoff, B. (1990). Has iron deficiency been shown to cause altered behavior in infants? In J. Dobbing (Ed.), *Brain, behaviour, and iron in the infant diet* (pp. 107-131). London: Springer-Verlag.

Lozoff, B., Klein, N. K., Nelson, E. C., McClish, D. K., Manuel, M., and Chacon, M. E. (1998). Behavior of infants with iron-deficiency anemia. *Child Development, 69*, 24-36.

Martin, R. P., Foels, P., Clanton, G., and Moon, K. (2004). Season of birth is related to child retention rates, achievement, and rate of diagnosis of specific LD. *Journal of Learning Disabilities, 37*, 307-317.

McGrath, J. J. (2001). Does imprinting with low prenatal vitamin D contribute to the risk of various adult disorders? *Medical Hypotheses, 56*, 367-371.

Nakamura, K., Nashimoto, M., and Yamamoto, M. (2000). Summer/winter differences in the serum 25-hydroxyvitamin D3 and parathyroid hormone levels of Japanese women. *International Journal of Biometeorology, 44*, 186-189.

Need, A. G., Morris, H. A., Horowitz, M., and Nordin, B. E. C. (1993). Effects of skin thickness, age, body fat, and sunlight on serum 25-hydroxyvitamin D: integral components of the vitamin D endocrine system. *American Journal of Clinical Nutrition, 58*, 882-885.

Norman, A. W. (1998). Sunlight, season, skin pigmentation, vitamin D, and 25-hydroxyvitamin D: integral components of the vitamin D endocrine system. *American Journal of Clinical Nutrition, 67*, 1108-1110.

Ong, P. Y., Ohtake, T., Brandt, C., Strickland, I., Boguniewicz, M., Ganz, T., Gallo, R. I., and Leung, D. Y. (2002). Endogenous antimicrobial peptides and skin infections in atopic dermatitis. *New England Journal of Medicine, 347*, 1151-1160.

Polizzi, N., Martin, R. P., and Dombrowski, S. (2007). Season of birth of students receiving special education services under a diagnosis of emotional and behavioral disorders. *School Psychology Quarterly. 22*, 44-57.

Raloff, J. (November, 2006). The antibiotic vitamin: deficiency in vitamin D may predispose people to infection. *Science News, 170*, 312-317.

Ramakrishnan, U., Manjrekar, R., Rivera, J., Gonzales-Cossio, T. and Martorell, R. (1999). Micronutrients and pregnancy outcome: a review of the literature. *Nutrition Research, 19*, 103-159.

Rao, R., and Georgieff, M. K. (2000). Early nutrition and brain development. In C. A. Nelson (Ed.), *The effects of early adversity on neurobehavioral development: The Minnesota Symposia on Child Development, Vol. 31*. Mahway, N.J.: Erlbaum

Rao, R., De Ungria, M., Sullivan, D., Wu, P., Wobken, J., Nelson, C. A. et al. (1999). Perinatal brain iron deficiency increases the vulnerability of the rat hippocampus to hypoxic-ischemic injury. *Journal of Nutrition, 129*, 199-206.

Rothman, K. J., Moore, L. L., Singer, M. R., Nguyen, U.D.T., Mannino, S., and Milunsky, A. (1995). Teratogenicity of high vitamin A intake. *New England Journal of Medicine, 333*, 1369-1373.

Schwartz J., and Weiss, S. T. (1990). Dietary factors and their relation to respiratory symptoms. *American Journal of Epidemiology, 132*, 67-76.

Seouw, W. K. (2003). Diagnosis and management of unusual dental abscesses in children. *Australian Dental Journal, 48*, 156-168.

Smithells, D. (1996). Vitamins in early pregnancy. *British Medical journal, 313*, 128-129.

St. Clair, D., Xu, M., Wang, P., Yu, Y., Fang, Y., Zhang, F. et al. (2005). Rates of adult schizophrenia following prenatal exposure to the Chinese famine of 1959-1961. *Journal of the American Medical Association, 294*, 557-562.

Strauss, R. S., and Dietz, W. H. (1998). Growth and development of term children born with low birth weight: effects of genetics and environmental factors. *Journal of Pediatrics, 133*, 67-72.

Susser, E., and Lin, S. P. (1992). Schizophrenia after prenatal exposure to the Dutch hunger winter of 1944-1945. *Archives of General Psychiatry, 49*, 983-988.

Thomas, M. K., Lloyd, J. D., Thadhani, R. I., Shaw, A. C., Deraska, D. J., and Kitch, B. T. (1998). Hypovitaminosis in medical inpatients. *New England Journal of Medicine, 338*, 777-783.

United States National Center for Health Statistics (1979). Food consumption profiles for white and black persons aged 1-74 years: United States, 1971-1974. Hyattsville, MD: National Center for Health Statistics, 47-48.

Waldie, K. E., Poulton, R., Kirk, I. J., and Silva, P. A. (2000). The effects of pre- and post-natal sunlight exposure on human growth: evidence from the Southern Hemisphere. *Early Human Development, 60*, 35-42.

Willer, C. J., Dyment, D. A., Sadovnick, A. D., Rothwell, P. M., Murray, T. J., and Ebers, G. D. (2005). Timing of birth and risk of multiple sclerosis: population based study. *British Medical Journal, 330*, 1-20.

Willhite, C. C., Hill, R. M., and Irving, D. W. (1986). Isotretinoin-induced craniofacial malformations in humans and hamsters. *Journal of Craniofacial Genetics and Developmental Biology (Supplement 2)*, 193-209.

Wohlfahrt, J., Melbye, M., Christens, P., Anderson, A. N. and Hjalgrim, H. (1998). Secular and seasonal variation of length and weight at birth. *Lancet, 352,* 2-6.

Yip, R., Parvanta, I., Scanlon, K., Borland, E. W., Russell, C. M., and Trowbridge, F. L. (1992). Pediatric nutrition surveillance system—United States, 1980-1991. *Morbidity and Mortality Weekly Report, 41,* 1-24.

Chapter 8

Abrams, S. M., Field, T., Scafidi, F., and Prodromidis, M. (1995). Newborns of depressed mothers. *Infant Mental Health Journal, 16,* 233-239.

Adler, N. E., and Snibbe, A. C. (2002). The role of psychosocial processes in explaining the gradient between socioeconomic status and health. *Current Trends in Psychological Science, 12, 119-123.*

Baker, G., Irani, M., Byrom, N. A., Naqvekar, N. M., Wood, R. J., Hobbs, J. R. et al. (1985). Stress, cortisol concentrations and lymphocye subpopulations. *British Medical Journal, 270,* 1110-1112.

Barker, D. J. P. (1998). In utero programming of chronic disease. *Clinical Science, 95,* 115-128.

Braungart, J., Plomin, R., DeFries, J. C., and Fulker, P. (1992). Genetic influence on tester rated infant temperament as assessed by Bayley's Infant Behavior Record: nonadoptive and adoptive siblings and twins. *Development Psychology, 28,* 40-47.

Bridge, L. R. Little, B. C., Hayworth, J., Dewhurst, J., and Priest, R. G. (1985). Psychometric antenatal predictors of postnatal depressed mood. *Journal of Psychosomatic Research, 29,* 325-331.

Brouwer, E. P. M., van Baar, A. L., and Pop, V. J. M. (2001). Maternal anxiety during pregnancy and subsequent infant development. *Infant Behavior and Development, 24,* 95-106.

Carlson, D., and LaBarba, R. (1979). Maternal emotionality during pregnancy and reproductive outcomes: A review of the literature. *International Journal of Behavioral Development, 2,* 343-376.

Clarke, A. S., Soto, A., Bergholz, T., and Schneider, M. L. (1996). Maternal gestational stress alters adaptive and social behavior in adolescent rhesus monkey offspring. *Infant Behavior and Development, 19,* 451-461.

Cohen, S., Tyrrell, D., and Smith, A. (1991). Psychological stress and susceptibility to the common cold. *New England Journal of Medicine, 325,* 606-612.

DiPietro, J. A., Hilton, S. C., Hawkins, M., Costigan, K. A., and Pressman, E. K. (2002). Maternal stress and affect influence fetal neurobehavioral development. *Developmental Psychology, 38,* 659-668.

DiPietro, J. A., Hodgson, D. M., Costigan, K. A., Hilton, S. C., and Johnson, T. R. B. (1996a). Fetal neurobehavioral development. *Child Development, 67,* 2553-2567.

DiPietro, J. A., Hodgson, D. M., Costigan, K. A., Hilton, S. C., and Johnson, T. R. B. (1996b). Development of fetal movement-fetal heart rate coupling from 20 weeks through term. *Early Human Development, 44,* 139-151.

Fride, E., and Weinstock, M. (1984). The effects of prenatal exposure to predictable or unpredictable stress on early development in the rat. *Developmental Psychobiology, 17,* 651-660.

Fujioka, T., Fujioka, A., Tan, N., Chowdhury, G., Mouri, H., Sakata, Y., and Nakamura, S. (2001). Mild prenatal stress enhances learning performance in the non-adopted rat offspring. *Neuroscience, 103,* 301-307.

Gennero, S., and Fehder, W. (1996). Stress, immune function, and relationship to pregnancy outcome. *Nursing Clinics of North America, 31,* 293-303.

Gitau, R., Cameron, A., Fisk, N., and Glover, V. (1998). Fetal exposure to maternal cortisol. *Lancet, 352,* 707-708.

Grant, K. E., Compas, B. E., Stuhlmacher, A., Thurm, A. E., McMahon, S., and Halpert, J. (2003). Stressors and child/adolescent psychopathology: Moving from markers to mechanisms of risk. *Psychological Bulletin, 129*, 447-466.

Hansen, D., Lou, H. C., and Olsen, J. (2000). Serious life events and congenital malformations: A national study with complete follow-up. *Lancet, 356*, 875-880.

Hepper, P. G., and Shahidullah, S. (1990). Fetal response to maternal shock. *Lancet, 336*, 1068.

Hobel, C. J., Dunkel-Schetter, C., Roesch, S. C., Castro, L. C., and Arora, C. P. (1999). Maternal plasma corticotropin-releasing hormone associated with stress at 20 weeks gestation in pregnancies ending in preterm delivery. *American Journal of Obstetrics and Gynecology, 180*, S257-S263.

Huizink, A. C., Robles de Medina, P. R., Mulder, E. J. H., Visser, G. H. A., and Buitelaar, J. K. (2002). Psychological measures of prenatal stress as predictor of infant temperament. *Journal of the American Academy of Child and Adolescent Psychiatry, 41*, 1078-1085.

Huizink, A. C., Robles de Medina, P. R., Mulder, E. J. H., Visser, G. H. A., and Buitelaar, J. K. (2003). Stress during pregnancy is associated with developmental outcome in infancy. *Journal of Child Psychology and Psychiatry, 44*, 810-818.

Huizink, A. C., Mulder, E. J. H., and Buitelaar, J. K. (2004). Prenatal stress and risk of psychopathology: Specific effects or induction of general susceptibility. *Psychological Bulletin, 130*, 115-142.

Huttunen, M. O., and Niskanen, P. (1978). Prenatal loss of father and psychiatric disorders. *Archives of General Psychiatry, 35*, 429.

Jarrah-Zedeh, A., Kane, F., Van de Castle, R., Lachenbruch, P., and Ewing, J. (1969). Emotional and cognitive changes in pregnancy and early puerperium. *British Journal of Psychiatry, 115*, 811-825.

Kemeny, M. E. (2003). The psychobiology of stress. *Current Trends in Psychological Science, 12, 124-129.*

Kurki, T., Hiilesmaa, V., Raitasalo, R., Mattila, H., and Ylikorkala, O. (2000). Depression and anxiety in early pregnancy and risk for preeclampsia. *Obstetrics and Gynecology, 95, 487-490.*

Lazarus, R. S., and Folkman, S. (1984). *Stress, appraisal, and coping.* New York: Springer.

Leckman, J. F., Dolnansky, E. S., Hardin, M. T., Clubb, M., Walkup, J. T., Stevenson, J., and Pauls, D. L. (1990). Perinatal factors in the expression of Tourette's syndrome: an exploratory study. *Journal of the American Academy of Child & Adolescent Psychiatry, 29*, 220-226.

Lederman, R. P. (1995). Relationship of anxiety, stress, and psychosocial development to reproductive health. *Behavioral Medicine, 21*, 101-112.

Leifer, M. (1980). *Psychological effects of motherhood: A study of first pregnancy.* New York: Praeger.

Linn, B., Linn, M., and Klimas, N. (1988). Effects of psychophysical stress on surgical outcome. *Psychosomatic Medicine, 50*, 230-234.

Lips, H. M (1985). A longitudinal study of the reporting of emotional and somatic symptoms during and after pregnancy. *Social Science and Medicine, 21, 631-640.*

Lubin, B., Gardener, S. H., and Roth, A. (1975). Mood and somatic symptoms during pregnancy. *Psychosomatic Medicine, 37*, 136-146.

Luoma, I., Tamminen, T., Kaukonen, P., Laippala, P., Puura, K., Salnelin, R., and Almqvist, F. (2001). Longitudinal study of maternal depressive symptoms and child well-being. *American Academy of Child and Adolescent Psychiatry, 40*, 1367-1374.

Martin, R. P., Noyes, J., Wisenbaker, J., and Huttunen, M. O. (1999). Prediction of early childhood negative emotionality and inhibition from maternal distress during pregnancy. *Merrill-Palmer Quarterly, 45*, 370-391.

Montagu, A. (1962). *Prenatal influences.* Springfield, IL: Thomas.

Neiderhofer, H., and Reiter, A. (2000). Maternal stress during pregnancy, its objectivation by ultrasound observation of fetal intrauterine movements and child's temperament at 6 months and 6 years of age: A pilot study. *Psychological Reports, 86*, 526-528.

O'Connor, T. G., Heron, J., Golding, J., Beveridge, M., and Glover, V. (2002). Maternal antenatal anxiety and behavioural problems in early childhood. *British Journal of Psychiatry, 180,* 520-508.

Ottinger, D. R., and Simmons, J. E. (1964). Behavior of human neonates and prenatal maternal anxiety. *Psychological Reports, 17,* 22-27.

Oyemade, U., Cole, O., Johnson, A., Knight, E., Westney, O., Laryea, H., et al. (1994). Prenatal predictors of performance on the Brazelton Neonatal Behavioral Assessment Scale. *Journal of Nutrition, 124,* 1000S-1005S.

Plomin, R. (1990). *Nature and nurture: An introduction to human behavior genetics.* Pacific Grove, CA: Brooks/Cole.

Rofe, Y., Blittner, M., and Lewin, I. (1993). Emotional experiences during the three trimesters of pregnancy. *Journal of Clinical Psychology, 49,* 3-12.

Rondo, P. H., Ferreira, R. F., Nogueira, F., Ribeiro, M. C., Lobert, H., and Artes, R. (2003). Maternal psychological stress and distress as predictors of low birth weight, prematurity and intrauterine growth retardation. *European Journal of Clinical Nutrition, 57,* 266-272.

Schneider, M. L. (1992). The effect of mild stress during pregnancy on birthweight and neuromotor maturation in Rhesus monkey infants (Macaca mulatta). *Infant Behavior and Development, 15,* 389-401.

Schneider, M. L., Roughton, E. C., Koehler, A. J., and Lubach, G. R. (1999). Growth and development following prenatal stress exposure in primates: An examination of ontogenetic vulnerability. *Child Development, 70,* 263-274.

Schneider, M. L., Roughton, E. C., and Lubach, G. R. (1997). Moderate alcohol consumption and psychological stress during pregnancy induce attention and neuromotor impairments in primate infants. *Child Development, 68,* 747-759.

Segerstrom, S. C., and Miller, G. E. (2004). Psychogical stress and the human immune system: A meta-analytic study of 30 years of inquiry. *Psychological Bulletin, 130,* 601-630.

Sjostrom, M., Valentin, L., Thelin, T., and Marsal, K. (1997). Maternal anxiety in late pregnancy and fetal hemodynamics. *European journal of Obstetrics and Gynecology, 74, 149-155.*

Spielberger, C. D., and Jacobs, G. A. (1979). Maternal emotions, life stress and obstetric complications. In L. Zichella and R. Pancheri (Eds.), *Emotion and reproduction* (pp. 12-22). London: Academic Press.

Sontag, L. W. (1941). The significance of fetal environmental differences. *American Journal of Obstetry and Gynaecology, 124,* 996-1003.

Standley, Soule, and Copans (1979). Dimensions of prenatal anxiety and their influence on pregnancy outcome, *American Journal of Obstetrics and Gynecology, 135,* 22-26.

Van den Bergh, B. R. H. and Marcoen, A. (2004). High antenatal maternal anxiety is related to ADHD symptoms, externalizing problems, and anxiety in 8- and 9-year-olds. *Child Development, 75,* 1085-1097.

Van den Bergh, B. R. H., Mulder, E. J. H., Visser, G. H. A., Poelmann-Weesjes, G., Bekedam, D. J., and Prechtl, H. F. R. (1989). The effect of (induced) maternal emotions on fetal behaviour: a controlled study. *Early Human Development, 19,* 9-19.

Van den Bergh, B. R. H. Vandenberghe, K., Daniels, H., Casaer, P., and Marcoen, A. (1989). The relationship between maternal emotionality during pregnancy and the behavioral development of the fetus and neonatus. In G. Genbnser, K. Marsal, N. Svenningen, and K. Lindstrom (Eds.), *Fetal and neonatal physiological measurements III* (pp. 359-363). Malmo, Denmark: Fenhags Trycheri.

Van Os, J., and Selton, J. (1998). Prenatal exposure to maternal stress and subsequent schizophrenia. *British Journal of Psychiatry, 172,* 324-326.

Vaughn, B. E., Bradley, C. F., Joffe, L. S., Seifer, R., and Barglow, T. (1987). Maternal characteristics measured prenatally are predictive of ratings of temperament 'difficulty' on the Carey Temperament Questionnaire. *Developmental Psychology, 23,* 152-161.

Welbert, L. A., and Seckl, J. R. (2001). Prenatal stress, glucocorticoids and the programming of the brain. *Journal of Neuroendocrinology, 13,* 113-128.

Weinstock, M. (2001). Alternations induced by gestational stress in brain morphology and behavior of the off-spring. *Progress in Neurobiology, 65*, 427-451.

Wehr, T. A., Duncan, W. C., Sher, L., Aeschbach, D., Schwartz, P. J., Turner, E. H. et al. (2001). A circadian signal of change of season in patients with seasonal affective disorder. *Archives of General Psychiatry, 58*, 1108-1114.

Zuckerman, B., Bauchner, H., Parker, S., and Cabral, H. (1990). Maternal depressive symptoms during pregnancy, and newborn irritability. *Journal of Developmental and Behavioral Pediatrics, 11*, 190-194.

Section D: Maternal Use of Recreational Drugs

Chapter 9

Abel, E., and Hannigan, J. (1996). Alcohol and the developing child. In Spohr and Steinhausen (Eds.), *Risk factors and pathogenesis* (pp. 63-75). Cambridge, MA: Cambridge University Press.

Adams, J. (2003). Statement of the Public Affairs Committee of the Teratology Society on the importance of smoking cessation during pregnancy. *Birth Defects Research Part A: Clinical and Molecular Teratology, 67*, 895-899.

Aligne, C., and Stoddard, J. (1997). Tobacco and children. *Archives of Pediatric and Adolescent Medicine, 151*, 648-653.

American Academy of Pediatrics Committee on Environmental Health (1997). Environmental tobacco smoke: A hazard to children. *Pediatrics, 99*, 639-642.

Astrup, P., Olson, H. M., Trolle, D., and Kjeldsen, K. (1972). Effects of carbon monoxide exposure on fetal development. *Lancet, 2*, 1220-1222.

Bakoula, C., Kafritsa, Y., Kavadias, G., and Lazopoulou, D. (1995). Objective passive-smoking indicators and respiratory morbidity in young children. *Lancet, 346*, 280-281.

Batstra, L., Hadders-Algar, M., and Neeleman, J. (2003). Effect of antenatal exposure to maternal smoking on behavioral problems and academic achievement in childhood; prospective evidence from a Dutch birth cohort. *Early Human Development, 75*, 21-33.

Bauman, K., Flewelling, R., and LaPrelle, J. (1991). Parental cigarette smoking and cognitive performance of children. *Health Psychology, 10*, 282-288.

Beeber, S. J. (1996). Parental smoking and childhood asthma. *Journal of Pediatric Health Care, 10*, 58-62.

Bonham, G. S., and Wilson, R. W. (1981). Children's health in families with cigarette smokers: *American Journal of Public Health, 71*, 290-293.

Brennan, P. A., Grekin, E. R. and Mednick, S. A. (1999). Maternal smoking during pregnancy and adult male criminal outcomes. *Archives of General Psychiatry, 56*, 223-224.

Brennan, P. A., Grekin, E. R., Mortensen, E. L., and Mednick, S. A. (2002). Relationship of maternal smoking during pregnancy with criminal arrest and hospitalization for substance abuse in male and female adult offspring. *American Journal of Psychiatry, 159*, 48-54.

Breslau, N., Paneth, N., Lucia, V. C., and Paneth-Pollack, R. (2005). Maternal smoking during pregnancy and offspring IQ. *International Journal of Epidemiology, 34*(5), 1047-1053.

Brook, J. S., Brook, D. W., and Whiteman, M. (2000). The influence of maternal smoking during pregnancy on the toddler's negativity. *Archives of Pediatrics and Adolescent Medicine 154*, 381–385.

Butler, N. R., and Goldstein, H. (1973). Smoking in pregnancy and subsequent child development. *British Medical Journal, 4*, 573-575.

Centers for Disease Control (2004). Smoking During Pregnancy—United States, 1990-2002. *Morbidity and Mortality Weekly Report, 53*(39), 911-915.

Charlton, A. (1994) Children and passive smoking: a review. *Journal of Family Practice, 38*, 267-277.

Cherry, N., and Kiernan, K. (1976). Personality scores and smoking behavior - a longitudinal study. *British Journal of Preventive and Social Medicine, 30*, 123-121.

Chilmoncyzk, B., Salmun, L., Megathlin, K., Neveux, L., Palomaki, G., Knight, G., Pulkkinen, A., and Haddow, J. (1993). Association between exposure to environmental tobacco smoke and exacerbations of asthma in children. *New England Journal of Medicine, 328*, 1665-1669.

Colley, J. R. R., Holland, W. W., and Corkhill, R. T. (1974). Influence of passive smoking and parental phlegm on pneumonia and bronchitis in early childhood. *Lancet, 1*, 529-532.

Committee on Nutritional Status and Weight Gain During Pregnancy, National Science Foundation, (1990). *Nutrition during pregnancy*. Washington, D.C.,: National Science Foundation.

Cornelius, M. D., Ryan, C. M., Day, N. L., Goldschmidt, L., and Willford, J. A. (2001). Prenatal tobacco effects on neuropsychological outcomes among preadolescents. *Journal of Development and Behavioral Pediatrics, 22*, 217-225.

Cunningham, J., Dockery, D., and Speizer, F. (1994). Maternal smoking during pregnancy as a predictor of lung function in children. *American Journal of Epidemiology, 139*, 1139-1152.

Day, N. L., Richardson, G. A., Goldschmidt, L., and Cornelius, M. D. (2000). Effects of prenatal tobacco exposure on preschoolers' behavior. *Journal of Developmental and Behavioral Pediatrics, 21*, 180-188.

Denson, R., Nanson, J. L., and McWatters, M. A. (1975). Hyperkinesis and maternal smoking: *Canadian Psychiatric Association Journal, 20*, 183-187.

DiFranza, J. R. and Lew, R. A. (1995). Effects of maternal cigarette smoking on pregnancy complications and sudden infant death syndrome. *Journal of Family Practice, 40*, 385-394.

Dombrowski, S. C., Martin, R. P., and Huttunen, M. O. (2005). Gestational exposure to cigarette smoke imperils the long term physical and mental health of offspring. *Birth Defects Research Part A: Clinical and Molecular Teratology, 73*, 170-176.

Dunn, H. G., McBurney, A. K., Ingram, S., and Hunter, C. M. (1977). Maternal cigarette smoking during pregnancy and the child's subsequent development. II: Neurological and intellectual maturation to the age of 6½ years. *Canadian Journal of Public Health, 68*, 43-45.

Ernst, M., Moolchan, E. T., and Robinson, M. L. (2001). Behavioral and neural consequences of prenatal exposure to nicotine. *Journal of the American Academy of Child & Adolescent Psychiatry, 6*, 630–641.

Ernester, V. L. (1993) Woman and smoking. *American Journal of Public Health, 83*, 1202-1204.

Eysenck, H. (1991). *Smoking, personality, and stress*. New York: Springer-Verlag.

Fergusson, D., Horwood, J., and Lynskey, M. (1993). Maternal smoking before and after pregnancy: effects of behavioral outcomes in middle childhood. *Pediatrics, 92*, 815-822.

Fergusson, D. M., Woodward, L. J., and Horwood, L. J. (1998). Maternal smoking during pregnancy and psychiatric adjustment in late adolescence. *Archives of General Psychiatry, 55*, 721-727.

Fielding, J. E. (1985). Smoking: health effects and control. *New England Journal of Medicine, 313*, 491-498.

Fingerhut, L. A., Kleinman, J. C., and Kendrick, J. S. (1990). Smoking before, during, and after pregnancy. *American Journal of Public Health, 80*, 541-544.

Floyd, R. L., Rimer, B. K., Giovino, G. A., Mullen, P. D., and Sullivan, S. E. (1993). A review of smoking in pregnancy: effects on pregnancy outcomes and cessation efforts. *Annual Review of Public Health, 14*, 379-411.

Fogelman, K. R. (1980). Smoking in pregnancy and subsequent development of the child. *Child: Care, Health and Development, 6*, 233-249.

Fogelman, K. R., and Manor, O. (1988). Smoking in pregnancy and development into early adulthood. *British Medical Journal, 297*, 1233-1235.

Fried, P. A., and Makin, J. E. (1987). Neonatal behavioral correlates of prenatal exposure to marihuana, cigarettes and alcohol in a low-risk population. *Neurotoxicology and Teratology, 9*, 1-7.

Fried, P. A., and Watkinson, B. (1988). 12- and 24-month neurobehavioral follow-up of children prenatally exposed to marijuana, cigarettes, and alcohol: cognitive and language assessment. *Neurotoxicology and Teratology, 16*, 305-313.

Fried, P. A., and Watkinson, B. (1990). 36- and 48-month neurobehavioral follow-up of children prenatally exposed to marijuana, cigarettes, and alcohol. *Developmental and Behavioral Pediatrics, 11*, 49-58.

Fried, P. A., Watkinson, B., Dillon, R. F., and Dulberg, C. S. (1987). Neonatal neurological status in a low-risk population after prenatal exposure to cigarettes, marijuana, and alcohol. *Developmental and Behavioral Pediatrics, 11*, 49-58.

Fried, P. A., Watkinson, B., and Gray, R. (1992b). A follow-up study of attentional behavior in six-year-old children exposed prenatally to marijuana, cigarettes and alcohol. *Neurotoxicology*, 505-529.

Fried, P. A., Watkinson, B., and Gray, R. (2003). Differential effects on cognitive functioning in 12- to 16-year-olds prenatally exposed to cigarettes and marihuana. *Neurotoxicology and Teratology, 25*, 427-436.

Graham, H. (1995). Women, smoking and disadvantage. In K. Slama (Ed.), *Smoking and health*. New York: Plenum.

Grunberg, N.E. (1990). The inverse relationship between tobacco use and body weight. In L. T. Kozlowski, H. M. Annis, H. D. Cappel, F. B. Glaser, M. S. Goodstadt, Y. Israel, H Kalunt, E. M. Sellers, and E. R. Vingilis (Eds.), *Research advances in alcohol and drug problems: Vol. 10* (pp. 273-316). New York: Plenum.

Grunberg, N. E., Winders, S. E., and Wewers, M. E. (1991). Gender differences in tobacco use. *Health Psychology, 10*, 143-153.

Gunnar, M. R., Porter, F. L., Wolf, C. M., Rigatuso, J., and Larson, M. C. (1995). Neonatal stress reactivity: predictions to later emotional temperament. *Child Development, 66*, 1-13.

Gusella, J. L., and Fried, P. A. (1984). Effects of maternal social drinking and smoking on off-spring at 13 months. *Neurobehavioral Toxicology and Teratology, 6*, 13–17.

Hanrahan, J., Tager, I., Segal, M., Tosteson, T., Castile, R., Van Vunakis, H., Weiss, S., and Speizer, F. (1992). The effect of maternal smoking during pregnancy on early infant lung function. *American Review of Respiratory Disease, 145*, 1129-1135.

Hardy, J. B., and Mellitis, D. D. (1972). Does maternal smoking during pregnancy have a long-term effect on the child? *Lancet, 2*, 1332.

Harlap, S., and Davies, A. M. (1974). Infant admissions to hospital and maternal smoking. *Lancet, 1*, 529-532.

Hill, C. (1995). Trends and implications of tobacco use. Lessons from the French experience. In K. Slama (Ed.), *Tobacco and health* (pp. 121-127). New York: Plenum.

Hinton, A. E. (1989). Surgery for otitis media with effusion in children and its relationship to parental smoking. *Journal of Laryngol Otology, 103*, 559-561.

Hirschman, R. S., Leventhal, H., and Glynn, K. (1984). The development of smoking behavior. *Journal of Applied Social Psychology, 14*, 184-206.

Huizink, A. C., Mulder, E. J. H., and Buitelaar, J. K. (2004). Prenatal stress and risk for psychopathology: Specific effects or induction of general susceptibility? *Psychological Bulletin, 130*, 115-142.

Hunt, C. E., and Hauck, F. R. (2006). Sudden infant death syndrome. *Canadian Medical Association Journal, 174*, 1861-1869.

Isohanni, M., Oja, H., Moilanen, I., Koiranen, M., and Rantakallio, P. (1995). Smoking or quitting during pregnancy: associations with background and future social factors. *Scandinavian Journal of Social Medicine, 23*, 32-38.

Jacobson, S. W., Fein, G. G., Jacobson, J. L., Schwartz, P., and Dowler, J. (1984). Neonatal correlates of prenatal exposure to smoking, caffeine and alcohol. *Infant Behavior and Development, 7*, 253-265.

Jin, C., and Rossignal (1993). Effects of passive smoking on respiratory illness from birth to age eighteen months in Shanghai, People's Republic of China. *Journal of Pediatrics, 123*, 553-558.

Jones, K. L. (1989). Effects of chemical and environmental agents. In R. K. Creasy and R. Resnik (Eds.), *Maternal-fetal medicine: principles and practice* (2nd ed., pp. 180-192). Philadelphia, PA: Saunders.

Kallen, K. (2000). Multiple malformations and maternal smoking. *Paediatric Perinatology and Epidemiology, 14*, 227-33.

Kemppainen, L., Jokelainen, J., Isohanni, M., Jarvelin, M., and Rasanen, P. (2002). Predictors of female criminality: Findings from the Northern Finland 1966 birth cohort. *Journal of the American Academy of Child & Adolescent Psychiatry*, 41, 854-859.

Kotimaa, A. J., Moilanen, I., Taanila, A., Ebeling, H., Smalley, S. L., McGough, J. J., Hartikainen, A., and Jarveling, M. (2003). Maternal smoking and hyperactivity in 8-year-old children. *Journal of the American Academy of Child & Adolescent Psychiatry, 42*, 826-833.

Kramer, M. S. (1987). Determinants of low birth weight: methodological assessment and meta-analysis. *Bulletin of the World Health Organization, 65*, 663-737.

Krapels, I. P., Zielhuis, G. A., Vroom, F., de Jong-van den Berg, L. T., Kuijpers-Jagtman, A. M., van der Molen, A. B., and Steegers-Theunissen, R. P. (2006). Periconceptional health and lifestyle factors of both parents affect the risk of live-born children with orofacial clefts. *Birth Defects Research, 76*(8), 613-620.

Kristjanson, E. A., Fried, P. A., and Watkinson, B. (1989). Maternal smoking during Pregnancy affects children's vigilance performance. *Drug and Alcohol Dependence, 24*, 11–19.

Kuzma, J. W., and Kissinger, D. G. (1982). Patterns of alcohol and cigarette use in pregnancy. *Neurobehavioral Toxicology and Teratology, 3*, 211-221.

Landesman-Dwyer, S., and Emanuel, I. (1979). Smoking during pregnancy. *Teratology, 19*, 119-126.

Law, K. L., Stroud, L. R., LaGasse, L. L., Niaura, R., Liu, J., and Lester, B. M. (2003). Smoking during pregnancy and newborn neurobehavior. *Pediatrics, 111*, 1318-1323.

Lebowitz, M. D., and Burrow, B. (1976). Respiratory symptoms related to smoking habits of family adults. *Chest, 69*, 48-50.

Lenz W. (1962). Thalidomide and congenital abnormalities. *Lancet 1*,1219.

Levin, E. D., and Slotkin, T. A. (1998). Developmental neurotoxicity of nicotine. In: Slikker, W., Chang, L. W. (Eds.), *Handbook of Developmental Neurotoxicity* (pp.587-615). New York: Academic Press.

Lichtensteiger, W., and Schlumpf, M. (1993). Prenatal nicotine exposure: biochemical and neuroendocrine bases of behavioral dysfunction. *Developmental Brain Dysfunction, 6*, 279-304.

Longo, L. (1977). The biological effects of carbon monoxide on the pregnant woman, fetus, and newborn infant. *American Journal of Obstetrics and Gynecology, 129*, 69-103.

Magee, B. D., Hattis, D., and Kivel, N. M. (2004). Role of smoking in low birth weight. *Journal of Reproductive Medicine, 49*, 23-27.

Makin, J., Fried, P. A., and Watkinson, B. (1991). A comparison of active and passive smoking during pregnancy: long term effects. *Neurological Toxicology, 13*, 5-12.

Martin, R. P., Dombrowski, S. C., Mullis, C., and Huttunen, M. O. (2006). Maternal smoking during pregnancy: Association with temperament, behavioral, and academics. *Journal of Pediatric Psychology, 31*, 490-500.

Martinez, F., Cline, M., and Burrows, B. (1992). Increased incidence of asthma in children of smoking mothers. *Pediatrics, 89*, 21-26.

Maughan, B., Taylor, A., Caspi, A., and Moffitt, T. E. (2004). Prenatal smoking and early childhood conduct problems. *Archives of General Psychiatry, 61*, 836-843.

Maughan, B., Taylor, C., Taylor, A., Butler, N., and Bynner, J. (2001). Pregnancy smoking and childhood conduct problems: A causal association? *Journal of Child Psychology and Psychiatry, and Allied Disciplines, 42*, 1021-1028.

McCartney, J. S., and Fried, P. A. (1993). Prenatal cigarette exposure and central auditory processing abilities in 6-11 year old children. *Teratology, 47*, 456-457.

McCartney, J. S., Fried, P. A., and Watkinson, B. (1994). Central auditory processing in school age children prenatally exposed to cigarette smoke. *Neurotoxicology and Teratology, 16*, 267-276.

Milberger, S., Bieberman, J., Farone, S. V., Chen, L., and Jones, J. (1996). Is maternal smoking during pregnancy a risk factor for attention-deficit hyperactivity disorder in children? *American Journal of Psychiatry, 153*, 1138-1142.

Mindell, J. (1995a). Smoking prevalence in pregnant women in Southern Derbyshire, UK in 1992. In K. Slama (Ed.), *Tobacco and health* (pp. 797-798). New York: Plenum.

Montreaux, M. C., Blacker, D., Biederman, J., Fitzmaurice, G., and Buka, S. L. (2006). Maternal smoking during pregnancy and offspring overt and covert conduct problems: a longitudinal study. *Journal of Child Psychology and Psychiatry, 47*, 883-890.

Mortensen, E. L., Michaelsen, K. F., Sanders, S. A., Reinisch, J. M., and Machover, J. (2005). A dose-response relationship between maternal smoking during late pregnancy and adult intelligence in male offspring. *Paediatric and Perinatal Epidemiology, 19*(1), 4-11.

Naeye, R. L., and Peters, E. C. (1984). Mental development of children whose mothers smoked during pregnancy. *Obstetrics and Gynecology, 64*, 601-609.

Nichols, P. L. (1977). *Minimal brain dysfunction: Association with perinatal complications*. Paper presented to the Society for Research in Child Development, New Orleans.

Nugent, J. K., Lester, B. M., Greene, S. M., Wieczorek-Deering, D., and O'Mahony, P. (1996). The effects of maternal alcohol consumption and cigarette smoking during pregnancy on acoustic cry analysis. *Child Development, 67*, 1806-1816.

O'Campo, P. O., Faden, R. R., Brown, H., and Gielen, A. C. (1992). The impact of pregnancy on women's prenatal and postpartum smoking behavior. *American Journal of Preventative Medicine, 8*, 8-13.

Ojima, T., Uehara, R., Watanabe, M., Tajimi, M., Oki, I., and Nakamura, Y. (2004). Population attributable fraction of smoking to low birth weight in Japan. *Pediatrics International, 46*, 264-267.

Olds, D. L., Henderson, C. R., and Tatelbaum (1994). Intellectual impairment in Children of women who smoke cigarettes during pregnancy. *Pediatrics, 93*, 221-227.

Olshan, A. F., and Faustman, E. M. (1993). Male-mediated developmental toxicity. *Annual Review of Public Health, 14*, 159-181.

Orlebeke, J. F., Knol, D. L., and Verhulst, F. C. (1999). Child behavior problems increased by maternal smoking during pregnancy. *Archives of Environmental Health, 54*, 15-19.

Owen, M. J. Baldwin, C. D., Swank, P. R., Pannu, A. K., Johnson, D. L. and Howie, V. M. (1993). Relation of infant feeding practices, cigarette smoke exposure, and group child care to the onset and duration of otitis media with effusion in the first two years of life. *Journal of Pediatrics, 123*, 702-711.

Picone, T. A., Allen, L. H., Olsen, P. N., and Ferris, M. E. (1982). Pregnancy outcome in North American women. II. Effects of diet, cigarette smoking, stress, and weight gain on placentas, and on neonatal physical and behavioral characteristics. *The American Journal of Clinical Nutrition, 36*, 1214-1224.

Polanski, K., Hanke, W., and Sobala, W. (2005). Smoking relapse one year after delivery among women who quit smoking during pregnancy. *International Journal of Occupational Medicine and Environmental Health, 18*, 159-165.

Pratt, T. C., McGloin, J. M., and Fearn, N. E. (2006). Maternal cigarette smoking during pregnancy and criminal/deviant behavior. A meta-analysis. *International Journal of Offender Therapy and Comparative Criminology, 50*, 672-690.

Ramsey, D. S., Bendersky, M. I., and Lewis, M. (1996). Effects of prenatal alcohol and cigarette exposure on two- and six-month-old infants: adrenocortical reactivity to stress. *Journal of Pediatric Psychology, 7*, 833-840.

Rantakallio, P. (1983). A follow-up study to the age of 14 of children whose mothers smoked during pregnancy. *Acta Paediatrica Scandinavica, 72*, 747-753.

Rantakallio, P., Laara, E., Isohanni, M., and Moilanen, I. (1992). Maternal smoking during pregnancy and delinquency of the offspring: as association without causation? *International Journal of Epidemiology, 21*, 1106-1113.

Savitz, D. A., Schwingle, P. J., and Keels, M. A. (1991). Influence of paternal age, smoking, and alcohol consumption on congenital anomalies. *Teratology, 44*, 429-440.

Saxton, D. (1978). The behavior of infants whose mothers smoke in pregnancy. *Human Development, 2,* 263–269.

Schmitz, M., Denardin, D., Silva, T. L., Pianca, T., Hutz, M. H., Faraone, S., and Rohde, L. A. (2006). Smoking during pregnancy and attention-deficit/hyperactivity disorder, predominantly inattentive type: A case-control study. *Journal of the American Academy of Child & Adolescent Psychiatry, 45,* 1338-1345.

Sexton, M., Fox, N. L., and Hebel, J. R. (1990). Prenatal exposure to tobacco. II. Effects on cognitive functioning at age 3. *International Journal of Epidemiology, 19,* 72-77.

Shah, T., Sullivan, K., and Carter, J. (2006). Sudden infant death syndrome and reported maternal smoking during pregnancy. *American Journal of Public Health, 96,* 1757-1759.

Shenassa, E. D., and Brown, M. J. (2004). Maternal smoking and infantile gastrointestinal dysregulation: The case of colic. *Pediatrics, 114,* 497–505.

Silberg, J. L., Parr, T., Neale, M. C., Rutter, M., Angold, A., and Eaves, L. J. (2003). Maternal smoking during pregnancy and risk to boys' conduct disturbance: An examination of the causal hypothesis. *Society of Biological Psychiatry, 53,* 130-135.

Silverstein, B., Feld, S. and Kozlowski, L. T. (1980). The availability of low-nicotine cigarettes as a cause of cigarette smoking among teenage females. *Journal of Health and Social Behavior, 21,* 383-388.

Simpson, W. J. (1957). A preliminary report on cigarette smoking and the incidence of prematurity. *American Journal of Obstetrics and Gynecology, 73,* 808-815.

Sondergaard, C., Henriksen, T. B., Obel, C., and Wisborg, K. (2001). Smoking during pregnancy and infantile colic. *Pediatrics, 108,* 342-346.

Spira, A., Spira, N., Goujard, J., and Schwartz, D. (1975). Smoking during pregnancy and placental weight: a multivariate analysis on 3759 cases. *Journal of Perinatal Medicine, 3,* 237-241.

Stein, Z. and Kline, J. (1983). Smoking, alcohol and reproduction. *American Journal of Public Health, 73,* 1154-1156.

Tager, I. B., Weiss, S. T., Rosner, B., and Speizer, F. E. (1979). Effect of parental cigarette smoking on the pulmonary function of children. *American Journal of Epidemiology, 100,* 15-26.

Thapar, A., Fowler, T., Rice, F., Scourfield, J., van den Bree, M., Thomas, H., Harold, G., and Hay, D. (2003). Maternal smoking during pregnancy and attention-deficit hyperactivity disorder symptoms in offspring. *The American Journal of Psychiatry, 160,* 1985-1989.

Tolson, C. M., Seidler, F. J., McCook, E. C., and Slotkin, T. A. (1995). Does concurrent or prior nicotine exposure interact with neonatal hypoxia to produce cardiac cell damage? *Teratology, 52,* 298-305.

United States Department of Health and Human Services (1980). *The health consequences of smoking for women: a report of the surgeon general.* Washington, D.C.: United States Department of Health and Human Services.

Wakschlag, L. S. and Hans, S. L. (2002). Maternal smoking during pregnancy and conduct problems in high risk youth: A developmental framework. *Development Psychopathology, 14,* 351-369.

Wakschlag, L. S., Lahey, B. B., Loeber, R., Green, S. M., Gordon, R. A., and Leventhal, B. L. (1997). Maternal smoking during pregnancy and the risk of conduct disorder in boys. *Archives of General Psychiatry, 54,* 670-676.

Weitzman, M., Gortmaker, S., Walker, D. K., and Sobel, A. (1990). Maternal smoking and childhood asthma. *Pediatrics, 85,* 505-511.

Williams, J. G., and Covington, C. J. (1997). Prediction of cigarette smoking among adolescents. *Psychological Reports, 80,* 481-482.

Wojtacki, J., and Dziewulsha-Bokiniec, A. (1995). Benign breast disease and active smoking: a case-control study. In K. Slama (Ed.), *Smoking and Health* (pp. 525-527). New York: Plenum.

Chapter 10

Abel, E. L. (1984). *Fetal alcohol syndrome and fetal alcohol effects*. New York: Plenum

Abel, E. L., and Hannigan, J. H. (1996). Risk factors and pathogenesis. In H. L. Spohr and H. C. Steinhausen (Eds.), *Alcohol and the developing child* (pp 63-75). Cambridge, MA: Cambridge University Press.

Abel, E. L., and Sokol, R. J. (1987). Incidence of fetal alcohol syndrome and economic impact of FAS-related anomalies. *Drug and Alcohol Dependence, 19*, 51-70.

Abel E. L., Kruger M. L., and Friedl, J. (1998). How do physicians define "light," "moderate," and "heavy" drinking?. *Alcoholism: Clinical and Experimental Research. 22*: 979-84, 1998

Assadi, F. K., and Ziai, M. (1986). Zinc status of infants with fetal alcohol syndrome. *Pediatric Research, 20*, 551-554.

Autti-Ramo, I., and Granstrom, M. L. (1991). The psychomotor development during the first year of life of infants exposed to intrauterine alcohol of various duration. *Neuropediatrics, 22*, 59-64.

Baer, J. S., Sampson, P. D., Barr, H. M., Connor, P. D., and Streissguth, A. P. (2003). A 21-year longitudinal analysis of the effects of prenatal alcohol exposure on young adult drinking. *Archives of General Psychiatry, 60*, 377-385.

Boyd, T. A., Ernhart, C. B., Greene, T. H., Sokol, R. J., and Martier, S. (1991). Prenatal alcohol exposure and sustained attention in the preschool years. *Neurotoxicology and Teratology, 13*, 49-55.

Burden, M. J., Jacobson, S. W., Sokol, R. J., and Jacobson, J. L. (2005). Effects of prenatal alcohol exposure on attention and working memory at 7.5 years of age. *Alcoholism: Clinical and Experimental Research, 29*, 443-452.

Carmichael-Olsen, H., Feldman, J. J., Streissguth, A. P., and Gonzalez, R. D. (1992). Neuropsychological deficits and life adjustment in adolescents and adults with fetal alcohol syndrome. *Alcoholism: Clinical and Experimental Research, 16*, 380.

Carmichael-Olsen, H., Streissguth, A. P., Sampson, P. D., Barr, H. M., Bookstein, F. L., and Thiede, K. (1997). Association of prenatal alcohol exposure with behavioral and learning problems in early adolescence. *Journal of the American Academy of Child & Adolescent Psychiatry, 36*, 1187-1194.

Centers for Disease Control and Prevention Alcohol consumption amount pregnant woman and childbearing-aged women. United States, 1991 and 1995. *MMWR Morbidity and Mortality Weekly Report, 1997, 46*, 346-350.

Coles, C. D., Brown, R. T., Smith, I. E., Platzman, K. A., Erickson, S., and Falek, A. (1991). Effects of prenatal alcohol exposure at school age. I. Physical and cognitive development. *Neurotoxicology and Teratology, 13*, 357-367.

Davis, P. J. M., Partridge, J. W., and Storrs, C. N. (1982). Alcohol consumption in pregnancy: how much safe? *Archives of Disease in Childhood, 57*, 940-943.

Diav-Citrin, O., and Ornoy, A. (2000). Adverse environment and prevention of early pregnancy disorders. *Early Pregnancy, 4*, 5-18.

Ernhart, C. B., Morrow-Tlulack, M., Sokol, R. J., and Martier, S. (1988). Underreporting of alcohol use in pregnancy. *Alcoholism: Clinical Experimental Research, 12*, 506-511.

Fried, P. A. and Watkinson, B. (1990). 36- and 48-month neurobehavioral follow-up of children prenatally exposed to marijuana, cigarettes, and alcohol. *Journal of Developmental and Behavioral Pediatrics, 11*, 49-58.

Fried, P. A., O'Connell, C. M., and Watkinson, B. (1992a). 60- and 72-month follow-up of children prenatally exposed to marihuana, cigarettes, and alcohol: cognitive and language assessment. *Journal of Developmental and Behavioral Pediatrics, 13*, 383-391.

Goldschmidt, L., Richardson, G. A., Cornelius, M. D., and Day, N. L. (2004). Prenatal marijuana and alcohol exposure and academic achievement at age 10. *Neurotoxicology and Teratology, 26*, 521-532.

Gray, J. K, and Streissguth, A. P. (1990). Memory deficits and life adjustment in adults with fetal alcohol syndrome: A case control study. *Alcoholism: Clinical and Experimental Research, 14,* 294.

Green, J. H. (2007). Fetal alcohol spectrum disorders: understanding the effects of prenatal alcohol exposure and supporting students. *Journal of School Health, 77,* 103-108.

Hankin, J. R. and Sokol, R. J. (1995). Identification and care of problems associated with alcohol ingestion in pregnancy. *Seminars in Perinatology, 19,* 286-292

Hill, S. Y., Lowers, L., Locke-Wellman, J., and Shen, S. A. (2000). Maternal smoking and drinking during pregnancy and the risk for child and adolescent psychiatric disorders. *Journal of Studies on Alcohol, 6,* 661-668.

Howell, K. K., Lynch, M. E., Platzman, G., Smith, H., and Coles, C. D. (2006). Prenatal alcohol exposure and ability, academic achievement, and school functioning in adolescence: A longitudinal follow-up. *Journal of Pediatric Psychology, 21,* 116-126.

Huizink, A. C., and Mulder, E. J. H. (2006). Maternal smoking, drinking or cannabis use during pregnancy and neurobehavioral and cognitive functioning in human offspring. *Neuroscience and Biobehavioral Reviews, 30, 24-41.*

Jones, K. L. and Smith, D. W. (1973). Recognition of the fetal alcohol syndrome in early infancy. *Lancet, 2,* 999-1001.

Jones, K. L., Smith, D. W., Ulleland, C. N., and Streissguth, A. P. (1973). Pattern of malformation in offspring of chronic alcoholic mothers. *Lancet, 1,* 1267-1271.

Julien, R. M. A. (1998). *A primer of drug action, a concise, non-technical guide to the actions, uses and side effects of psychoactive drugs* (8th ed., pp. 64-78). New York: Freeman and Company.

Kalberg, W. O., Provost, B., Tollison, S. J., Tabachnick, B. G., Robinson, L. K., Hoyme, H. E., Trujillo, P. M., Buckley, D., Aragon, A. S., and May, P. A. (2006). Comparison of Motor Delays in Young Children With Fetal Alcohol Syndrome to Those With Prenatal Alcohol Exposure and With No Prenatal Alcohol Exposure. *Alcoholism: Clinical and Experimental Research, 30,* 2037–2045.

Kelly, S. J., Day, N., and Streissguth, A. P. (2000). Effects of prenatal alcohol exposure on social behavior in humans and other species. *Neurotoxicology and Teratology, 22,* 143-149.

Kyllerman, M., Aronson, M., Sabel, K-G, Karlberg, E., Sandin, B., and Olegard, R. (1985). Children of alcoholic mothers: Growth and motor performance compared to matched controls. *ACTA Paediatrica Scandinavica, 74,* 20-26.

Landesman-Dwyer, S., and Ragozin, A. S. (1981). Behavioral correlates of prenatal alcohol exposure: a four-year follow-up study. *Neurobehavioral Toxicology and Teratology, 3,* 187-193.

Leech, S. L., Richardson, G. A., Goldschmidt, L., and Day, N. L. (1999). Prenatal substance exposure: effects on attention and impulsivity of 6-year-olds. *Neurotoxicology and Teratology, 21*(2), 109-118.

Lemoine, P., Harousseau, H., Borteyru, J. P., and Menuet, J. C. (1968). Les enfants de parents alcooliques: Anomalies observes. A propos de 127 cas [Children of alcoholic parents: Abnormalities observed in 127 cases]. *Quest Medical, 21,* 476-482.

Lynch, M. E., Coles, C. D., Corley, T., and Falek, A. (2003). Examining delinquency in adolescents differentially prenatally exposed to alcohol: The role of proximal and distal risk factors. *Journal of Studies on Alcohol, 64,* 678-686.

Marbury, M. C., Linn, S., Monson, R. R., Schoenbaum, S., Stubblefield, P. G. and Ryan K. J. (1983). The association of alcohol consumption and outcome of pregnancy. *American Journal of Public Health, 73,* 1165-1168.

Mattson, S. N., Goodman, A. M., Caine, C., Delis, D. C., and Riley, E. P. (1999). Executive functioning in children with heavy prenatal alcohol exposure. *Alcoholism: Clinical Experimental Research, 23,* 1808-1815.

Mattson, S. N., and Riley, E. P. (1998). A review of the neurobehavioral deficits in children with fetal alcohol syndrome or prenatal exposure to alcohol. *Alcoholism: Clinical and Experimental Research, 22,* 279-294.

Mattson, S., and Riley, E. (1999). Implicit and explicit memory functioning in children with heavy prenatal alcohol exposure. *Journal of International Neuropsychological Society, 5,* 462–471.

Mattson, S. N., and Riley, E. P. (2000). Parent ratings of behavior in children with heavy prenatal alcohol exposure and IQ-matched controls. *Alcoholism: Clinical and Experimental Research, 22*, 226-231.

Mattson, S. N., Riley, E. P., Delis, D. C., Stern, C., and Jones, K. L. (1996). Verbal learning and memory in children with fetal alcohol syndrome. *Alcoholism: Clinical and Experimental Research, 20*, 810-816.

Nanson, J. L., and Hiscock, M. (1990). Attention-deficitis in children exposed to alcohol prenatally. *Alcoholism: Clinical and Experimental Research, 14*, 656-661.

O'Connor, M. J., Shah, B., Whaley, S., Cronin, P., Gunderson, B., and Graham, J. (2002). Psychiatric illness in a clinical sample of children with prenatal alcohol exposure. *American Journal of Drug and Alcohol Abuse, 28*, 743-754.

Olson, H. C., Streissguth, A. P., Sampson, P. D., Barr, H. M., Bookstein, F. L., and Thiede, K. (1997). Association of prenatal alcohol exposure with behavioral and learning problems in early adolescence. *Journal of the American Academy of Child & Adolescent Psychiatry, 36*, 1187-1194.

Paley, B., O'Connor, M. J., Kogan, N., and Findlay, R. (2005). Prenatal alcohol exposure, child externalizing behavior, and maternal stress. *Parenting: Science and Practice, 5*, 29-56.

Rasmussen, C. (2005) Executive Functioning and Working Memory in Fetal Alcohol Spectrum Disorder. *Alcoholism: Clinical and Experimental Research, 29*, 8.

Richardson, G. A., Ryan, C., Willford, J., Day, N. L., and Goldschmidt, L. (2002). Prenatal alcohol and marijuana exposure: effects on neuropsychological outcomes at 10 years. *Neurotoxicology and Teratology, 24*, 309-320.

Riikonen, R., Salonen, S. N., Partanen, K., and Verho, S. (1999). Brain perfusion SPECT and MRI in fetal alcohol syndrome. *Developmental Medicine and Child Neurology, 42*, 652-659.

Riley, J. C. M., and Behrman, H. R. (1991). Oxygen radicals and reactive oxygen species in reproduction. *Proceedings of the Society for Experimental Biology and Medicine, 198*, 781-791.

Roebuck, T. M., Mattson, S. N., and Riley, E. P. (1999). Prenatal exposure to alcohol: Effects on brain structure and neuropsychological functioning. In J. H. Hannigan and L. P. Spear (Eds.), *Alcohol and alcoholism: Effects on brain and development* (pp. 1-16). Mahwah, NJ: Lawrence Erlbaum Associates, Inc.

Rosett, H. L., Weiner, L., Lee, A., Zuckerman, B., Dooling, E. and Oppenheimer, E. (1983). Patterns of alcohol consumption and fetal development. *Obstetrics Gynecology 61*, 539-546.

Schonfeld, A. M., Mattson, S. N., Riley, E. P. (2005). Moral maturity and delinquency after prenatal alcohol exposure. *Journal of Studies on Alcohol, 66*, 545-554.

Soby, J. M. (1994). *Prenatal Exposure to drugs/alcohol*. Springfield, IL: Charles C. Thomas.

Sokol R. J., Delaney-Black V., and Nordstrom B. (2003). Fetal alcohol spectrum disorder. *Journal of the American Medical Association, 290*, 2996-2999.

Sood, B., Delaney-Black, V., Covington, C., Nordstrom-Klee, B., Ager, J., Templin, T., Janisse, J., Martier, S., and Sokok, R. J. (2001). Prenatal alcohol exposure and childhood behavior at age 6 to 7 years. I. Dose-response effect. *Pediatrics, 108*, e34.

Sowell, E. R., Mattson, S. N., Thompson, P. M., Jernigan, T. L., Riley, E. P., and Toga, A. W. (2001). Mapping callosal morphology and cognitive correlates: effects of heavy prenatal alcohol exposure. *Neurology, 57*, 235-244.

Spohr, H. L., and Steinhausen, H. C. (1996). *Alcohol, pregnancy and the developing child*. New York: Cambridge University Press.

Steinhausen, H-C., Willaims, J., and Sphor, H-L. (1993). Correlates of psychopathology and intelligence in children Stoler with fetal alcohol syndrome. *Journal of Child Psychology and Psychiatry, 35*, 323-331.

Streissguth A. P., Martin D. C., Martin, J. C., Barr, H. M. (1981).: The Seattle Longitudinal Prospective study on alcohol and pregnancy. *Neurobehavior, Toxicology and Teratology, 3*, 223-233.

Streissguth, A. P. (1986). Smoking and drinking during pregnancy. In M. Lewis, *Learning disabilities and prenatal risk* (pp. 28-67). Chicago: University of Illinois Press.

Streissguth, A. P., Aase, J. M., Clarren, S. K., Randels, S. P., LaDue, R. A., and Smith, D. F. (1991). Fetal alcohol syndrome in adolescents and adults. *Journal of the American Medical Association, 265,* 1961-1967.

Streissguth, A. P., Barr, H. M., Bookstein, F. L., Sampson, P. D., and Olson, H. C. (1999). The long-term neurocognitive consequences of prenatal alcohol exposure: a 14-year study. *Psychological Science, 10,* 186-190.

Streissguth, A. P., Barr, H. M., Kogan, J., and Bookstein, F. L. (1997). Primary and secondary disabilities. In A. P. Streissguth, and J. Kanter (Eds.), *Fetal alcohol syndrome in the challenge of fetal alcohol syndrome: Overcoming secondary disabilities* (pp. 25-39). Seattle: University of Washington Press.

Streissguth, A. P., Barr, H. M., and Sampson, P. D. (1990). Moderate prenatal alcohol exposure: effects on child IQ and learning problems at age 7.5 years. *Alcoholism: Clinical and Experimental Research, 14,* 662-669.

Streissguth, A., Bookstein, F., Sampson, P., and Barr, H. (1989). Neurobehavioral effects of prenatal alcohol: Part III. PLS analyses of neuropsychologic tests. *Neurotoxicology and Teratology, 11,* 493-507.

Streissguth, A. P., Randels, S. P., and Smith, D. F. (1991b). A test-retest study of intelligence in patients with fetal alcohol syndrome: Implications for care. *Journal of the American Academy of Child & Adolescent Psychiatry, 30,* 584-587.

Streissguth, A. P., Sampson, P. D., and Barr, H. M. (1989). Neurobehavioral dose-response effects of prenatal alcohol exposure in humans from infancy to adulthood. *Annals New York Academy of Science, 562,*145-158.

Stoler, J. M., and Holmes, L. B. (1999). Under-recognition of prenatal alcohol effects in infants of known alcohol abusing women. *Journal of Pediatrics, 135,* 430–436.

Testa, M., Quigley, B. M., and Eiden, R. D. (2003). The effect of prenatal alcohol exposure on infant mental development: a meta-analytic review. *Alcohol and Alcoholism, 38,* 295-304.

Thomas, S. E., Kelly, S. J., Mattson, S. N., and Riley, E. P. (1998). Comparison of social abilities of children with fetal alcohol syndrome to those of children with similar IQ scores and normal controls. *Alcoholism: Clinical and Experimental Research, 22,* 528-533.

Willford, J. A., Richardson, G. A., Leech, S. L., and Day, N. L. (2004). Verbal and visuospatial learning and memory function in alcohol exposure. *Alcoholism: Clinical and Experimental Research, 28,* 497-507.

Yates, W. R., Cadoret, R. J., Troughton, E. P., Stewart, M., and Giunta, T. S. (1998). Effect of fetal alcohol exposure on adult symptoms of nicotine, alcohol, and drug dependence. *Alcoholism: Clinical and Experimental Research, 22,* 914-920.

Chapter 11

Accornero, V. H., Morrow, C. E., Bandstra, E. S., Johnson, A. L., and Anthony, J. C. (2002). Behavioral outcomes of preschoolers exposed prenatally to cocaine: Role of maternal behavioral health. *Journal of Pediatric Psychology, 27*(3), 259-256.

Arendt, R., Short, E., Singer, L. T., Minnes, S., Hewitt, J., Flynn, S., Charlson, L., Min, M. O., Klein, N., and Flannery, D. (2004). Children prenatally exposed to cocaine: developmental outcomes and environmental risks at seven years of age. *Journal of Development of Behavioral Pediatrics, 25,* 83-90.

Arria, A. M., Deraug, C., LaGasse, L. L., Grant, P., Shah, R., Smith, L., Haning, W., Huestis, M., Strauss, A., Grotta, S. D., Liu, J., and Lester, B. (2006). Methamphetamine and other substance use during pregnancy: preliminary estimates from the infant development, environment, and lifestyle (IDEAL) study. *Maternal and Child Health Journal, 10,* 293-302.

Bandstra, E. S., Morrow, C. E., Anthony, J. C., Accornero, V. H., and Fried, P. A. (2001). Longitudinal investigation of task persistence and sustained attention in children with prenatal cocaine exposure. *Neurotoxicology and Teratology, 23,* 545-559.

Bays, J. (1990). Substance abuse and child abuse: Impact of addiction on the child. *Pediatric Clinics of North America, 37*, 881-904.

Behnke, M., Davis E. F., Duckworth, W. T., Wilson, G., C., Hou, W., and Wobei, K. (2006). Outcome from a prospective, longitudinal study of prenatal cocaine use: Preschool development at 3 years of age. *Journal of Pediatric Psychology, 31*(1), 41-49.

Billing, L.., Eriksson, M., Jonsson, B., Steneroth, G., and Zetterstrom, R. (1994). The influence of environmental factors on behavioral problems in 8-year-old children exposed to amphetamine during fetal life. *Child Abuse and Neglect, 18*, 3-9.

Billing, L., Eriksson, M., Steneroth, G., and Zetterstrom, R. (1988). Predictive indicators for adjustment in 4-year-old children whose mothers used amphetamine during pregnancy. *Child Abuse and Neglect, 12*, 503-507.

Bingol, N., Fuchs, M., Diaz, V., Stone, R. K. and Gromish, D. S. (1987). Tertatogenicity of cocaine in humans. *Journal of Pediatrics, 110*, 93-96.

Bureau, A. (1895). Aechoucement d'une morphinomane: prevue chumique du passage de la morphine a travers le placenta: reflexions. *Bulletin of Members of the Society of Obstetericians and Gynecologists*, 356-362.

Cernerud, L., Eriksson, M., Jonsson, B., Steneroth, G., Zetterstrom, R. (1996). Amphetamine addiction during pregnancy: 14-year follow-up of growth and school performance. *ACTA Paediatrica, 85*(2), 204-208.

Chasnoff, I. J., Anson, A., Hatcher, R., Stenson, H., Iaukea, K., and Randolph, L. A. (1998). Prenatal exposure to cocaine and other drugs. Outcome at four to six years. *Annals of the New York Academy of Child and Adolescent Psychiatry, 36*(7), 971-979.

Chiriboga, C. A. (2003). Fetal alcohol and drug effects. *The Neurologist, 9*(6), 267-279.

Church, M., Overbeck, G., and Andrezejczak, A. (1990). Prenatal cocaine exposure in the Long-Evans rat: I. Dose-dependent effects on gestation, mortality and postnatal maturation. *Neurotoxicology and Teratology, 12*, 327-334.

Connors, C. (1989). *Manual for Conners Rating Scales*. Toronto: MultiHealth Systems.

Dalterio, S., and Bartke, A. (1979). Perinatal exposure to cannabinoids alters male reproductive function in mice. *Science, 205*, 1420-1422.

Day, N., Cornelius, M., Goldschmidt, L., Richardson, G., Robles, N., and Taylor, P. (1992). The effects of prenatal tobacco and marijuana use on offspring growth from birth through 3 years of age. *Neurotoxicology and Teratology, 14*, 407-414.

Delaney-Black, V., Covington, C., Templin, T., Ager, J., Nordstrom-Klee, B., Martier, S., Leddick, L., Czerwinski, R. H., and Sokol, R. J. (2000). Teacher-assessed behavior of children prenatally exposed to cocaine. *Pediatrics, 106*(4), 782-791.

DeCristofaro, J. D., and LaGamma, E. F. (1995). Prenatal exposure to opiates. *Mental Retardation and Developmental Disabilities Research and Reviews, 1*, 177-182.

Dreher, M. C. (1997). Cannabis and pregnancy. In *Cannabis in Medical Practice: A Legal, Historical and Pharmacological Overview of the Therapeutic Use of Marijuana*. Edited by M. L. Mathre, Jefferson, NC: McFarland.

Dreher, M. C., Nugent, K., and Hudgins, R. (1994). Prenatal marijuana exposure and neonatal outcomes in Jamaica: An ethnographic study. *Pediatrics, 93*, 254-260.

Ericksson, M., and Zetterstrom, R. (1994). Amphetamine addiction during pregnancy: 10-year follow-up. *ACTA Paediatrica Supplement, 404*, 27-31.

Ericksson, M., Billing, L., Steneroth, G., and Zetterstrom, R. (1989). Health and development of 8-year-old children whose mothers abused amphetamine during pregnancy. *ACTA Paediatrica Scandinavica, 78*(6), 944-949.

Ericksson, M., Larsson, C., Windbladh, B., Zetterstrom, R. (1978). The influence of amphetamine addiction on pregnancy and the newborn infant. *ACTA Paediatrica Scandinavica, 67*, 95-99.

Frank, D. A., Augustyn, M., Knight, W. G., Pell, T., and Zuckerman, B. (2001). Growth, development, and behavior in early childhood following prenatal cocaine exposure: a systematic review. *Journal of the American Medical Association, 285*, 1613-1626.

Fried, P. A. (1980). Marihuana use by pregnant women: Neurobehavioral effects in neonates. *Drug and Alcohol Dependence, 6*, 415-424.

Fried, P. A. (1982). Marihuana use by pregnant women and effects on offspring: An up-date. *Neurotoxicology and Teratology, 4,* 451-454.

Fried, P. A. (2002). Conceptual issues in behavioral teratology and their application in determining long-term sequelae of prenatal marihuana exposure. *Journal of Child Psychology and Psychiatry, 43,* 81-102.

Fried, P. A., James, D. S., and Watkinson, B. (2001). Growth and pubertal milestones during adolescence in offspring prenatally exposed up to cigarettes and marihuana. *Neurotoxicology and Teratology, 23,* 431-436.

Fried, P. A., and Makin, J. E. (1987). Neonatal behavioural correlates of prenatal exposure to marihuana, cigarettes and alcohol in a low risk population. *Neurotoxicology and Teratology, 9,* 1-7.

Fried, P. A., O'Connell, C. M., and Watkinson, B. (1992). 60-and 72-month follow-up of children prenatally exposed to marijuana, cigarettes and alcohol: Cognitive and language assessment. *Journal of Developmental and Behavioral Pediatrics, 13,* 383-391.

Fried, P. A., and Smith, A. (2001). A literature review of the consequences of prenatal marihuana exposure. An emerging theme of a deficiency in aspects of executive function. *Neurotoxicology and Teratology, 23,* 1-11.

Fried, P. A., and Watkinson, B. (1988). 12-and 24-month neurobehavioural follow-up of children prenatally exposed to marihuana, cigarettes and alcohol. *Neurotoxicology and Teratology, 10,* 305-313.

Fried, P. A., and Watkinson, B. (2000). Visuoperceptual functioning differs in 9-to 12-year olds prenatally exposed to cigarettes and marihuana. *Neurotoxicology and Teratology, 22,* 11-20.

Fried, P. A., and Watkinson, B. (2001). Differential effects on facets of attention in adolescents prenatally exposed to cigarettes and marihuana. *Neurotoxicology and Teratology, 23, 421-430.*

Fried, P. A., Watkinson, B., and Gray, R. (1999). Growth from birth to early adolescence in offspring prenatally exposed to cigarettes and marihuana. *Neurotoxicology and Teratology, 21,* 513-525.

Fried, P. A., Watkinson, B., and Gray, R. (2003). Differential effects on cognitive functioning in 13- to 16-year olds prenatally exposed to cigarettes and marihuana. *Neurotoxicology and Teratology, 25, 427-436.*

Glass, N., Dragunow, M., and Faull, R. L. M. (1997). Cannabinoid receptors in the human brain: a detailed anatomical and quantitative autoradiographic study in the fetal, neonatal, and adult human brain. *Neuroscience, 77,* 299-318.

Goldschmidt, L., Day, N. L., and Richardson, G. A. (2000). Effects of prenatal marijuana exposure on child behavior problems at age 10. *Neurotoxicology and Teratology, 22,* 325-336.

Hamill, R. W., and LaGamma, E. F. (1992). Autonomic nervous system development. In Bannister R. (ed): Autonomic Failure: A Textbook of Clinical Disorders of the Autonomic Nervous System. New York: Oxford Press, pp. 13-35.

Harvey, J. A., Romano, A. G., Gabriel, M., Simansky, K. J., Du, W., Aloyo, V. J., and Friedman, E. (2003). Effects of prenatal exposure to cocaine on the developing brain: anatomical, chemical, physiological and behavioral consequences. *Neurotoxicology Research, 3,* 117-1143.

Hayes, J., Dreher, M., and Nugent, K. (1988). Newborn outcomes with maternal use in Jamaican woman. *Pediatric Nursing, 14,* 107-110.

Hingson, R., Alpert, J. J., Day, N., Dooling, E., Kayne, H., Morelock, S., Oppenheimer, E., and Zuckerman, B. (1982). Effects of maternal drinking and marijuana use on fetal growth and development. *Pediatrics, 70,* 539-546.

Hulse, G. K., English, D. R, Milne, E., Holman, C. D. J., and Bower, C. I., (1997). Maternal cocaine use and low birth weight newborns: a meta-analysis. *Addiction, 92*(11), 1561-1570.

Hulse, G. K., Milne, E., English, D. R., and Holman, C. D. J. (1997). The relationship between maternal use of heroin and methadone and infant birth weight. *Addiction, 92,* 1571-1579.

Kilbride, H. W., Castor, C. A., and Fuger, K. L. (2006). School-age outcome of children with pre-natal cocaine exposure following early case management. *Developmental and Behavioral Pediatrics, 27*(3), 181-187.

Leech, S. L., Richardson, G., Goldschmidt, L., and Day, N. L. (1999). Prenatal substance exposure: Effects on attention and impulsivity of 6-year-olds. *Neurotoxicology and Teratology, 21,* 109-118.

Lester, B., and Dreher, B. M. (1989). Effects of marihuana use during pregnancy on newborn cry. *Child Development, 60,* 765-771.

Lester, B. M., LaGasse, L. L. and Seifer R. (1998). Cocaine exposure and children: the meaning of subtle effects. *Science, 282*(5389), 633-634.

Lester, B. M., Tronick, E. Z., LaGasse, L. L., Seifer, R., Bauer, C. R., and Shankaran, S., Bada HS. Wright LL. Smeriglio VL. Lu J. Finnegan LP. Maza PL. (2002). The maternal lifestyle study (MLS): effects of substance exposure during pregnancy on one-month neurodevelop-mental outcome. *Pediatrics, 110,* 1182-1192.

Lidow, M. S. (1995). Prenatal cocaine exposure adversely affects development of the primate cer-ebral cortex. *Synapse, 21,* 332-341.

Lidow, M. S. (2003). Consequences of prenatal cocaine exposure in nonhuman primates. *Developmental Brain Research, 147,* 23-36.

Lifschitz, M. H., and Wilson, G. S. (1991). Patterns of growth and development in narcotic-exposed children. In M. M. Kilbey and K. Asghar (Eds.). *Methodological Issues in Controlled Studies on Effects of Prenatal Exposure to Drug Abuse.* NIDA Research Monograph, 114, pp. 323-339.

Linares, T. F., Singer, L. T., Kirchner, H. L., Short, E. J., Meeyoung, M. O., Hussey, P., and Minnes, S. (2005). Mental health outcomes of cocaine-exposed children at 6 years of age. *Journal of Pediatric Psychology, 31,* 85-97.

Linn, S., Schoenbaum, S. C., Monson, R. R., Rosner, R., Stubblefield, P. C., and Ryan, K. J. (1983). The association of marijuana use with outcome of pregnancy. *American Journal of Public Health, 73,* 1161-1164.

Lutiger, B., Graham, K., Einarson, T. R., and Koren, G. (1991). Relationship between gestational cocaine use and pregnancy outcome. *Teratology, 44,* 405-414.

McCarthy, P. (1972). *McCarthy Scales of children's Abilities.* New York: The Psychological Corporation.

Messinger, D. S., Bauer, C. R., Abhik, D., Seifer, R., Lester, B. M., Lagasse, L. L., Wright, L. L., Shankaran, S., Bada, H. S., Smeriglio, V. L., Langer, J. C., Beeghly, M., and Poole, W. K. (2004). The maternal lifestyle study: Cognitive, motor, and behavioral outcomes of cocaine-exposed and opiate-exposed infants through three years of age. *Pediatrics, 113*(6), 1677-1685.

Middaugh, L. D. (1989). Prenatal amphetamine effects on behavior: possible mediation by brain monoamines. *Annals of New York Academy of Sciences, 562,* 308-318.

O'Connell, C. M. and Fried, P. A. (1991). Prenatal exposure to Cannabis: a preliminary report of postnatal consequences in School-age children. *Neurotoxicology and teratology, 13,* 631-639.

Qazi, Q. H., Mariano, E., Milman, D. H., Beller, E., and Crombleholme, W. (1985). Abnormalities in offspring associated with prenatal marihuana exposure. *Developmental Pharmacology and Therapeutics, 8,* 141-148.

Richardson, G. A. (1998). Prenatal cocaine exposure: A longitudinal study of development. *Annals of the New York Academy of Science, 846,* 144-152.

Richardson, G. A., and Day, N. L. (1998). Epidemiologic studies of the effects of prenatal cocaine exposure on child development and behavior. In: Sliker Jr., W., Chang, L. W. (Eds.), Handbook of Developmental Neurotoxicology. Academic Press, San Diego, CA, pp. 487-496.

Richardson, G., Day, N., and Taylor, P. (1989). The effect of prenatal alcohol, marijuana, and tobacco exposure on neonatal behavior. *Infant Behavioral Development, 12,*199-209.

Richardson, G. A., Ryan, C., Willford, J., Day, N. L., Goldschmidt, L. (2002). Prenatal alcohol and marijuana exposure: effects on neuropsychological outcomes at 10 years. *Neurotoxicology and Teratology, 24,* 309-320.

Rodriguez de Fonseca, F., Cebeira, M. Fernandez-Ruiz, J. J., Navarro, M., and Ramos, J. A. (1991). Effects or pre- and perinatal exposure to hashish extracts on the ontogeny of brain dopaminergic neurons. *Neuroscience, 43,* 713-723.

Smith, A. M., Fried, P. A., Hogan, M. J., and Cameron, I. (2004). Effects of prenatal marijuana on response inhibition: an fMRI study of young adults. *Neurotoxicology and Teratology, 26,* 533-542.

Smith, L., Yonekura, M. L., Wallace, T., Berman, N., Kuo, N., Berkowitz, C. (2003). Effects of prenatal methamphetamine exposure on fetal growth and drug withdrawal symptoms in infants born at term. *Developmental and Behavioral Pediatrics, 24,* 17-23.

Tennes, K., Avitable, N., Blackard, C., Boyles, C., Hassoun, B., Holmes, L., and Kreye, M. (1985). Marijuana: Prenatal and postnatal exposure in the human. In *Current Research on the Consequences of Maternal Drug Abuse.* Edited by T. M. Pinkert. NIDA Research Monograph No. 59. Rockville: United States Department of Human Health and Services.

Thorndike, R. L., Hagan, E., and Sattler, J. (1986). *The Stanford-Binet Intelligence Scale: 4th ed.* Chicago: Riverside Publishing.

Vardaris, R. M., Weisz, D. J., Fazel, A., and Rawitch, A. B. (1976). Chronic administration of delta-9-tetrahydrocannabinol to pregnant rats: Studies of pup behavior and placental transfer. *Pharmacology, Biochemistry and Behavior, 4,* 249-254.

Zagon, I. S. (1985). Opioids and development: New lessons from old problems. *NIDA Research Monograph, 60,* 58-77.

Zagon, I. S., McLaughlin, P. J., Weaver, D. J., and Zagon, E. (1982). Opiates, endorphins and the developing organism: A comprehensive bibliography. *Neuroscience Biobehavioral Reviews, 6,* 439-479.

Section E: Pollutants and the Development of the Human Fetus: An Introduction

Adgate, J. L., Church, T. R., Ryan, A. D., Ramachandran, G., Fredrickson, Stock, T. H. et al. (2004). Outdoor, indoor, and personal exposure to VOC's in children. *Environmental Health Perspectives, 112,* 1386-1392.

Colburn, T. (2004). Neurodevelopment and endocrine disruption. *Environmental Health Perspectives, 112,* 944-949.

Colburn, T., and Clement, C. (1992). *Chemically induced alterations in sexual and functional development: the wildlife/human connection.* Princeton, NJ: Princeton Scientific.

Cone, M. *Silent snow: The slow poisoning of the arctic.* Los Angeles: Grove Press.

Daston, G., Faustman, E., Ginsberg, G., Fenner-Criso, P., Olin, S., Sonawane, B., Bruckner, J., and Breslin, W. (2004). A framework for assessing risks to children from exposure to environmental agents. *Environmental Health Perspectives, 112,* 238-256.

Faustman, E. M., Lewandowski, T. A., Hoelt, J. A., Bartelli, S. M., Wong, E. Y., and Griffith, W. C. (2003). Biomarkers for children's health: developing biologically based risk assessment models for linking exposure and health effects. *Institute of Risk Analysis Risk Communication, 3,* 1-25.

Ginsberg, B. L., Harris, D., Sonawane, B., Russ, A., Banati, P., Koziak, M. et al. (2002). Evaluation of child/adult pharmacokinetic differences from a database derived from the therapeutic drug literature. *Toxicological Science, 66,* 185-200.

Marshall, J. (2005). Megacity, megamess. *Nature, 437, September 15,* 312-314.

Short, P. and Colburn, T (1999). Pesticide use in the United States and policy implications: a focus on herbicides. *Toxicological Industrial Health, 15,* 240-275.

United States Census Bureau (2006). *Statistical abstract of the United States: 2006.* Springfield, VA: National Technical Information Service.

Woolf, A. D. (2005). Childhood lead poisoning in 2 families associated with spices used in food preparation. *Pediatrics, 8,* 314.

Chapter 12

Adgate, J.L., Kukowski, A., Stroebel, C., Shubat, P. J., Morrell, S., Quackenboss, J. J. et al. (2000). Pesticide storage and use patterns in Minnesota households with children. *Exposure Analysis and Environmental Epidemiology, 10,* 159-167.

Adriani, W., Seta, D. D., Dessi-Fulgheri, F., Farabollini, F., and Laviola, G. (2003). Altered profiles of spontaneous novelty seeking, impulsive behavior, and response to D-Amphetamine in rats perinatally exposed to Bisphenol A. *Environmental Health Perspectives, 111,* 395-401.

Aldridge, J. E., Meyer, A., Seidler, F. J., and Slotkin, T. A. (2005). Synaptic activity in adhulthood after prenatal or neonatal chlorpyrifos exposure. Environmental Health Perspectives, 113, 1027-1031.

Atanassova, N., McKinnell, C., Turner, K. J., Walker, M., Fisher, J. S., Morley, M. et al., (2000). Comparative effects of neonatal exposure of male rats to potent and weak environmental estrogens on spermatogenesis at puberty and the relationship to adult testis size and fertility: evidence for stimulatory effects of low estrogen levels. *Endocrinology, 141,* 3898-3907.

Barone, S., Das, K. P., Lassiter, T. L., and White, L. D. (2000). Vulnerable processes of nervous system development: a review of markers and methods. *Neurotoxicology, 21,* 15-36.

Barnes, K.K., Kolpin, D.W., Furlong, E.T., Zaugg, S.D., Meyer, M.T., Barber, L.B., and Focazio, M.J. (2004). Pharmaceuticals, hormone, and other organic wastewater contaminants in ground water resources. In Proceedings of Groundwater Foundation Annual Conference and Groundwater Guardian Designation, Groundwater and Public Health—-Making the Connection, Washington, D.C., November 4-5, 2004: Groundwater Foundation, p. 24-30.

Berkowitz, G. S., Obel, J., Deych, E., Lapinski, R., Godbold, J.G, Liu, Z. et al. (2003). Exposure to indoor pesticides during pregnancy in a multiethnic, urban cohort. *Environmental Health Perspectives, 111,* 79-84.

Berkowitz, G. S., Wolff, M. S., Janevic, T. M., Holzman, I Rl, Yehuda, R., and Landrigan, P. J. (2003). The World Trade Center Disaster and intrauterine growth restriction. *Journal of the American Medical Association, 290,* 2943.

Bobach, M. (2000). Outdoor air pollution, low birth weight, and prematurity. *Environmental Health Perspectives, 108,* 173-176.

Bove, F., Shim, Y., and Zeitz, P. (2002). Drinking water contaminants and adverse Pregnancy outcomes: a review. *Environmental Health Perspectives, 110,* 61-74.

Bradman, A., and Whyatt, R. M. (2005). Characterizing exposures to nonpersistent pesticides during pregnancy and early childhood in the National Children's Study: a review of monitoring and measurement methodologies. *Environmental Health Perspectives, 113,* 1092-1099.

Carlsen, E., Giwercman, A., Keiding, N., and Skakkedaek, N. E. (1992). Evidence for the decreasing quality of semen during the past 50 years. *British Medical Journal, 305,* 609-612.

Clean Air Act Amendments (1990). Part A, Section 112, Public law 101-548.

Clegg, D. J., and van Gemert, M. (1999a). Determination of the reference dose of chlorplyrifos: proceedings of an expert panel. *Journal of Toxicology and Environmental Health, 2,* 257-279.

Clegg, D. J., and van Gemert, M. (1999b). Expert panel report of human studies of chlorpyrifos and other organophosphate exposures. *Journal of Toxicology and Environmental Health, 2,* 257-279.

Colborn, T. (2006). A case for revisiting the safety of pesticides: a closer look at neurodevelopment. *Environmental Health Perspectives, 114,* 10-17.

Dohm, M. R., Mautz, W. J., Andrade, J. A., Gellert,.K. S., Salas-Ferguson, L.J., Nicolaisen, N. et al. (2005). Effects of ozone exposure on nonspecific phagocytic capacity of pulmonary macrophages from an amphibian. *Environmental Toxicology and Chemistry, 24,* 1-8.

Dolk, H., Vrijheid, M., Armstrong, B., Abramsky, L., Bianchi, F., Garne, E., et al. (1998). Risk of congenital anomalies near hazardous-wast landfill sites in Europe: The EUROHAZCON study. *Lancet, 352,* 423-427.

Garcia, S. J., Seidler, F., and Slotkin, T. A. (2003). Developmental neurotoxicity elicited by prenatal or postnatal chlorpyrifos exposure: Effects on neurospecific proteins indicate changing vulnerabilities. *Environmental Health Perspectives, 111*, 297-303.

Garry, V. F., Harkins, M. E., Erickson, L. L., Long-Simpson, L. K., Holland S. E., and Burroughs, B. L. (2002). Birth defects, season of conception, and sex of children born to pesticide applicators living in the Red River Valley of Minnesota, USA. *Environmental Health Perspectives, 110 (supplement 3)*. 441-449.

Guillette, L. J. J., Pickford, D. B., Crain, D. A., Rooney, A. A., and Percival, H. F. (1996). Reduction in penis size, and testosterone concentration in juvenile alligators living in a contaminated environment. *General and Comparative Endocrinology, 101*, 32-42.

Hutchinson, J. B. (1997). Gender-specific steroid metabolism in neural differentiation. *Cellular and Molecular Neurobiology, 17*, 603-626.

Hwang, B. F., Magnus, P., and Jaakkolal, J. J. K. (2002). Risk of specific birth defects in relation to chlorination and the amount of natural organic matter in the water supply *American Journal of Epidemiology, 156*, 374-382.

Infante-Rivard, C. (2004). Drinking water contaminants, gene polymorphisms, and fetal growth. *Environmental Health Perspectives, 112*, 1213-1216.

Jedrychowski, W., Bendkowskia, I., Flak, E., Penar, A., Jecek, R., Kaim, I. et al. (2004). Estimated risk of altered fetal growth resulting from exposure to fine particles during pregnancy: An epidemiologic prospective cohort study in Poland. *Environmental Health Perspectives, 112*, 1398-1402.

Klepeis, N. E., Nelson, W. C., Ott, W. R., Robinson, J. P., Tsang, A. M. Switzer, P. et al. (2001). The national human activity pattern survey (NHAPS): a resource for assessing exposure to environmental pollutants. *Journal of Exposure Analysis and Environmental Epidemiology, 11*, 231-252.

Kersemaekers, W. M., Roeleveld, N., Zielhuis, G. A., and Gabreels, F. J. (1997). Neurodevelopment of offspring of hairdressers. *Developmental Medicine and Child Neurology, 39*, 358-362.

Kim, S. Y., Lee, J. T., Hong, Y. C., Ahn, K. J., and Kim, H. (2004). Determining the threshold effect of ozone on daily mortality: an analysis of ozone and mortality in Seoul, Korea, 1995-1999. *Journal of Environmental Research, 94*, 113-119.

King, W., Dobbs, L., Armson, B. A., Allen, A. C., Fell, D. B., and Nimrod, C. (2004). Exposure assessment in epidemiologic studies of adverse pregnancy outcomes and disinfection byproducts. *Journal of Exposure Analysis and Environmental Epidemiology, 14*, 466-472.

Lederman, S. A., Rauh, V., Weiss, L., Stein, J. L., Hoepner, L. A., Becker, M., and Perera, F. P. (2004). The effects of the World Trade Center event on birth outcomes among term deliveries at three lower Manhattan hospitals. *Environmental Health Perspectives, 112*, 1772-1778.

Lee, B. E., Ha, E. H., Park, H. S., Kim, Y. J., Hong, Y. C., Kim, H., and Lee, J. T. (2003). Exposure to air pollution during different gestational phases contributes to risks of low birth weight. *Human Reproduction, 18*, 638-643.

Lin, M., Chen, Y., Villeneuve, P. J., Burnett, R. T., Lemyre, L., Hertzman, C., McGrail, K. M., and Krewski, D. (2004). Gaseous air pollutants and asthma hospitalization of children with low household income in Vancouver, British Columbia, Canada. *American Journal of Epidemiology, 159*, 294-303.

Maisonet, M., Bush, T. J., Correa, A., and Jaakkola, J. J. K. (2001). Relation between ambient air pollution and low birth weight in the Northeastern United States. *Environmental Health Perspectives, 109* (supplement), S351-S356.

Mendola, P. (2005). Get article. *American Journal of Epidemiology* (reference in September 3, science news) pg. 168.

Munger, R., Isacson, P., Hu, S., Burns, T., Hanson, J., Lynch, C. F., Cherryholmes, K., VanDorpe, P., and Hausier, W. J. (1997). Intrauterine growth retardation in Iowa communities with herbicide-contaminated drinking water supplies. *Environmental Health Perspectives, 105*, 308-314.

Palmer, S. R., Dunstan, F. D. J., Fielder, H., Fone, H., Higgs, D. L., Higgs, G., and Senior, M. L. (2005). Risk of congenital anomalies after the opening of landfill sites. *Environmental Health Perspectives, 113*, 1362-1365.

Peng, R. D., Dominick, F., Pastor-Barriuso, R., Zegler, S. L., and Samet, J. M. (2005) Seasonal analyses of air pollution and mortality in 100 United States Cities. *American Journal of Epidemiology, 161*, 585-594.

Perera, F. P., Rauh, V., Tsai, W.Y., Kinney, P., Cammann, D. Barr, D.. (2003). Effects of transplacental exposure to environmental pollutants on birth outcomes in a multiethnic population. *Environmental Health Perspectives, 111*, 201-205.

Perera, F. P., Rauh, V., Whyatt, R. M., Tsai, W. Y., Barnert, J. T., Tu, Y. H. et al. (2004). Molecular evidence of an interaction between prenatal environmental exposures and birth outcomes in a multiethnic population. *Environmental Health Perspectives, 111*, 201-205.

Raloff, J. (February 6, 2006). A little less green? Studies challenge the benign image of pyrethroid insecticides. *Science News, 169*, 74-76.

Richter, A., Burrows, J. P., Nuss, H, Granier, C., and Niemeier, U. (2005). Increase in tropospheric nitrogen dioxide over China observed from space. *Nature, 437, (September 1)* 129-132.

Ritz, B., Yu, F., Fruin, S., Chapa, G., Shaw, G. M. and Harris, J. A. (2002). Ambient air pollution and risk of birth defects in Southern California. *American Journal of Epidemiology, 155*, 17-24.

Rubes, J., Selevan, S. G., Evenson, D. P., Zudova, D., Vozdova, M., Zudova, Z. et al (2005). Episodic air pollution is associated with increased DNA fragmentation in human sperm without other changes in semen quality. *Human Reproduction, 20*, 2776-2783.

Shi, L., and Chia, S. E. (2001). A review of studies on maternal occupational exposures and birth defects, and the limitations associated with these studies. *Occupational Medicine, 51*, 230-244.

Sokol, R. Z., Kraft, P., Fowler, I. M., Mamet, R., Kim, E. and Berhane, K. T. (2005). Exposure to environmental ozone alters semen quality. *Environmental Health Perspectives, 114, 360-365.*

Somers, C. M., McCarry, B. E., Malek, F., and Quinn, J. S. (2004). Reduction of particulate air pollution lowers the risk of heritable mutations in mice. *Science, 304*, 1008-1010.

Somers, C. M., Yau,k, C. L., White, P. A., Parfett, C. L. J., Quinn, J. S. (2002). Air pollution induces heritable DNA mutations. *Proceedings of the National Academy of Sciences of the United States of America, 99*, 15904.

Sonnenfeld, N., Hertz-Piccioto, I., and Kaye, W. E. (2001). Tetrachloroethylene in drinking water and birth outcomes at the United States Marine Corps base at Camp Lejeune, North Carolina. *American Journal of Epidemiology, 154*, 902-908

Sram, R., Binkova, B., Dejnela, J., and Bobak, M. (2005). Ambient air pollution and pregnancy outcomes: a review of the literature. *Environmental Health Perspectives, 113*, 375-382.

Storrs, S. L., and Kiesecker, J. M. (2004). Survivorship patterns of larval amphibians exposed to low concentrations of atrozine. *Environmental Health Perspectives, 112*, 1054-1057.

Toledano, M. B., Nieuwenhuijsen, M. J., Best, N., Whitaker, H., Hambly, P., de Hoogh, C., et al. (2005). Relation of trihalomethane concentrations in public water supplies to stillbirth and birth weight in three water regions in England. *Environmental Health Perspectives, 113*, 225-232.

Urch, B., Silverman, F., Corey, P., Brook, R., Lukic, K. Z., Rajagopalan, S. et al. (2005). Acute blood pressure responses in healthy adults during controlled air pollution exposure. *Environmental Health Perspectives, 113*, 1052-1055.

Wang, X., Ding, H., Ryan, L., and Xu, X. (1997). Association between air pollution and low birth weight: a community-based study. *Environmental Health Perspectives, 105*, 514-520.

Whyatt, R. M., Camann, D. E., Kinney, P., Reyes, A., Ramirez, J., Dietrich, J. (2002). Residential pesticide use during pregnancy among a cohort of urban minority women. *Environmental Health Perspectives, 110*, 507-514.

Wilhelm, M., and Ritz, B. (2003). Residential proximity to traffic and adverse birth outcomes in Los Angeles County, California 1994-1996. *Environmental Health Perspectives, 111*, 200-216.

Yang, C. Y., Chen, Y. S., Yang, C. H., and Ho, S. C. (2004). Relationship between ambient air pollution and hospital admissions for cardiovascular diseases in Kaohsiung, Tiawan. *Journal of Toxicology and Environmental Health, 67*, 483-493.

Chapter 13

Adgate, J. L., Church, R. R., Ryan, A. D., Ramachandran, G., Fredrickson, W., Stock et al. (2004). Outdoor, indoor, and personal exposure to VOC's in children. *Environmental Health Perspectives, 112*, 1386-1392.

Anderson, A. C., Pueschel, S. M., and Linakis, J. G. (1996). Pathophysiology of lead poisoning. In S. M Pueschel, J. G. Linakis, and A. C. Anderson (eds), *Lead poisoning in childhood* (pp. 75-96). Baltimore, Maryland: Brooks.

Cernichiari, C., Brewer, R., Myers, G. J., March, D. O., Lapham, L. W., Cox, C., et al. (1995). Monitoring methylmercury during pregnancy: maternal hair predicts fetal brain exposure. *Neurotoxicology, 16*, 705-710.

Chen, A., Dietrich, K. N., Ware, J. H., Radcliffe, J., and Rogan, W. J. (2005). IQ and blood lead from 2 to 7 years of age: Are the blood lead levels of 7 year-old children the residual of high blood lead concentrations at 2 years-of-age? *Environmental Health Perspectives, 113*, 597-601.

Cox, C., Clarkson, T. W., Marsh, D. O., Amin-Zaki, L., Tikriti, S., and Myers, G. G. (1989). Dose-response analysis of infants prenatally exposed to methyl mercury: An application of a single compartment model to single-strand hair analysis. *Environmental Research, 49*, 318-332.

Dallaire, F., Dewailly, E., Muckle, C., Vezina, C., Jacobson, S. W., Jacobson, J. L. et al. (2004). Acute infections and environmental exposure to organochlorines in Inuit infants fron Nanavik. *Environmental Health Perspectives, 112*, 1359-1364.

Delville, Y. (1999). Exposure to lead during development alters aggressive behavior in golden hamsters. *Neurotoxicology and Teratology, 21*, 445-449.

Dietrich, K. N. (1996). Low-level lead exposure during pregnancy and its consequences for fetal and child development. In S. M. Pueschel, J. G. Linakis, and A. C. Anderson (eds.), *Lead poisoning in childhood* (pp. 117-139). Baltimore, Maryland: Brookes.

Duty, S. M., Silva, M. J., Barr, D. B., Brock, J. W., Ryan, L. Chen, Z, et al. (2003). Phthalate exposure and human semen parameters. *Epidemiology, 14*, 269-277.

Foster, P. M. D., Mylchreest, E., Gaido, K. W. and Sar, M. (2001). Effects of phthalate esters on the developing reproductive tract of male rates. *Human Reproductive Update, 7*, 231-235.

Gladen, B., and Rogan, W. (1991). Effects of perinatal polychlorinated biphenyls and dichlorodiphenyl dichloroethane on later development. *Journal of Pediatrics, 119*, 58-63.

Goldstein, G. (1990). Lead poisoning and brain cell function. *Environmental Health Perspectives, 89*, 91-94.

Grandjean, P., Weihe, P., White, R. F., and Debes, F. (1998). Cognitive performance of children prenatally exposed to 'safe' levels of methylmercury. *Environmental Research, 77*, 165-172.

Gray, L. E., Ostby, J., Furr, J., Prince, M., Veeramachaneni, D. N. and Parks, L. (2000). Perinatal exposure to the phthalates DEHP, BBP, and DINP, but not DEP, DMP, or DOTP, alters sexual differentiation of the male rate. *Toxicological Science, 58*, 350-365.

Gulson, B. L., Jameson, C. W., Mahaffey, K. R., Mizon, K. J., Korsch, M. J. and Vimpani, G. (1997). Pregnancy increase mobilization of lead from maternal skeleton. *Journal of Laboratory and Clinical Medicine, 130*, 51-62.

Gulson, B. L., Mizon, K. J., Palmer, J. M., Taylor, M.. and Mahaffey, K. R. (2005). Blood lead changes during pregnancy and postpartum with calcium supplementation. *Environmental Health Perspectives, 112*, 1499-1507.

Harada, M. (1995). Minamata disease: Methylmercury poisoning in Japan caused by environmental pollution. *Critical Reviews in Toxicology, 25*, 1-24.

Hightower, J. M., and Moore, D. (2003). Mercury levels in high-end consumers of fish. *Environmental Health Perspectives, 111*, 604-608.

Hubbs-Tait, L., Nation, J. R., Krebs, N. F., and Bellinger, D. C. (2005). Neurotoxicants, micronutrients, and social environments: individual and combined effects on children's development. *Psychological Science in the Public interest, 6*, 57-121.

Huisman, M., Koopman-Esseboom, C., Fidler, V., Hadders-Algra, M., van der Paauw, C. G., Tuinstra, L. G. M., et al. (1995a). Perinatal exposure to polychlorinated biphenyls and dioxins and its effect on neonatal neurological development. *Early Human Development, 41*, 111-127.

Huisman, M., Koopman-Esseboom, C., Lanting, C. I., van der Paauw, C. G., Tuinstra, L. G. M., Fidler, V. et al. (1995b). Neurological conditions in 18 months-old children perinatally exposed to polychlorinated biphenyls and dioxins. *Early Human Development, 41*, 165-176.

Jacobson, J. L.., and Jacobson, S. W. (1997). Teratogen update: polychlorinated biphenyls. *Teratology, 55, 538-532.

Jacobson, S. W., and Jacobson, J. L. (2000). Teratogenic insult and neurobehavioral function in infancy and childhood. In C. A. Nelson (Ed.), *The effects of early adversity on neurobehavioral development (The Minnesota Symposia on Child Psychology, Vol. 31, pp.* 61-113). Mahwah, NJ: Erlbaum.

Klepeis, N. E., Nelson, W. C., Ott, W. R., Robinson, A. M., Tsang, A. M., Switzer, P. et al. (2001). The national human activity pattern survey (NHAPS): a resource for assessing exposure to environmental pollutants. *Journal of Exposure Analysis and Environmental Epidimiology, 11*, 231.

Koger, S. M., Schettler, T., and Weiss, B. (2005). Environmental toxicants and developmental disabilities: A challenge for psychologists. *American Psychologist, 50*, 243-255.

Koopman-Esseboom, C., Huisman, M., Weisglas-Kuperus, N., Van der Pasuw, C. G., Tuinstra, L. G., Boersma, E. R., and Sauer, P. J. J. (1994). PCB and dioxin levels in plasma and human milk of 418 Dutch women and their infants: predictive value of PCB congener levels in maternal plasma for fetal and infant's exposure to PCB's and dioxin. *Chemosphere, 9*, 1721-1732.

Lee, M. G. Chun, O. K., and Song, W. O. (2005). Determinants of the blood lead level of United States women of reproductive age. *Obstretics and Gynecology Survey, 60*, 625-626.

Lau, C., Thibodeaux, J. R., Hanson, R. G., Rogers, J. M., Grey, B. E., Stanton, M. E., Butenhoff, J. L., and Stevenson, L. A. (2003). Exposure to perfluorooctane sulfonate during pregnancy in rat and mounse.II: postnatal evaluation. *Toxicological Science, 74*, 382-392.

Lai, T. J., Liu, X., Guo, Y. L., Guo, N. W. et al. (2002). A cohort study of behavioral problems and intelligence in children with high prenatal polychlorinated biphenyl exposure. *Archives of General Psychiatry, 59*, 1061-1066.

Lanting, C. I., Patandin, S., Fidler, V., Weisglas-Kuperius, N., Sauer, P. J. J., Boersma, E. R., et al., (1998). Neurological condition in 42-month-old children in relation to pre- and postnatal exposure in polychlorinated biphenyls and dioxins. *Early Human Development, 50*, 283-292.

Latini, G., De Felice, C., Presta, G., Del Vecchio, A., Paris, I., Ruggieri, F. et al. (2003). In utero exposure to di (2-ethylhexyl) phthalate and duration of human pregnancy. Environmental Health Perspectives, 111, 1783-1785.

Li, W., Han, S., Greeg, T. R., Kemp, F. W., Davidow, A. L., Louria, D. B., Siegel, A., and Bogden, J. D. (2003).Lead exposure potentiates predatory attack behavior in the cat. *Environmental Research, 92, 197-206.

McDowell, M. A., Dillon, C. F., Osterioh, J., Bolger, P. M., Pellizzari, E. et al., (2004). Hair mercury levels in United States children and women of childbearing age: reference range data form NHANES 1999-2000. Environmental Health Perspectives, 112, 1165-1171.

Mokhtar, G., Hossny, E., El-Awady, M., and Zekry, M. (2002). In utero exposure to cadmium pollution in Cairo and Giza governorates of Egypt. *Eastern Mediterranean Health Journal, 8*, 254-260.

Nation, J. R., Cardon, A. L., Heard, H. M., Valles, R., and Bratton, G. R. (2003). Perinatal lead exposure and relapse to drug-seeking behavior in the rat: a cocaine reinstatement study. *Psychopharmacology, 168*, 236-243.

Newland, M. C., and Rasmussen, E. B. (2003). Behavior in adulthood and during aging is affected by contaminant exposure in utero. *Current Directions in Psychological Science, 12*, 212-217.

Newland, M. C., Ng, W., Baggs, R. B., Gentry, G. D., Weiss, B., and Miller, R. K. (1986). Operant behavior in transition reflects neonatal exposure to cadmium. *Teratology, 34*, 231-241.

Opler, M.G.A., Brown, A. S., Graziano, J., Desai, M., Zheng, W., Schaefer, C., et al., (2004). Prenatal lead exposure, delta-amino-levulinic acid, and schizophrenia. *Environmental Health Perspective, 112*, 548-552.

Patandin, S., Lanting, C. I., Mulder, P. G. H., Boersma, E. R., Sauer, P. J. J., Weisglas-Kuperus, N. (1999). Effects of environmental exposure to polychlorinated biphenyls and dioxins on cognitive abilities in Dutch children at 42 month of age. *Journal of Pediatrics, 134*, 33-41.

Pirkle, J. L., Brody, D. J., Gunter, E. W., Kramer, R. A., Paschal, D. C., Flegal, K. M., and Matte, T. D. (1994). The decline in blood lead levels in the United States. The National Health and Nutrition Examination Surveys (NHANES). *Journal of the American Medical Association, 272*, 277-283.

Pueschel, S. M., Linakis, J. G., and Anderson, A. C. (1996). Chapter 1: lead poisoning: a historical perspective. In S. M. Pueschel, J. G. Linakis, and A. C. Aneierson (eds.), *Lead poisoning in childhood* (pp. 1-14). Baltimore, Maryland: Brookes.

Raloff, J. (October 25, 2003). New PCBX: Throughout life, our bodies accumulate flame retardants, and scientists are starting to worry. *Science News, 164*, 266-267.

Rocha, A., Valles, R., Cardon, A. L., Bratton, G. R., and Nation, J. R. (2005). Enhanced acquisition of cocaine self-administration in rats developmentally exposed to lead. *Neuropsychopharmacology, 30*, 2058-2064.

Schantz, S. L., Widholm, J. J., and Rice, D. C. (2003). Effects of PCB exposure on neuropsychological functioning in children. *Environmental Health Perspectives, 111*, 357-376.

Sharpe, R. M., and Skakkebaek, N. E. (1993). Are oestrogens involved in falling sperm counts and disorders of the male reproductive tract. *Lancet, 341*, 1392-1395.

Schell, L. M., Denham, M., Stark, A. D., Gomez, M., Ravenscroft, J., Parsons, P.J. (2003). Maternal blood lead concentration, diet during pregnancy, and anthropometry predict neonatal blood lead in a socioeconomically disadvantaged population. *Environmental Health Perspectives, 111*, 195-200.

Silva, M. J., Barr, D. B., Reidy, J. A., Kato, K., Malek, N. A., and Hodge, C. C. (2004). Urinary levels of seven phthalate metabolites in the U. S. population from the National Health and Nutrition Examination Survey (NHANES) 1999-2000. *Environmental Health Perspectives, 112*, 331-338.

Steward, P., Reihman, J., Gump, B., Lonky, E., Darvill, T., and Pagano, J. (2005). Response inhibition at 8 and 9 ½ years of age in children prenatally exposed to PCBs. *Neurotoxicology and Teratology, 27*, 771-780.

Winter, D. D. N., and Koger, S. (2004). *The psychology of environmental problems*. Mahwah, N. J.: Erlbaum.

Yiin, L. M., Rhoads, G. G., and Lioy, P. J. (2000). Seasonal influences on childhood lead exposure. *Environmental Health Perspectives, 108*, 177-182.

Section F: Historical Perspective and the Future

Asbury, K., Dunn, J. F., and Plomin, R. (2006). Birthweight-discordance and differences in early parenting related to monozygotic twin differences in behaviour problems and academic achievement at age 7. *Developmental Science, 9*, 1-22.

DiPietro, J. A. (1998). The role of prenatal maternal stress in child development. *Current Direction in Psychological Science, 13*, 71-74.

Gregg, N. (1941). Congenital cataract following German measles in the mother. *Transactions of the American Ophthalmological Society, 3*, 35-45.

Harada, M. (1995). Minamata disease: Methylmercury poisoning in Japan caused by environmental pollution. *Critical Reviews in Toxicology, 25*, 1-24.

Kraeplin, E. (1919). *Dementia praecox and paraphrenia*. Edinburgh, Scotland: E and S Livingston.

Mattson, S. N., and Riley, E. P. (1998). A review of the neurobehavioral deficits in children with fetal alcohol syndrome or prenatal exposure to alcohol. *Alcoholism: Clinical and Experimental Research, 22*, 279-294.

Mednick, S. A., Machon, R. A., Huttunen, M. O., and Bonnett, D. (1988). Adult schizophrenia following prenatal exposure to an influenza epidemic. *Archives of General Psychiatry*, 45, 189-192.

Miller, S. P., Weiss, J., Barnwell, A., Ferriero, D. M., Latal-Hajnal, B., Ferrer-Rogers, A. et al. (2002). Seizure-associated brain injury in term newborns with perinatal asphyxia. *Neurology, 58*, 542-548.

Warkany, J. (1986). Teratogen update: Hyperthermia. *Teratology, 33*, 365-371.

Subject Index